PROGRESS IN CLINICAL AND BIOLOGICAL RESEARCH

Series Editors

RECENT TITLES

See pages following the index for previous titles in this series.

MOLECULAR BASIS OF CANCER

Part A: Macromolecular Structure, Carcinogens, and Oncogenes

MOLECULAR BASIS OF CANCER

Part A: Macromolecular Structure, Carcinogens, and Oncogenes

**Proceedings of the Conference held at
Roswell Park Memorial Institute, Buffalo, New York,
May 30–June 2, 1984**

Editor

Robert Rein

Roswell Park Memorial Institute
Department of Health
State of New York
Buffalo, New York

ALAN R. LISS, INC., NEW YORK

Address all Inquiries to the Publisher
Alan R. Liss, Inc., 41 East 11th Street, New York, NY 10003

Copyright © 1985 Alan R. Liss, Inc.

Printed in the United States of America.

Library of Congress Cataloging in Publication Data

Main entry under title

Molecular basis of cancer.

     Papers presented at the Conference on the Molecular Basis of Cancer, held under the auspices of the Roswell Park Memorial Institute and co-sponsored by the National Foundation for Cancer Research and others.
     Includes bibliographies and index.
     Contents: pt. A. Macromolecular structure, carcinogens, and oncogenes—pt. B. Macromolecular recognition, chemotherapy, and immunology.
     1. Cancer—Congresses. 2. Molecular biology—Congresses. I. Rein, Robert. II. Conference on the Molecular Basis of Cancer (1984: Roswell Park Memorial Institute) III. Roswell Park Memorial Institute. IV. National Foundation for Cancer Research. [DNLM: 1. Medical Oncology—congresses. 2. Molecular Biology—congresses. W1 PR668E v.172 pt.A-B/QZ 200 M7183]
RC261.A2M65 1985   616.99'4'071   84-23430
ISBN 0-8451-5022-7 (set)
ISBN 0-8451-0186-2 (pt. A)
ISBN 0-8451-0187-0 (pt. B)

Contents

I. NUCLEIC ACIDS: STRUCTURE, REACTIVITY, AND FUNCTION

II. STRUCTURE AND REACTIVITY OF CARCINOGENS AND DNA LESIONS

x / Contents

Contributors

Marianna Abramovich, Department of Chemistry, University of Illinois at Chicago, Chicago, IL 60680 **[217]**

James L. Alderfer, Biophysics Department, Roswell Park Memorial Institute, Buffalo, NY 14263 **[199, 249]**

Leland C. Allen, Department of Chemistry, Princeton University, Princeton, NJ 08544 **[87]**

Russell J. Athay, Molecular Modeling Group, Evans & Sutherland Computer Corporation, Salt Lake City, UT 84108 **[319]**

Lee E. Babiss, Rockefeller University, New York, NY 10021 **[489]**

K. Balasubramanian, Department of Chemistry, Arizona State University, Tempe, AZ 85287 **[263]**

Paul Bates, Department of Biochemistry, University of Queensland, Brisbane, QLD 4067, Australia **[409]**

Robert Benezra, Department of Human Genetics and Development, Columbia University College of Physicians and Surgeons, New York, NY 10032 **[3]**

Harold C. Box, Biophysics Department, Roswell Park Memorial Institute, Buffalo, NY 14263 **[199]**

Henri Broch, Biophysics Laboratory, IPM, Nice University, Nice 06034 Cédex, France **[525]**

Suse Broyde, Department of Biology, New York University, New York, NY 10003 **[153]**

Jonathan J. Burbaum, Department of Chemistry, Massachusetts Institute of Technology, Boston, MA 02139 **[187]**

J. Caldwell, Department of Pharmaceutical Chemistry, School of Pharmacy, University of California, San Francisco, CA 94143 **[173]**

Charles R. Cantor, Department of Human Genetics and Development, Columbia University College of Physicians and Surgeons, New York, NY 10032 **[3]**

M. Charlier, Centre de Biophysique Moléculaire, Centre National de Recherche Scientifique, Orléans 45045, France **[401]**

Fu-Ming Chen, Department of Chemistry, Tennessee State University, Nashville, TN 37203 **[207]**

Janet Cicariello, Department of Chemistry, Rutgers University, New Brunswick, NJ 08903 **[109]**

F. Culard, Centre de Biophysique Moléculaire, Centre National de Recherche Scientifique, Orléans 45045 France **[401]**

Roger S. Davis, Molecular Modeling Group, Evans & Sutherland Computer Corporation, Salt Lake City, UT 84108 **[319]**

Charles DeLisi, Laboratory of Mathematical Biology, National Cancer Institute, National Institutes of Health, Bethesda, MD 20205 **[431, 443]**

Khang D. Do, Department of Chemistry, Rutgers University, New Brunswick, NJ 08903 **[109]**

The number in brackets is the opening page number of the contributor's article.

Josef Dommen, Department of Chemistry, ETH, Zurich, Switzerland **[187]**

Paul Elvin, Department of Anatomy and Experimental Pathology, University of St. Andrews, St. Andrews, Fife KY16 9TS, Scotland, UK **[537]**

Clive W. Evans, Department of Anatomy and Experimental Pathology, University of St. Andrews, St. Andrews, Fife KY16 9TS, Scotland, UK **[537]**

Paul B. Fisher, Department of Microbiology, Cancer Center/Institute of Cancer Research, Columbia University College of Physicians and Surgeons, New York, NY 10032 **[489]**

Y. Flashner, Department of Biochemistry, Israel Institute for Biological Research, Ness-Ziona 70450, Israel **[19]**

Barbara L. Gaffney, Department of Chemistry, Rutgers University, New Brunswick, NJ 08903 **[369]**

Arthur P. Grollman, Department of Pharmacological Sciences, State University of New York at Stony Brook, Stony Brook, NY 11794 **[389]**

P.C. Hariharan, Department of Chemistry, The Johns Hopkins University, Baltimore, MD 21218 **[263]**

Ronald G. Harvey, Ben May Laboratory for Cancer Research, University of Chicago, Chicago, IL 60637 **[217]**

Stephen C. Harvey, Department of Biochemistry, University of Alabama in Birmingham, Birmingham, AL 35294 **[123]**

Karen Haydock, Department of Chemistry, Princeton University, Princeton, NJ 08544 **[87]**

G. Hazel, Biophysics Department, Roswell Park Memorial Institute, Buffalo, NY 14263 **[249]**

Henry Hermo, Jr., Department of Microbiology, Cancer Center/Institute of Cancer Research, Columbia University College of Physicians and Surgeons, New York, NY 10032 **[489]**

I. Hertman, Israel Institute for Biological Research, Ness-Ziona 70450, Israel **[19]**

Brian Hingerty, Health & Safety Research Division, Oak Ridge National Laboratory, Oak Ridge, TN 37830 **[153]**

Stephen R. Holbrook, Chemical Biodynamics Division, Lawrence Berkeley Laboratory, University of California, Berkeley, CA 94720 **[143]**

A.J. Hopfinger, Department of Medicinal Chemistry, Searle Research & Development, Skokie, IL 60077 **[277]**

Robert C. Hopkins, Division of Sciences, University of Houston—Clear Lake, Houston, TX 77058 **[299]**

Jane Houldsworth, Division of Biology, California Institute of Technology, Pasadena, CA 91125 **[409]**

Keerthi Jayasuriya, Department of Chemistry, University of New Orleans, New Orleans, LA 70148 **[227]**

Roger A. Jones, Department of Chemistry, Rutgers University, New Brunswick, NJ 08903 **[369]**

Neville R. Kallenbach, Department of Biology, University of Pennsylvania, Philadelphia, PA 19104 **[99]**

Alexander N. Kalos, Department of Chemistry, Case Western Reserve University, Cleveland, OH 44106 **[287]**

Minoru Kanehisa, Laboratory of Mathematical Biology, National Cancer Institute, National Institutes of Health, Bethesda, MD 20205 **[431, 443]**

Joyce J. Kaufman, Department of Chemistry, The Johns Hopkins University, Baltimore, MD 21218 **[263]**

Thomas Kieber-Emmons, Unit of Theoretical Biology, Roswell Park Memorial Institute, Buffalo, NY 14263 **[357, 453]**

Sung-Hou Kim, Department of Chemistry, University of California, Berkeley, CA 94720 **[143]**

Petr Klein, Laboratory of Mathematical Biology, National Cancer Institute, National Institutes of Health, Bethesda, MD 20205 [431]

Gilles Klopman, Department of Chemistry, Case Western Reserve University, Cleveland, OH 44106 [287]

Peter Kollman, Department of Pharmaceutical Chemistry, School of Pharmacy, University of California, San Francisco, CA 94143 [173]

Walter S. Koski, Department of Chemistry, The Johns Hopkins University, Baltimore, MD 21218 [263]

Hubert Kranck, Biophysics Laboratory, IPM, Nice University, Nice 06034 Cédex, France [525]

Sharad Kumar, Department of Biochemistry, University of Queensland, Brisbane, QLD 4067, Australia [409]

János J. Ladik, Chair for Theoretical Chemistry, Laboratory of the National Foundation for Cancer Research, Universität Erlangen-Nürnberg, D-8520 Erlangen, Federal Republic of Germany [343]

Patricia R. Laurence, Department of Chemistry, University of New Orleans, New Orleans, LA 70148 [227]

Martin F. Lavin, Department of Biochemistry, University of Queensland, Brisbane, QLD 4067, Australia [409]

Pierre R. LeBreton, Department of Chemistry, University of Illinois at Chicago, Chicago, IL 60680 [217]

Kirk J. Leister, Research Affiliate, Department of Experimental Biology, Roswell Park Memorial Institute, Buffalo, NY 14263 [513]

Wen-Shing Liaw, Department of Microbiology, Cancer Center/Institute of Cancer Research, Columbia University College of Physicians and Surgeons, New York, NY 10032 [489]

Ronald E. Loomis, Department of Oral Biology, State University of New York at Buffalo, Buffalo, NY 14214 [249]

T. Lybrand, Department of Pharmaceutical Chemistry, School of Pharmacy, University of California, San Francisco, CA 94143 [173]

Rong-Ine Ma, Department of Biology, University of Pennsylvania, Philadelphia, PA 19104 [99]

Marcos F. Maestre, Biology and Medicine Division, Lawrence Berkeley Laboratory, Berkeley, CA 94220 [99]

Luis A. Marky, Department of Chemistry, Rutgers University, New Brunswick, NJ 08903 [369]

Nancy L. Marky, Department of Chemistry, Rutgers University, New Brunswick, NJ 08903 [109]

Kenneth A. Marx, Department of Chemistry, Dartmouth College, Hanover, NH 03755 [131]

J.C. Maurizot, Centre de Biophysique Moléculaire, Centre National de Recherche Scientifique, Orléans 45045, France [401]

J. Andrew McCammon, Department of Chemistry, University of Houston, Houston, TX 77004 [123]

Joseph McDonald, Unit of Theoretical Biology, Roswell Park Memorial Institute, Buffalo, NY 14263 [453]

Robert J. McDonald, Department of Microbiology, Cancer Center/Institute of Cancer Research, Columbia University College of Physicians and Surgeons, New York, NY 10032 [489]

L. David Meeker, Department of Mathematics, University of New Hampshire, Durham, NH 03824 [379].

Kenneth J. Miller, Department of Chemistry, Rensselaer Polytechnic Institute, Troy, NY 12181 [187]

Rahmah Mohamed, Department of Biochemistry, University of Queensland, Brisbane, QLD 4067, Australia **[409]**

Randall H. Morse, Department of Human Genetics and Development, Columbia University College of Physicians and Surgeons, New York, NY 10032 **[3]**

Krishnan Namboodiri, Department of Chemistry, Case Western Reserve University, Cleveland, OH 44106 **[287]**

Timothy E. O'Connor, Associate Institute Director for Scientific Affairs, Roswell Park Memorial Institute, Buffalo, NY 14263 **[467]**

Wilma K. Olson, Department of Chemistry, Rutgers University, New Brunswick, NJ 08903 **[109]**

David A. Pearlman, Department of Chemistry, University of California, Berkeley, CA 94720 **[143]**

Matthew R. Pincus, Department of Pathology, Columbia College of Physicians and Surgeons, New York, NY 10032 **[419]**

Isabel M. Pinto, Department of Microbiology, Cancer Center/Institute of Cancer Research, Columbia University, College of Physicians and Surgeons, New York, NY 10032 **[489]**

David Pirkle, Department of Chemistry, University of California, Berkeley, CA 94720 **[143]**

M. Prabhakaran, Department of Biochemistry, University of Alabama in Birmingham, Birmingham, AL 35294 **[123]**

Arungundrum S. Prakash, Department of Chemistry, University of Illinois at Chicago, Chicago, IL 60680 **[217]**

Peter Politzer, Department of Chemistry, University of New Orleans, New Orleans, LA 70148 **[227]**

Alberte Pullman, Department of Theoretical Biochemistry, Institut de Biologie Physico-Chimique, Paris 75005, France **[71]**

Bernard Pullman, Department of Theoretical Biochemistry, Institut de Biologie Physico-Chimique, Paris 75005, France **[55]**

S. Rao, Department of Pharmaceutical Chemistry, School of Pharmacy, University of California, San Francisco, CA 94143 **[173]**

Milan Randić, Department of Mathematics and Computer Science, Drake University, Des Moines, IA 50311; Ames Laboratory—DOE, Iowa State University, Ames, IA 50011 **[309]**

Robert Rein, Unit of Theoretical Biology, Roswell Park Memorial Institute, Buffalo, NY 14263 **[xxi, xxv, 19, 357, 453]**

Christopher A. Reynolds, National Foundation for Cancer Research Project, Chemistry Department, University of St. Andrews, St. Andrews KY16 9ST, Scotland, UK **[239]**

Marie Agnès Rix-Montel, Biophysics Laboratory, IPM, Nice University, Nice 06034 Cédex, France **[525]**

George C. Ruben, Department of Pathology, Dartmouth Medical School, Hanover, NH 03756 **[131]**

Eric Savant-Ros, Biophysics Laboratory, IPM, Nice University, Nice 06034 Cédex, France **[525]**

Nadrian C. Seeman, Department of Biological Sciences, State University of New York at Albany, Albany, NY 12222 **[99]**

A. Shafferman, Department of Biochemistry, Israel Institute for Biological Research, Ness-Ziona 70450, Israel **[19]**

Minoti Sharma, Biophysics Department, Roswell Park Memorial Institute, Buffalo, NY 14263 **[199, 249]**

Masayuki Shibata, Unit of Theoretical Biology, Roswell Park Memorial Institute, Buffalo, NY 14263 **[357]**

U.C. Singh, Department of Pharmaceutical Chemistry, School of Pharmacy, University of California, San Francisco, CA 94143 **[173]**

M. Spodheim-Maurizot, Centre de Biophysique Moléculaire, Centre National de Recherche Scientifique, Orléans 45045, France **[401]**

Annankoil R. Srinivasan, Department of Chemistry, Rutgers University, New Brunswick, NJ 08903 **[109]**

Akira Suyama, Department of Physics, Faculty of Science, University of Tokyo, Tokyo 113 Japan **[37]**

László V. Szentpály, Institut für Theoretische Chemie, Universität Stuttgart, D-7000 Stuttgart 80, Federal Republic of Germany **[327]**

Masaru Takeshita, Department of Pharmacological Sciences, State University at Stony Brook, Stony Brook, NY 11794 **[389]**

Eric R. Taylor, Department of Chemistry, Rensselaer Polytechnic Institute, Troy, NY 12181 **[187]**

Henry J. Thompson, Department of Animal and Nutritional Sciences, University of New Hampshire, Durham, NH 03824 **[379]**

Colin Thomson, National Foundation for Cancer Research Project, Department of Chemistry, University of St. Andrews, St. Andrews KY16 9ST, Scotland, UK **[239]**

L. David Tomei, Comprehensive Cancer Center, Ohio State University, Columbus, OH 43210 **[513]**

V.S. Vaidhyanathan, Department of Biophysical Sciences, State University of New York at Buffalo, Buffalo, NY 14214 **[549]**

Harjeet Van der Keyl, Department of Pharmacological Sciences, State University at Stony Brook, Stony Brook, NY 11794 **[389]**

Dan Vasilescu, Biophysics Laboratory, IPM, Nice University, Nice 06034 Cédex, France **[525]**

Akiyoshi Wada, Department of Physics, Faculty of Science, University of Tokyo, Tokyo 113 Japan **[37]**

Robert D. Wells, Department of Biochemistry, University of Alabama in Birmingham, Birmingham, AL 35294 **[47]**

Charles E. Wenner, Department of Experimental Biology, Roswell Park Memorial Institute, Buffalo, NY 14263 **[513]**

Irene S. Zegar, Department of Chemistry, University of Illinois at Chicago, Chicago, IL 60680 **[217]**

Theresa J. Zielinski, Unit of Theoretical Biology, Roswell Park Memorial Institute, Buffalo, NY 14263; and Department of Chemistry, Niagara University, Niagara, NY 14109 **[357]**

Contents of Part B: Macromolecular Recognition, Chemotherapy, and Immunology

III. ONCOGENES

A. RELATION TO MUTAGENS, CARCINOGENS, AND ACTIVATION MECHANISMS

B. STRUCTURE OF ONCOGENE PROTEINS

C. FUNCTION OF ONCOGENE PROTEINS, MEMBRANE REACTIONS, AND CELL TRANSFORMATIONS

Preface

Molecular Basis of Cancer combines, in two volumes, over seventy articles dealing with current interdisciplinary studies on the molecular aspects of cancer. These articles represent the contents of most of the invited talks and a few selected posters from the conference on the "Molecular Basis of Cancer: An Interdisciplinary Discussion on Basic and Applied Aspects of Cancer" held at Roswell Park Memorial Institute in Buffalo, New York on May 29—June 2, 1984. The collection of research reports and mini-reviews contained in these volumes provides a broad overview of the role of the major biological macromolecules (eg, nucleic acids and proteins) in the process of mutagenesis and carcinogenesis, as well as their role as targets in cancer chemotherapy. Further topics include: oncogene activation and the biochemical and biological mechanisms of oncogene products in cell regulation and transformation; and mechanisms of cellular activation of the immune system. A strong emphasis is given to the description of research methodologies and, in particular, to the integration of physical, chemical, and theoretical methods with those of molecular and cellular biology.

The most outstanding feature of this book is the broad interdisciplinary range of its content on the one hand, and the cohesiveness of its topics on the other. The interdisciplinary character is emphasized with respect to the reported research topics, and the methods and techniques used in the studies. Cohesiveness between the topics provides for a synthesis of the processes into an integrated overview on how cancer progresses from an initial insult to the genetic system to tumorogenesis and metastatic spread. To illustrate these features, the relation between the various articles focusing on chemical carcinogens can be considered. Studies of nucleic acid structure and stability by methods of physical chemistry—such as the thermodynamics of melting, NMR and optical spectroscopy—supplemented by theoretical studies, serve to identify the most reactive sites on DNA susceptible for covalent attack by such typical carcinogens as polycyclic aromatic hydrocarbons, nitrosamines, halogenated olefin epoxides, and other alkylating agents. Quantum chemical methods are used to study the reaction mechanisms and chemical intermediates involved in the attack of these agents on the macromolecular targets. Perturbation of nucleic acid structure in precarcinogenic lesions induced either by covalent attack or formation of non-covalent complexes by intercalation are investigated by a combination of theoretical conformational analysis and molecular interaction theory and various forms of NMR and optical spectroscopy. The fate of the precarcinogenic lesions (eg, repair or incorporation into nucleic acids through replication) are further considered, based on genetic data on the one side and thermodynamic stability measurements and theoretical considerations on the other. The important issue of the relation between the biological endpoints of mutation and carcinogenesis is analyzed by considering the effect of mutational loads necessary for oncogene activation. The role of carcinogens in genetic rearrangement and transposition is studied by methods of molecular biology and genetics, to assess the mutational frequencies and the role of these processes in carcinogenesis. Methods of plasmid biology are used to study the role of palindromes in DNA excision repair mechanisms. The synergetic effects of chemical carcinogens and adenoviruses in cell transformation are reported based on studies of cell culture systems. Another interesting mechanism is studied in the model of UV induced derepression. A study of genetic rearrangement and insertion mutation induced by AAF enlightens yet another interesting connection between cancer and mutations.

Molecular Basis of Cancer is organized in six chapters appearing in two volumes. Broadly speaking, the articles fall into three categories: original research reports; reviews of the authors' own work; or mini-reviews on specific topics. In this last category of particular significance are O'Connor's mini-review of oncogenes, Fischer and co-workers' discussion of cellular transformation, Wenner et al's overview of tumor promoters, and Box's discussion of NMR methodologies as applied to nucleic acid structural studies.

Nucleic Acids: Cancer is essentially a disease caused by defects in genetic regulation mechanisms. The underlying basic knowledge necessary for understanding and possibly intervening in this disorder is the relation between nucleic acid structure and genetic control. The reports in this section provide a good insight into the structural principles governing the physical and chemical properties of DNA, and its biological and genetic function. The collection of papers on this topic features reports on chromatin structure (Cantor), palindromic instabilities and DNA repair (Shafferman), DNA stability in relation to gene control (Wada), biological properties of Z-DNA (Wells), origin of specificity in nucleic acid reactions (B. Pullman), steric and electronic factors in reactivity of tRNA (A. Pullman), and nucleic acid junctions in solutions (Seeman). Several papers report on calculations of nucleic acid structure and energetics (Olson, Kollman, Miller, Lavery, Kothekar, Sandorfy, Del Re, and Scheiner).

Molecular Principles of Drug Activity in Cancer Chemotherapy: Many of the drugs used in cancer chemotherapy form complexes with nucleic acids and are cytostatic agents. The sequence specificity and the stability of these complexes are of central interest. Thus, several articles address the question of drug-DNA interactions. Dabrowiak reports on the DNAse I footprinting method for identification of the DNA region interacting with a drug. Neidel's report discusses rational cancer drug design via structural studies and drug-DNA interactions. Sundaralingam and others report on the mechanisms of interaction of Pt and related metal complexes with DNA. Krugh and coworkers report on their NMR studies of the interaction of the potent antitumor antibiotics anthramycin and oligodeoxyribonucleotide sequences. Marky, Curry, and Breslauer's comprehensive thermodynamic study deals with the nature of the binding of netropsin to DNA. An alternative approach in cancer chemotherapy utilizes enzyme inhibitors in metabolic pathways in the synthesis of nucleic acid precursors. Cody reports on a computer graphics study of dihydrofolate reductase inhibitors. Duax's article discusses the structure and mechanism of the action of estrogens and antiestrogens. Vasilescu et al analyze the interaction between radioprotective agents with lipids and with DNA. Mayhew and Rustum discuss the use of liposomes as carriers for selective delivery of antitumor agents. Sieber reports on merocyanine 540 mediated photosensitization of tumor cells. Fiel's analysis of DNA interactive porphyrins is relevant both in the context of strand scission and photosensitization. Bloch's paper explores the use of DNA-specific agents to induce proliferating cancer cells that are arrested at various stages of their differentiation to mature to a nonproliferating state. Korytnyk uses computerized molecular modelling to design glycosidase inhibitors. Several papers deal with structure/activity relations for drug design. Hopfinger's QSAR analysis, Klopman's artificial intelligence approach, and Randić's graph theoretical method fall into this category. Liebman uses an ingenious topological approach in the form of distance matrix partitioning to identify biological activity in the structure activity analysis. He uses this method to study spindle poisons related to colchicine and vinblastine. Another group of papers reports on analysis of protein nucleic acid recognition models (Loew, Kumar). These model studies are forming the basis for the rational design of drugs via agents controlling gene expression.

Oncogenes: Mechanisms of oncogene activation are considered by Ladik and by Rein et al. Ladik's emphasis is on possible mechanisms in LTR's enhancing oncogene expression. Rein's paper deals with spontaneous and carcinogen-induced point mutation mechanisms. Papers by DeLisi, Kanehisa, Pincus, and Kieber-Emmons consider oncogene protein structure. O'Connor's mini-review is concerned with biochemical and biological mechanisms of the action of oncogene protein and their key role in cellular transformation. Wenner and coworkers present an overview of the role of promoters, membrane associated alterations, and intracellular processes.

Immunological Recognition: The paper by Stollar et al considers helical shape specific DNA antibodies, with special emphasis on Z-DNA. Schwartz analyzes the recognition aspects of cellular receptors with immunogenes and the major histocompatability antigen system in T-lymphocyte activation. Kohler et al discuss the use of idiotypes (internal images); and HLA-DR antigen production is reported by Liao et al. Papers by Hopp, Fraga, and Singh describe theoretical approaches in identification of antigenic determinants.

In summary, this treatise is of significance to those who are interested in obtaining an overview of the current state of ideas, methodologies, and unifying principles of molecular and cellular biology, biophysics, and biochemistry of cancer. The biologically oriented reader benefits from an exposure to the ever increasing use of computer based theoretical methods in molecular sciences. By the same token, physical scientists and theoreticians are exposed to a comprehensive overview of cancer biology. This is of the utmost importance for developing a better intuition and recognition for a judicious choice of biologically relevant topics to be modelled. Those interested in medicinal chemistry, pharmacology, and cancer drug design will benefit from exposure to a wealth of structural information on the two principal biomacromolecules and their adducts on one hand, and consideration of membrane and membrane surface phenomena on the other. This will provide conceptual insight into possible mechanisms that can be utilized for specific targeting of antitumor drugs. The reader will also benefit from a comprehensive exposure to the rapidly evolving field of oncogenes.

Robert Rein

Foreword

Over seventy papers presented at the Conference on the Molecular Basis of Cancer between May 30—June 2, 1984 are included in this and the accompanying volume. The conference was held under the auspices of Roswell Park Memorial Institute and co-sponsored by the National Foundation for Cancer Research, National Cancer Institute, Occidental Chemical Corporation, Hoffman-La Roche Incorporated, Bristol-Myers Company, International Society of Quantum Biology, Schering Corporation, Searle Research and Development, the Upjohn Company, Evans & Sutherland Computer Corporation, S. Leslie Misrock of Pennie and Edmonds, and Alfred Roach of TII Industries Incorporated.

On behalf of my colleagues on the organizing committee—Timothy O'Connor, Harel Weinstein, Bernard Pullman, Charles DeLisi, and Per-Olov Lowdin, I would like to express my gratitude to the sponsors, participants, and contributors to the conference. The editor is deeply indebted to the authors for their outstanding contributions to these volumes. My special thanks are also due to Deborah Raye and Kimberley Ruhl whose help in compiling these volumes was invaluable.

Robert Rein

I. NUCLEIC ACIDS: STRUCTURE, REACTIVITY, AND FUNCTION

Molecular Basis of Cancer, Part A: Macromolecular
Structure, Carcinogens, and Oncogenes, pages 3–18
© 1985 Alan R. Liss, Inc.

TORSIONAL PROPERTIES OF DNA IN CHROMATIN

Charles R. Cantor, Randall H. Morse,
        Robert Benezra
Department of Human Genetics and Development,
Columbia University College of Physicians and
Surgeons, 701 West 168 Street, New York,
NY10032

POSSIBLE FUNCTIONAL AND STRUCTURAL CONSEQUENCES OF
SUPERCOILING

In the past few years it has become evident
that DNA has accessible a wide range of helical
structures (Cantor 1981). The most dramatic of
these is left handed Z-DNA (Wang et al. 1979).
There is considerable evidence for other DNA
structural changes from short duplexes of known
crystal structure (Dickerson, Drew 1981), from
solution physico-chemical studies (Marini et al.
1982; Vorlickova et al. 1982), and from the
unexpected sequence specificity of many agents that
cleave DNA (Lomonossoff et al. 1981; Keene, Elgin
1981; Horz, Altenberger 1981; Dingwall et al. 1981;
Cartwright, Elgin 1982; Pope, Sigman 1984). These
alternate DNA structures may have great functional
importance. For example, unusual DNA structures
present an attractive way in which proteins that
regulate gene expression can show class-specific
responses. The search for principles that govern
how cells exploit the structural polymorphism of
DNA in gene expression will occupy molecular
biologists for years to come.

Various DNA structures differ in the number of
base pairs per turn (Rhodes, Klug 1981; Peck, Wang
1981). Thus the relative stability of these
structures can be altered greatly by changing the

torsional tension (Benham 1981). For example, sequences with Z-DNA potential can be driven into the Z-form in a closed circular duplex plasmid by increasing the superhelical density (Stirdivant et al. 1982; Peck et al. 1982). Highly supercoiled DNA can also untwist into other unusual DNA structures such as cruciform loops, if appropriate sequences are present (Mizuuchi et al. 1982; Lilly 1980). Since supercoiling will favor some structures at the expense of others, it could act to coordinate events at different places along the DNA.

In bacteria an elaborate system exists to regulate the average superhelical density. It includes at least two topoisomerases and other control proteins (Gellert et al. 1983). The activity of various genes is affected differently by changes in supercoiling (Smith et al. 1978). The genome of E. coli consists of a single circular chromosome segregated into about 50 independent supercoiled domains, averaging 50 kb in length (Pettijohn 1982). The functional significance of this arrangement is unknown although in principle it allows for independent regulation of the superhelical density of different regions of the genome. In vivo the bacterial chromosome and bacterial plasmids behave as highly supercoiled molecules and thus one can expect to find alternate DNA structures favored by high torsional tension. Even linear bacteriophage DNA behaves as though it contains torsional tension in vivo (Sinden, Pettijohn 1982).

In eukaryotic cells, chromosomal DNAs are usually linear molecules. However, attachment to the nuclear matrix or chromosomal scaffolding apparently restricts the free rotation of DNAs. The result is that each DNA is segregated into topologically independent domains ranging in size from typical E. coli domains to about 10 fold larger (Benyajati, Worcel 1976; Paulson, Laemmli 1977). There are indications that each domain is one replicon (Buongiorno et al. 1982; Vogelstein et al. 1980). Most eukaryotic DNA is packaged into nucleosomes resulting in 1.75 left hand supercoils per particle (Klug et al. 1980). When nucleosomes are removed from chromosomes without disruption of the scaffold, the remaining DNA is highly supercoiled. However, in native chromatin the DNA behaves as though there were little or no torsional tension (Sinden et al. 1980). Thus, the supercoils are sequestered into the nucleosomes.

We would like to understand how nucleosomes and alternate DNA structures interact in helping to regulate gene expression: Can the torsional tension within the nucleosome be exploited to modulate the binding of other proteins to DNA such as regulatory molecules or RNA polymerases? Does the presence of nucleosomes encourage or discourage the formation of alternate DNA structures? Are there domains of supercoil density trapped between nucleosomes or in small clusters of nucleosomes that are important in gene expression?

There are a few tantalizing hints that supercoiling is still felt by the DNA in chromatin. An S1 hypersensitive site in globin chromatin is also S1 hypersensitive when the globin gene is present in a nucleosome-free supercoiled plasmid DNA but not when that DNA is relaxed (Weintraub et al. 1981). If the S1 hypersensitivity is the result of torsional tension where did that tension come from in the supposedly relaxed globin chromatin? One of the most likely possibilities is shown schematically in Figure 1. There is evidence that nucleosomes may transiently dissociate from supercoiled DNA (Weintraub 1983). This leads to free supercoiled DNA. If rotational diffusion of the DNA region is constrained, a local supercoiled domain may persist long enough to drive a conformation change in a section of the DNA contained within it. This could produce an S1 hypersensitive alternate structure (Schon et al. 1983; Nickol, Felsenfeld 1983). That unusual structure might serve as the recognition site for a regulatory protein or a polymerase.

There is some evidence that supercoiling is important for gene expression in eukaryotes. The superhelical density of a plasmid isolated from yeast carrying mating locus genes is more negative in strains in which these genes are repressed

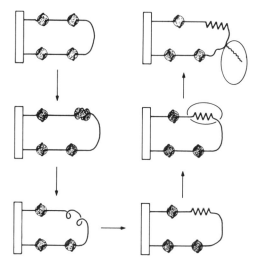

Fig.1. Schematic illustration of possible stages in
t.ie activation of a gene on a domain of chromatin.
Shown, counter clockwise, starting from upper left
are: inactive chromatin, a nucleosome with altered
structure, loss of a nucleosome, conversion of
local torsional energy to an altered DNA structure,
binding of a regulatory protein, and initiation of
transcription.

(Abraham et al. 1983). This could mean that fewer
nucleosomes are bound to the plasmid when the gene
is active or that supercoiling somehow is part of
the regulation process. Circular plasmids injected
into Xenopus oocytes have much higher
transcriptional activity than linear plasmids
(Hurland et al. 1983). Torsional tension is the
most likely way in which circles and linear
molecules will differ in vivo. Control experiments
rule out such obvious artifacts as differential
survival of linear and circular minichromosomes.
The transcription of 5S rRNA genes in Xenopus
oocytes is linked to a dynamic form of chromatin.
This form is relaxed, and transcription abolished,
by novobiocin, a drug that is known to inhibit
prokaryotic DNA gyrases (Ryogi, Worcel 1984)

     Here we will explore, briefly, several aspects
of the possible relationship between DNA

supercoiling and gene expression in higher
eukaryotes. If the schematic picture in Figure 1
bears any relationship to reality, we might expect
to see differences in the numbers, placement, and
structures of nucleosomes on actively transcribed
genes. We might also expect to see evidence that
small supercoiled domains might be restricted from
diffusion in chromatin. Such domains could
conceivably contain sufficient stored free energy
to drive DNA structural changes. The findings
discussed below are preliminary but they provide
support for all of these expectations.

NUCLEOSOME STRUCTURE IN ACTIVELY TRANSCRIBED GENES.

It has been known for some time that the
structure of chromatin in actively transcribed
genes is different from that of bulk chromatin.
Various nucleases preferentially digest the DNA of
active chromatin. Most evidence suggests that these
differences in accessibility to nucleases do not
represent the complete absence of nucleosomes.

We have examined the structure of nucleosomes
on heavily transcribed genes coding for ribosomal
RNA (Prior et al. 1983). In Physarum polycephalum
(and certain other simple organisms) the ribosomal
genes are located on relatively small palindromic
DNAs in the nucleolus. Isolated nucleoli provide a
highly enriched sample of active chromatin. This
can be further fractionated by direct digestion
with restriction nucleases and subsequent sucrose
gradient separation of different sized
nucleoprotein fractions. In this way relatively
pure samples of nucleosomes from actively
transcribed genes were prepared. They have the same
four histones as normal nucleosomes. However they
differ from the nucleosomes of bulk chromatin in
several important aspects. Additional proteins are
present, most likely the Physarum equivalent of HMG
proteins seen in nuclease sensitive chromatin from
active genes of higher organisms (Weisbrod et al.
1980). The hydrodynamic properties of nucleosomes
from active genes indicate a much more extended or
open structure. This is confirmed by their
appearance in the electronmicroscope. In normal
nucleosomes the conserved cysteine residues at

position 11Ø of histone H3 are inaccessible under physiological conditions. However, in the nucleosomes from Physarum ribosomal chromatin these cysteines are highly reactive to sulfhydryl reagents. Controls with stages of the organism in which ribosomal transcription is shut off show clearly that exposure of the cysteines occurs only in actively transcribed chromatin.

Little is known about the detailed structure of these active nucleosomes. However from our current picture of the structure of bulk nucleosomes it is difficult to see how one could expose cysteine 11Ø residues without changing the arrangement of the 8 histones and thus the winding of DNA on the protein core. Hence altered nucleosome structures can exist in active chromatin and these structures may be influenced by, or may influence the local superhelical density.

A more direct consequence of active genes could be loss of nucleosomes. This idea has been prevalent for some time fueled by the topological paradox of how one might transcribe a DNA molecule bound to a surface without penetrating that surface. We have recently undertaken a study of the arrangement of nucleosomes on the mouse beta major globin gene as a function of the potential of that gene for expression (Benezra et al. 1984). The experiments are straightforward in principle: nuclei were prepared from different cell lines and treated with the iron(II) complex of methidium-propyl-EDTA. This reagent has been shown to reveal the true positions of nucleosomes (Cartwright et al. 1983). It cuts DNA in the linker preferentially. More importantly, it shows little or no specificity on naked DNA even at very low degrees of digestion. Thus one can observe the footprint of the bound nucleosomes with little or no complications by convolution of the cleavage pattern with that of naked DNA.

Detection of the footprint of nucleosomes on single copy DNA of a higher eukaryote is done by indirect end labeling with appropriate cloned probes. The experiment requires probes at the highest obtainable specific activity, very long autoradiographic exposures, and photographic enhancement of the resulting films. When mouse L cells, and induced and uninduced Friend cells were examined, a clear result emerged. In the L cell, there is no potential for globin expression and the entire gene and flanking region is covered with nucleosomes. In the uninduced Friend cell which has the potential for expressing globin but is not actively transcribing it, the 3' region of the gene shows the same pattern of nucleosome positions as the L cell. The 5' region of the gene and the 5' flanking region show a complete loss of nucleosome footprint which we infer to mean that nucleosomes have either been rearranged or removed and replaced either by naked DNA or other bound proteins. When the Friend cell is activated to transcribe globin, there are further changes in the chromatin but these are more subtle than the changes already seen in the uninduced Friend cell. Thus an active single copy gene in higher eukaryotes has specific alterations in chromatin structure but nucleosomes are still present on at least part of the gene.

TORSIONAL PROPERTIES OF MINICHROMOSOMES.

The simplest way to examine topological aspects of DNA structure and gene expression is to use a small closed circular duplex plasmid. The number of supercoils can be measured by using gel electrophoretic techniques capable of resolving DNAs that differ by a single linking number (Wang 1979). The number of nucleosomes can be measured by counting them in the electron microscope. SV40 minichromosomes isolated either from cells or virions have been used for virtually all such studies in the past. A number of clear results have emerged along with many puzzles. SV40 contains a relatively sharp distribution of nucleosomes: 24 $\pm$ 2 for samples isolated at low salt and containing histone H1 and 21 $\pm$ 2 for samples that have been treated with higher salt and are lacking H1 (Keller et al. 1977; Germond et al. 1975; Muller et al. 1978). It was paradoxical that the DNA linker between nucleosomes failed to show the expected thermal dependence of DNA twist (Keller et al. 1977) and yet this DNA was clearly accessible to binding of various intercalators. We were curious whether this was some anomaly of the SV40 system or whether it was a general property of chromatin. If the latter, we would argue that the lack of thermal untwisting of DNA would imply both that the DNA is not free to twist on the surface of the nucleosome and that nucleosomes are restricted from rotating with respect to each other. This would mean that any small section of chromatin is a potential independent supercoiled domain.

There were several reasons for suspecting that SV40 chromatin might be anomalous. The linker DNA in SV40 is more irregular than most typical chromatin. Viral capsid proteins are present in all preparations and their effect on the structure is unknown. SV40 packs many functional sites into a small piece of DNA and the effect of all of this on the structure is unknown. Thus we decided to look at the effect of nucleosomes on DNA untwisting in reconstituted chromatin made from purified components. We knew, from previous work that it was possible to reconstitute different numbers of nucleosomes onto supercoiled closed circular DNA up to the densities of nucleosomes seen in natural chromatin (Germond et al. 1975). Such samples were prepared and treated with topoisomerase I at two different temperatures. Then both DNAs were returned to the same temperature and the difference in their linking number determined by standard gel electrophoretic procedures.

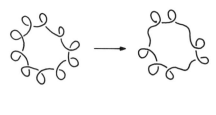

4°   37°

Fig. 2. Temperature dependence of the helical twist of DNA as revealed by changes in the number of supercoils in a closed circular DNA duplex.

The principle behind the method is shown for naked DNA in Figure 2. The most stable solution

structure of DNA gradually changes with
temperature. A net unwinding of approximately 1Ø
degrees per degree C per 1ØØØ bp is observed. This
works out to about 1 turn per 1Ø degrees C for a
3.7 Kb plasmid. The different twist of the DNA at
two temperatures will let topoisomerase I remove
different numbers of supercoils. The resulting DNA
will have a different linking number when the two
samples are compared at a constant temperature. One
then sees how the effect titrates with successive
additions of nucleosomes. If DNA were free to twist
on the surface of the nucleosome one might see no
effect of nucleosomes at all. If the DNA bound to
the protein core were restrained but the linker
were free, each nucleosome would remove the thermal
dependence of twist of 145 base pairs of DNA.

In fact what we actually observe is that each
nucleosome removes about 2ØØ base pairs of DNA
thermal twist (Morse, Cantor 1984). Thus not only
is the core DNA restrained from twisting, the
linker DNA is also. The mechanism of this restraint
is unknown. However previous work has shown that
the highly positively charged N-terminal regions of
histones are not needed to form core particles and
therefore may have little if any contact with core
DNA (McGhee, Felsenfeld 198Ø). However these tails
are presumably free to bind the DNA in the linker
regions of chromatin and such binding could clearly
lead to the kinds of torsional constraints we
observe. It is not clear how these results can be
reconciled with the observed binding of many
intercalators to chromatin since such binding
requires much greater unwinding of DNA than is
needed for thermal untwisting.

PROPERTIES OF SMALL SUPERCOILED DOMAINS.

If one removes one or two nucleosomes in
activating a gene, the resulting supercoiled domain
is much smaller than the typical supercoiled
plasmids studied in vitro. It is known that such
plasmids can contain enough stored energy that
localized regions may spontaneously untwist and
consequently reduce some of the energy stored in
DNA writhe (shown schematically in Figure 3).
Conversion of DNA sequences into left handed

helices would be particularly effective in releasing writhe energy since it would provide the maximum possible untwisting per base pair.

We wanted to see what the potential for torsionally driven structural changes would be in small supercoiled domains. The free energy of supercoiling increases as the square of the number

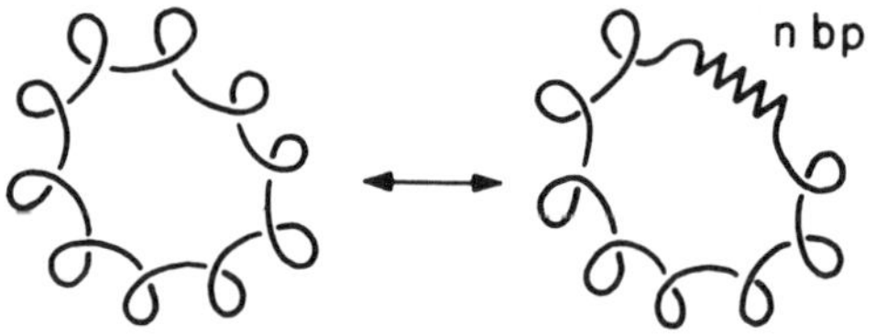

Fig. 3. Schematic illustration of a conformational change driven by torsional energy.

of supercoils according to the equation

$$G = Ki^2 \qquad\qquad -1-$$

where K is the supercoiling force constant and i is the number of supercoils, effectively the difference between the linking number of a particular DNA molecule and that of a relaxed DNA molecule under the same conditions. A relatively simple calculation shows that the free energy change when several supercoils exchange for an untwisted local DNA structure is

$$G = n^2 K f^2 + n(G_{gro} - 2Kif) + G_{nuc} \qquad -2-$$

where, f is the difference in twist per base pair between normal B DNA and the altered structure, n is the number of base pairs of altered structure, and G_{nuc} and G_{gro} are respectively the free energy of nucleating and the free energy per base pair of extending that altered structure. The quadratic form of the above equation means that there will be an optimal length of altered structure that will minimize the free energy (Cantor, Efstratiadis 1984).

The quadratic dependence of the supercoiling

free energy might lead one to believe that small
domains with few supercoils are low in energy.
However it turns out that the supercoiling force
constant is a very sensitive function of the size
of the domain and rises rapidly for domains less
than 2000 base pairs. This is illustrated in Figure
4 which summarizes the results of two different
laboratories (Shore, Baldwin 1983; Horowitz, Wang
1984). When equation -2- is evaluated for domains
as small as 200 to 400 base pairs it is clear that

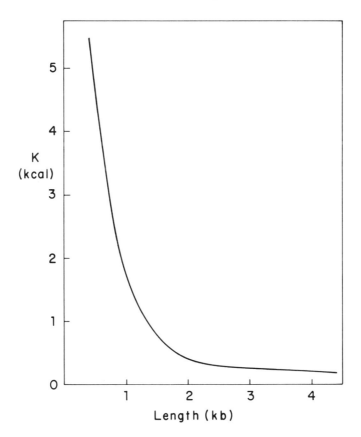

Fig. 4. Dependence of the torsional free energy,
defined in equation -1-, on the length of a closed
circular DNA duplex.

even a few supercoils in such a domain contain
enough torsional energy to drive DNA sequences from

B to Z helices or even melt DNA duplexes. Thus the
domains that will be generated by the loss of even
a single nucleosome contain sufficient torsional
free energy to lead to altered DNA structures.

We have shown several pieces of evidence,
largely circumstantial, that torsional free energy
is important in eukaryotes even though most of the
DNA supercoiling seems, at first glance, restrained
by the packaging of DNA into nucleosomes. The
relevance of supercoiling to the theme of this
conference, the molecular basis of cancer, is
purely a matter for speculation. However it is of
interest to note recent work showing that the
target of potent antitumor drugs is topoisomerase
II, one of the enzymes that can relax supercoils in
eukaryotes (Nelson et al. 1984). Thus DNA torsion
may or may not be important in the etiology of
cancer but it seems to play at least an indirect
role in its treatment.

Acknowledgement: Some of the work described in this
paper was supported by the NIH through research
grant CA 23767 and the NSF through research grant
PCM 83-02951. The cooperation of Richard Axel,
Argiris Efstratiadis, Christopher Prior, Vincent
Allfrey and Edward Johnson in various projects
mentioned in the article is gratefully
acknowledged.

REFERENCES

Abraham J, Feldman J, Nasmyth KA, Strathern JN,
    Klar, AJS, Broach JR, Hicks JB (1983). Sites
    required for position-effect regulation of
    mating-type information in yeast. Cold Spring
    Harbor Symp. Quant. Biol. 47:989.
Benezra R, Cantor CR, Axel R (1984). manuscript in
    preparation.
Benham CJ (1981). Theoretical analysis of
    competitive conformational transitions in
    torsionally stressed DNA. J. Mol. Biol. 150:43.
Benyajati C, Worcel A (1976). Isolation,
    characterization and structure of the folded
    interphase genome of Drosophila melanogaster.
    Cell 9:393.
Buongiorno-Nardelli M, Michelli G, Carri MT,

Marilley M (1982). A relationship between replicon size and supercoiled loop domains in the eukaryotic genome. Nature 298:100.

Cantor CR (1981). DNA choreography. Cell 25:293

Cantor CR, Efstratiadis A (1984). manuscript in preparation.

Cartwright IC, Elgin SCR (1982). Analysis of chromatin structure and DNA sequence organization: use of the 1,10-phenanthroline-cuprous complex. Nucleic Acids Res. 10:5835.

Cartwright IC, Hertzberg RP, Dervan PB, Elgin SCR (1983). Cleavage of chromatin with methidiumpropyl-EDTA iron (II). Proc. Natl. Acad. Sci. 80:3213.

Dingwall C, Lomonossoff GP, Laskey RA (1981). High sequence specificity of micrococcal nuclease. Acids Res. 9:2659.

Dickerson RE, Drew HR (1981). Kinetic model for B-DNA. Proc. Natl. Acad. Sci. 78:7318.

Gellert M, Menzel R, Mizuuchi K, O'Dea MH, Friedman DI (1983). Regulation of DNA supercoiling in Escherichia coli. Cold Spring Harbor Symp. Quant. Biol. 47:763.

Germond JE, Hirt B, Oudet P, Gross-Belard M, Chambon P (1975). Folding of the DNA double helix in chromatin-like structures from Simian virus 40. Proc. Natl. Acad. Sci. 72:1843.

Horowitz DS, Wang JC (1984). Torsional rigidity of DNA and length dependence of the free energy of DNA supercoiling. J. Mol. Biol. 173:75.

Horz W, Altenberger W (1981). Sequence specific cleavage of DNA by micrococcal nuclease. Nucleic Acids Res. 9:2643.

Hurland RM, Weintraub H, McKnight SL (1983). Transcription of DNA injected into Xenopus oocytes is influenced by template topology. Nature 302:38.

Keene MA, Elgin, SCR (1981). Micrococcal nuclease as a probe of DNA sequence organization and chromatin structure. Cell 27:57.

Keller W, Muller U, Eicken I, Wendel I, Zentgraf H (1977). Biochemical and structural analysis of SV40 chromatin. Cold Spring Harbor Symp. Quant. Biol. 42:227.

Klug A, Rhodes D, Smith J, Finch JT, Thomas JO (1980). A low resolution structure for the histone core of the nucleosome. Nature 287:509.

Lilly DMJ (1980). The inverted repeat as a recognizable structural feature in supercoiled

DNA molecules. Proc. Natl. Acad. Sci. 77:6468.
Lomonssoff GP, Butler PJG, Klug (1981).
Sequence-dependent variation in the conformation
of DNA. J. Mol. Biol. 149:745.
McGhee JD, Felsenfeld G (1980). Nucleosome
structure. Ann Rev. Biochem. 49:1115.
Marini JC, Levene SD, Crothers DM, Englund PT
(1982). Bent helical structure in kinetoplast
DNA. Proc. Natl. Acad. Sci. 79:7664.
Mizuuchi K, Mizuuchi M, Gellert M (1982). Cruciform
structures in palindromic DNA are favored by DNA
supercoiling. J. Mol. Biol. 156:229.
Morse RH, Cantor CR (1984). manuscript in
preparation.
Muller U, Zentgraf H, Eicken I, Keller W (1978).
Higher order structure of SV40 chromatin.
Science 201:406.
Nelson EM, Tewey KM, Liu, LF (1984). Mechanism of
antitumor drug action: poisoning of mammalian DNA
topoisomerase II on DNA by
4'-(9-acridinylamino)-methanesulfon-m-anisidide.
Proc. Natl. Acad. Sci. 81:1361.
Nickol JM, Felsenfeld G (1983). DNA conformation at
the 5' end of the chicken adult beta-globin gene.
Cell 35: 467.
Paulson JP, Laemmli UK (1977). The structure of
histone-depleted metaphase chromosomes. Cell
12:817.
Peck LJ, Nordheim A, Rich A, Wang JC (1982).
Flipping of the cloned $d(pCpG)_n \cdot d(pCpG)_n$ DNA
sequences from right- to left-handed helical
structure by salt, Co(III), or negative
supercoiling. Proc. Natl. Acad. Sci. 79: 4560.
Peck LJ, Wang JC (1981). Sequence-dependence of the
helical repet of DNA in solution. Nature
292:375.
Pettijohn DE (1982). Structure and properties of
the bacterial nucleoid. Cell 30:667.
Pope LE, Sigman DS (1984). Secondary structure
specificity of the nuclease activity of the
1,10-phenanthroline-copper complex. Proc. Natl.
Acad. Sci. 81:3.
Prior CP, Cantor CR, Johnson EM, Littau VC, Allfrey
VG (1983). Reversible changes in nucleosome
structure and histone H3 accessibility in
transcriptionally active and inactive states of
rDNA chromatin. Cell 34:1033.

Rhodes D, Klug A (1981). Sequence-dependent helical periodicity of DNA. Nature 292:378.

Ryoji M, Worcel A (1984). Chromatin assembly in Xenopus oocytes: in vivo studies. Cell 37:21.

Schon E, Evans T, Welsh J, Efstratiadis, E (1983). Conformation of promoter DNA: fine mapping of S1-hypersensitive sites. Cell 35:837.

Shore D, Baldwin RL (1983). Energetics of DNA twisting II. Topoisomer analysis. J. Mol. Biol. 170:983.

Sinden RR, Carlson JO, Pettijohn DE (1980). Torsional tension in the DNA double helix measured with trimethylpsoralen in living E. coli cells: analogous measurements in insect and human cells. Cell 21:773.

Sinden RR, Pettijohn DE (1982). Torsional tension in intracellular bacteriophage T4 DNA. Evidence that a linear DNA duplex can be supercoiled in vivo. J. Mol. Biol. 162:659.

Singleton CK, Wells, RD (1982). Relationship between superhelical density and cruciform formation in plasmid pVH51. J. Biol. Chem. 257:6292.

Smith CL, Kubo M, Imamoto F (1978). Promoter-specific inhibition of transcription by antibiotics which act on DNA gyrase. Nature 275:420.

Stirdivant SM, Klysik J, Wells RD (1982). Energetic and structural inter-relationship between DNA supercoiling andd the right- to left-handed Z helix transitions in recombinant plasmids. J. Biol. Chem. 257:10159.

Vogelstein B, Pardoll DM, Coffey DS (1980). Supercoiled loops and eucaryotic DNA replication. Cell 22:79.

Vorlickova M, Sedlacek P, Kypr J, Sponar J (1982). Conformationl transitions of poly(dA-dT).poly(dA-dT) in ethanolic solutions. Nucleic Acids Res. 10:6969.

Wang AH-J, Quigley GJ, Kolpak FJ, Crawford JL, van Boom JH, van der Marel G, Rich A (1979). Molecular structure of a left-handed double helical DNA fragment at atomic resolution. Nature 282:680.

Wang JC (1979). Helical repeat of DNA in solution. Proc. Natl. Acad. Sci. 76:200.

Weintraub H, Larsen A, Groudine M (1981).

β-Globin-gene switching during the development of chicken embryos:expression and chromatin structure. Cell 24:333.

Weintraub H (1983). A dominant role for DNA secondary structure in forming hypersensitive structures in chromatin. Cell 32:1191.

Weisbrod S, Groudine M, Weintraub H (1980). Interaction of HMG 14 and 17 with actively transcribed genes. Cell 19: 289.

Molecular Basis of Cancer, Part A: Macromolecular Structure, Carcinogens, and Oncogenes, pages 19–36
© 1985 Alan R. Liss, Inc.

DNA REPAIR IN THE IN VIVO SITE SPECIFIC EXCISION OF
PALINDROMIC SEQUENCES

A. Shafferman, Y. Flashner, I. Hertman and R. Rein

Department of Biochemistry
Israel Institute for Biological Research
P.O.Box 19, Ness-Ziona 70450, Israel

INTRODUCTION

Inverted repeat DNA sequences or palindromes have been
identified in DNA from many organisms. The prevalence of
palindromes at regulatory locations of such as transcription
initiation (Maniatis, et al. 1975), or termination signals
(Rosenberg, Court 1979), in DNA replication origins (Kolter,
Helinski]979) or at the ends of transposable DNA elements
in procaryotes or eucaryotes (Cold Spring Harbor, 43 Vol.1,
2 (1980)), has led to different speculations about their
possible biological significance. Such speculations were
guided by the realization (Platt 1955; Gierer 1966) that
palindromic DNA sequences can exist in two alternative structures: a regular DNA duplex with base pairing between strands
and a cruciform structure with intrastrand base pairing of
the self complementary sequence.

Thermodynamic as well as mechanical and statistical
mechanic calculations (Vologodskii, Frank-Kamenetskii 1982;
Benham 1982; Hsieh, Wang 1975) indicate that depending upon
the length and perfection of a palindromic sequence some
naturally occurring palindromes can form cruciforms at negative superhelicities that are typical of supercoiled DNAs
from natural sources. Mizuuchi et al. (1982) were able to
observe cruciform formation directly by electron microscopy
when a ring composed of very long inverted repeats was negatively supercoiled by DNA gyrase. It was also observed
(Lilley 1980; Panayotatos, Wells 1981; Singleton, Wells 1982),
that the single strand DNA specific nuclease S1 preferentially cleaves supercoiled DNAs at sites that are near the

dyads of palindromic sequences. These results were interpreted as a consequence of an attack at the single stranded
hairpin loop of the cruciform structure. All these observations together with indirect evidence that cellular processes might be influenced by DNA supercoiling (Cozzarelli
1980; Gellert 1981; Weisbard 1982; Larsen, Weintraub 1982)
imply again that cruciform structures may have intracellular
role. However, recent studies (Courey,Wang 1983; Gellert
et al. 1983; Sinden et al. 1983) suggest that while stable
cruciform structures in supercoiled DNA exist in-vitro
they rarely if at all exist in vivo. Nonetheless one cannot
exclude the possibility that such cruciform structures may
exist transiently in-vivo. Relevant to this point are the
numerous observations (Bolivar et al. 1977; Behnke et al.
1979; Collins 1980; Saedler et al. 1978; Brutlag et al.
1977; Collins et al. 1982; Gupta et al. 1983; Shafferman
et al. 1983), that there is a strong selection against long
inverted repeats which implies that topological effects
generating cruciforms are operative on DNA within a living
bacterium.

We have used the property of genetic instability of
inverted repeat sequences in bacteria as a research tool to
gain insight into the cellular state of palindromic DNA in
vivo. A limited sized 68bp perfect palindrome was constructed
(Shafferman, Helinski 1983; Shafferman et al. 1983) and inserted into various sites of a plasmid thereby generating
different plasmids each of which contains at different positions one copy of the palindrome (Fig. 1). The in vivo
fate of the palindrome in each plasmid derivatives was
followed by restriction enzyme analysis of plasmid DNA isolated from transformed bacteria. The palindrome possesses
a unique EcoRI site at its axis of symmetry, thus providing
a convenient way of determining whether or not the palindromic sequences were retained during their propagation in
vivo.

A detailed analysis of the fate of the 68bp palindromic
sequence in the various plasmids was reported recently
(Shafferman et al. 1983). Our main findings were:
a. Genetic instability of a given palindrome depends on its
    insertion locus.
b. Palindrome excision is driven by adjacent sequences which
    need be longer than 300bp from both sides of the palin-
    drome.

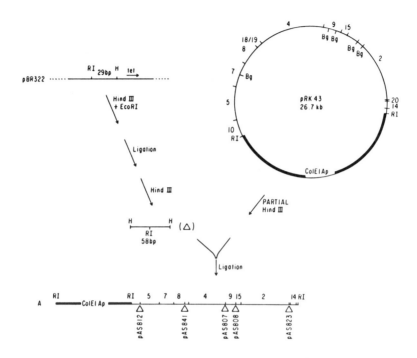

Fig. 1. Construction of pRK–43–derivatives which contain
an artificial 68bp palindrome at different sites. HindIII
sites are indicated and the fragments are numbered according
to Kolter and Helinski, 1978. Bg – refers to BglII sites on
the plasmid. A. Sites of the 68bp palindrome insertion are
indicated on the R6K sequences in pRK43. Any pRK43–derivative contains one copy of the palindrome.

c. Excision is independent of a functional host RecA gene
product but no excision is observed in a polA background.
Based on these observations a working model for in vivo excision of palindrome sequences was suggested. Here we report on our recent studies aimed at testing this working
model for the molecular events leading to palindrome instability in vivo.

DNA Sequence Analysis of Palindrome Deleted Plasmids

   To determine the DNA boundaries of the deletion associated with the loss of the palindromic EcoRI recognition
sequence (from its unstable configuration in pAS807) we have
analysed by restriction enzymes over 50 independent EcoRI-
deletion mutants designated pAS807-∇. Our ability to rege-
nerate the palindrome proximal HindIII DNA-fragments from
49 of the pAS807-∇ derivatives tested, suggests that sequences adjacent to the 68bp HindIII-palindrome are not
affected by the excision process. In addition at least one
of the two ClaI recognition sequence carried on the artificial 68bp palindrome is retained in any pAS807-∇ derivative tested by ClaI digestion. We conclude that in general
only palindromic sequences are being excised (from pAS807)
but that some of the palindrome sequences are still retained
in the resulting deleted pAS807-∇ plasmids. Ten pAS807-∇
were mapped more precisely for the extent of excision, and
in all of them, a deletion of about 50bp was found. Four
independent pAS807-∇ isolates were further subjected to DNA
sequence analysis. From such an analysis it turned out that
in all of the isolated pAS807-∇ 47bp of the original 68bp
palindrome were deleted (Fig. 2). The resulting pAS807-∇
plasmids still carry two inverted repeats of 9bp which are
separated by 3bp. It is in the context of the 3bp spacer
that these deletion isolates differ. Two isolates have a
GAT spacer sequence (deletion type I, Fig. 2) and two have
an ATC sequence (deletion type II). Interestingly, the spacer sequence of deletion type I is complementary to that of
deletion type II. This complementarity in the spacer region
and the fact that exactly the same number of bases are found
to be deleted in both deletion types, is suggestive of a
symmetrical event in the generation of these deletions, such
that may involve the two template strands of the parent palindromic molecule. But before we try to resolve the molecular events in the excision process, it is worth noting
that each of the 34bp inverted seuqences of the palindrome
possesses also two internal inverted repeats of 8bp, which
are identical to 8 out of 9bp in the inverted repeats found
in all pAS807-∇ derivatives. Furthermore, the 8bp internal
repeats of the 68bp palindrome are also separated by the
same 3bp bases (GAT or ATC) which separate the 9bp repeats
in the pAS807-∇ deletion mutants (Fig. 2). In Fig. 3, we
depict some of the possible secondary structures of the 68bp
palindrome taking into consideration the symmetry rules
stemming from the internal inverted repeats. From these

structures, it is easier to imagine how pAS807-∇ plasmids could have evolved upon replication. Without determining whether or not such structures stably exist in the cell or whether they are transient intermediates in the DNA replication process, it is clear that deletion type I or II in Fig. 2 are best explained either via an intermediate F structure (or its mirror image which is not depicted in Fig. 3) or via a G type structure.

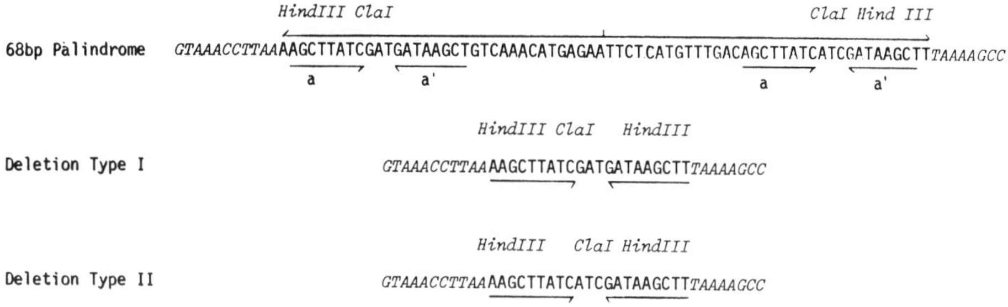

HindIII ClaI   ClaI Hind III

68bp Palindrome   GTAAACCTTAAAAGCTTATCGATGATAAGCTGTCAAACATGAGAATTCTCATGTTTGACAGCTTATCATCGATAAGCTTTAAAAGCC

           a   a'   a   a'

HindIII ClaI   HindIII

Deletion Type I   GTAAACCTTAAAAGCTTATCGATGATAAGCTTTAAAAGCC

HindIII   ClaI HindIII

Deletion Type II   GTAAACCTTAAAAGCTTATCATCGATAAGCTTTAAAAGCC

Fig. 2. Sequence of the intact 68bp palindrome in pAS807 and of the two types of deleted palindrome in pAS807-∇ plasmids. The R6K sequence bordering the palindrome are italicized. The 8bp palindrome internal inverted repeats are indicated by arrows above the letters a and a'.

Is a "Half Cruciform" Molecule a Stable Intermediate In Vivo?

In our working model (Shafferman et al. 1983) for the deletion of palindromic sequences, we have suggested that DNA polymerase I is able to replicate across stems and thereby produce "half cruciform" (or a hairpin molecule). A second round of DNA replication through hairpin can produce one copy of the observed deleted molecule. This simple model, which does not require DNA repair systems for the deletion of the palindrome, assumes that half cruciforms are stable intermediates in vivo. If indeed such intermediates are stable, then their presence can be revealed experimentally as described below.

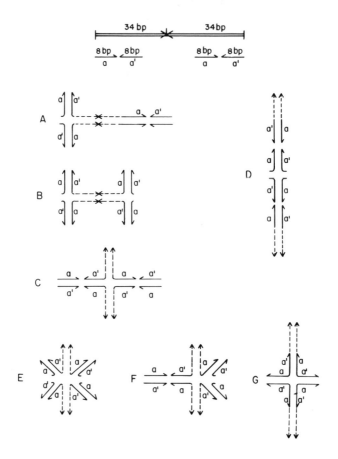

Fig. 3. Schematic presentation of possible secondary structures of the 68bp palindrome. The continuous arrows indicate the 8bp internal repeats (See Fig. 2), whereas the
interrupted arrows refer to the remaining repeat sequences
of the palindrome.

Both palindrome deleted molecules (pAS807-V) and half
cruciform molecules should exhibit resistance to EcoRI digestion of the palindrome sequence. The former molecule is
resistant simply because the EcoRI recognition sequence is

missing altogether while in the latter, the same sequence is present only in one strand (at the tip of the hairpin loop). However, the half cruciformic molecules may be converted to a DNA preparation which is susceptible to EcoRI (of the palindromic EcoRI site). This can be done by denaturation and annealing since in principle 50% of the half cruciforms represent either one of the parental palindromic strands. This expected behaviour of half cruciformic molecules served to test their possible existence.

A typical bacterial pAS807 transformant in which palindromes are being excised produces about 10% of palindrome deleted plasmid molecules when grown for 20 generations (Shafferman et al. 1983). Plasmid DNA preparation from such cultures show a characteristic pattern upon digestion with EcoRI. Instead of only 3 DNA fragments (1a, 1b and 2, Fig. 4) that should be generated by pAS807 plasmids carrying the complete palindrome, an additional band appears. This band (band - 1 in Fig. 4) originates from pAS807-∇ plasmids in which the palindromic EcoRI site is deleted. The molecular weight corresponding to DNA in band 1 is equal to that expected from the sum of DNA in band 1a and 1b. As explained above band 1 would also contain the EcoRI resistant half cruciform molecules if they exist. We therefore isolated the DNA from band 1. This DNA fragment was denatured and annealed, the 3' ends were labelled,then DNA was digested with EcoRI and finally applied to gel electrophoresis. If half cruciforms exist, some radioactive material will be recovered in positions corresponding to band 1a and 1b in addition to the radioactivity in band 1 which represents completely EcoRI deleted molecules. Following this protocol (Fig. 4), we were unable to detect radioactive material in position 1a and 1b (background was 100 cpm) and all the radioactivity was collected (10^6 cpm) in position 1.

Thus, the maximal ratio of DNA in band 1 to DNA in either band 1a or 1b is 10^4. This value is at least 20 fold higher than that expected if half cruciforms would have been stably maintained. (The frequency of excision is 10^{-4} per plasmid DNA replication round. Therefore after 20 cell generactions, at least $2 \times (20 \cdot 10^{-4})$ of the 10^6 counts found in a DNA representing deleted molecules (band 1, Fig. 4) would be expected to be found in DNA representing half cruciform structures (bands 1a+1b). In other words, in each of the bands 1a or 1b, we expect to find 2×10^3 cpm, yet experimental value is not higher than the background-10^2 cpm).

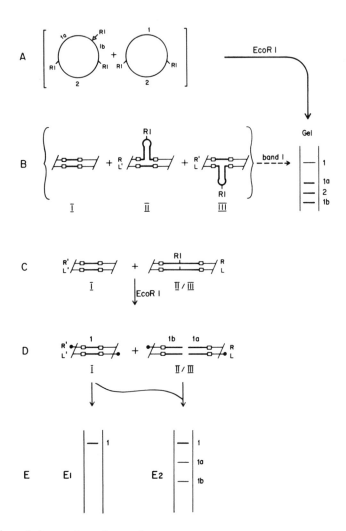

Fig. 4. Schematic plan of a test for half cruciforms.
A. The mixed plasmid DNA population (pAS807 & pAS807-∇) is
subjected to EcoRI digestion. B. The DNA is applied on agarose gel electrophoresis. Band 1 should contain three types
of DNA fragments: I-from pAS807 and II,III-from a fragment
containing a putative half cruciform structure. The palindromic sequences are presented by heavy lines. C. DNA is
isolated from band 1, denatured and annealed. The DNA is
then labelled at the 3' ends (by DNA PolI large fragment-
Klenow) and subjected again to EcoRI digestion. D. The ^{32}P

labelled DNA molecules are loaded on gel. E. After electrophoresis two pictures may emerge: E1 - If only palindrome
deleted molecule exist. E2 - Both palindrome deleted and half
cruciform molecules exist.
This may be revealed either by autoradiography or direct
measurement of the radioactivity.

In conclusion, this experiment suggests that if half
cruciforms are produced at all in the cell, they are very
short lived intermediates. Therefore, some DNA repair
mechanism is expected to be involved in the elimination of
hairpin structures during the process of generation of
palindrome deletions.

Incidence of Palindrome Loss in Bacteria Deficient in DNA
Repair Functions.

In a previous report (Shafferman et al. 1983), we have
shown that in a bacterial host which is wild type for DNA
repair functions, the 68bp palindrome is being lost from
pAS807 quite frequently. However, no loss of palindromic
sequences was detected in polA background. This phenomenon
can be used to prepare plasmid DNA which contains only pAS807
DNA without any detectable traces of pAS807-∇ plasmids. DNA
preparations of pAS807 isolated from polA bacteria is used
routinely for transformation of various bacterial strains in
which the frequency of excision of palindromes is to be determined. Very low DNA concentrations are used for all transformation experiments to minimize the effect of double transformation. DNA is isolated from transformed cells and monitored for the presence of palindromic EcoRI sequences, then
this DNA is used to retransform the same bacterial host from
which the DNA was isolated, and again DNA is extracted for
identification of palindrome deleted plasmid. Such double
cycles of transformation were carried out with many E. coli
mutants as summarized in Table 1. Whenever a process of excision of palindromic sequences occurs in a given strain (as
judged by the appearance of mixed plasmid DNA molecules ($\pm$
in Table 1)), then retransformation of this strain with the
plasmid DNA content from the isogenic strain yields about 15%
of clones which harbor palindrome deleted plasmids. Taking
into consideration the plasmid copy number in each strain (i.e.
15 to 30 copies(Shafferman, Helinski 1983; Shafferman et al.
1982) and the number of generations that have elapsed in
order to generate 15% of plasmid deleted molecules, we find

Table 1. Presence of Intact Palindrome in pAS807 –
Dependence on Various DNA Repair Functions

Transformed[a] Host	Presence of Palindrome[b]			No. of Clones Tested
	$-$	$\pm$	$+$	
Wild type	0	29	0	29
↓				
Wild type	3	24	0	27
polA1	0	0	27	27
↓				
polA1	0	0	24	24
polA (ex1)	0	0	26	26
↓				
polA (ex1)	0	0	15	15
lig(ts) (40°C)	0	0	24	24
↓				
lig(ts) (40°C)	0	0	12	12
endA	0	0	28	28
↓				
endA	0	0	24	24
recA13	0	19	0	19
↓				
recA13	4	15	0	19
uvrB	0	20	0	20
↓				
uvrB	2	16	0	18

a. The various transformed strains are as follows:
polA1 is C2110 (Kelley, Grindley 1976);polA(ex1) is
RS5052;lig(ts) is KS268; endA is YSI (Tomizawa et al.
1975); recA13 is HB101; uvrB is CSH71; wild type is C600,
and similar results were also obtained with LE392,
KS269 (isogenic partner of KS268) KS439b (isogenic partner of RS5052). The first cycle of transformation to any
of the mutants was done with pAS807 DNA (isolated from
polA) carrying the palindrome. Arrows indicate a second
cycle of transformation to any of the mutants.

b. Presence of palindrome was followed by EcoRI digestion
of plasmid DNA preparation from the indicated number of
independently isolated clones. +,–and $\pm$ refers to types
of plasmid population: intact palindrome, deleted palindrome and a mixed population, respectively.

that in bacteria wild type for DNA repair functions a frequency of deletion of 10^{-4} per round of plasmid DNA replication is obtained (Table 2). Similar frequencies are also obtained in bacterial strains deficient in functional RecA or uvrB gene products. These results suggest that the mechanism of excision of the inverted repeats does not depend upon homologous recA type recombination process or on the SOS type mechanism. In this sense, excision of the artificial palindromes resembles the independent transposition excision of transposons which depends on the presence of the right and left end inverted repeats of the transposons and which also occurs at frequencies of $3 \cdot 10^{-8}$ to 2×10^{-4} (Foster et al. 1981; Enger, Berg 1981).

Table 2. Excision Frequencies of Palindrome in Different DNA Repair Mutants.

Mutant	Enzyme or Function Defect	Frequency
Wild type	None	$\sim 10^{-4}$
polAl	DNA polymerization	$< 10^{-6}$
polAexl	$5' \rightarrow 3'$ exonuclease	$< 10^{-6}$
endA	ss and ds endonuclease	$< 10^{-6}$
lig(ts) $40°$	DNA ligation	$< 10^{-6}$
recAl3	DNA recombination, SOS repair	$\sim 10^{-4}$
uvrB	UV incision repair	$\sim 10^{-4}$

The fact that unlike other previously studied systems, in our system the artificial palindrome is cloned in a bifunctional replicon (pAS807 has both colE1 and R6K replication origins) that can be shuttled in between $polA^+$ or $polA$ background, allowed us to show that the excision of inverted repeats require DNA polymerase I. This is probably accomplished by the ability of PolI to replicate across stem structures (see below). Yet as a consequence of our failure to isolate the expected half cruciformic intermediate structures in a stable form, we have assumed that excision of palindromes involves in addition to DNA polymerization activity of PolI some other DNA repair enzymes. Indeed, it seems (Table 1 and 2) that endonuclease I, the PolI exonuclease $5' \rightarrow 3'$ and DNA ligase are also involved in the excision process.

Based on these studies and on the sequence analysis of palindrome deleted plasmids, we would like to suggest a model for excision of palindromic sequences in bacteria.

A Model for the Molecular Events Leading to Excision of Palindromes in Bacteria.

The model is depicted in Fig. 5. Our first assumption is that the presence of inverted repeats in a douplex DNA leads to formation of secondary structures such as cruciforms. When such structures are produced, either prior to DNA replication or as a consequence of DNA replication (by DNA unwinding and strand separation) these structures block further movement of the replication apparatus unless DNA polymerase I is available. It is known that unlike some DNA polymerases, such as E. coli PolII (Sherman, Gefter 1976; Challberg, Englund 1979), T4 or vaccinia DNA polymerase (Challberg, Englund 1979) which are stalled at secondary DNA structures, the E. coli PolI can efficiently traverse these structural barriers. It is possible that this property of PolI is a reflection of its unique ability to "strand switch" during displacement synthesis (Schildkraut et al. 1966). Strand switching is actually what is required in a replication across a double stranded stem structure. In the absence of DNA polymerization across the stem (as is suggested to be the case in polA mutants) incomplete DNA molecules will be produced and these may be degraded by cellular nucleases. This would explain the absence of palindrome deleted molecules in polA background. In other words, DNA carrying palindromes is not stabilized in polA, but rather any deletion event that commences in such a background is not recorded because the incomplete intermediate molecules are eliminated. This presumed lethal effect on the plasmid is not expected to lead to a concomitant decrease in plasmid copy number, since the excision event is not too frequent (10^{-4} per plasmid DNA replication round) to affect the copy number of pAS807. Indeed the plasmid copy number of pAS807 in polA is ~15 as found for wild type R6K (Shafferman et al. 1982).

Once DNA replication has proceeded through the stem (Stage 3, Fig. 5) a hairpin molecule should be produced and we would like to suggest that such an intermediate is a substrate for endonuclease I. The exact role of endonuclease I in the cell is still obscure, yet it is known (Kornberg 1982) that both double stranded and single stranded DNA can be attacked by endo I in vitro. It is therefore not unlikely that

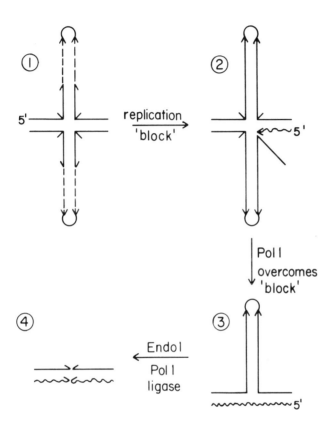

Fig. 5.   A model for molecular events involved in excision
of palindromes in bacteria (see text).

half cruciform like structures are legitimate substrate for
endonuclease I in vivo. Depending on the exact location of
endonucleolitic attack by endoI, again DNA polymerase I may
be required for both its 5'→3' exonuclease and its polymerization activities. Finally the DNA molecules are sealed up
by DNA ligase to produce the plasmid deleted molecules. This
sequence of events is compatible with all our observations.

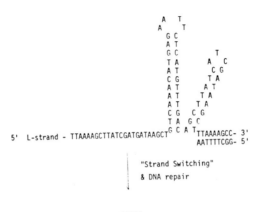

L- strand template: deletion type I.

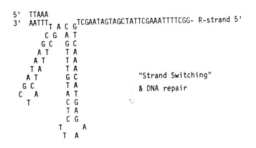

R-strand template: deletion type II

Fig. 6. Possible intermediate secondary structure of the 68bp palindrome which results in the observed two types of deletion mutants (Fig. 2), according to repair model in Fig. 5. The two types of deletion produce plasmids differing in the 3 bases of spacer region (marked by asterisks) separating the remaining inverted repeats.

In Fig. 6, we describe how the sequence of the palindrome in pAS807 can form the F structure depicted in Fig. 3, and how according to our model, the resulting deletion mutants can be generated depending on the template strand. The alternative simpler structure of a symmetrical cruciform (G in Fig. 3), can also generate the same deletion mutants. According to the model in Fig. 5, if endoI cleaves exactly at the base of the stem, no repair activity should follow the endonucleolitic attack, except that of the DNA ligase. However, we have shown that the exo 5'→3' activity of DNA PolI is essential for excision event. It follows then that either the strand switching by DNA polymerase requires the intactness of the complete DNA PolI molecule or more probably that the position of endonuclease action is not exactly at the base of the stem.

While our results are best explained by the presence of some transient cruciform structures, they provide no evidence for their stable existence. The cruciform state can be generated indirectly as a result of DNA replication either by strand separation and the folding of DNA through the intracomplementary sequences on one strand or as suggested in various cases of deletion between two direct repeats (Collins et al 1982; Farabaugh et al 1978) through the two internal 8bp direct repeats (a and a' in Fig. 2) of the 68bp palindrome. Nevertheless, if these secondary structures are just by products of DNA replication across a palindromic sequence, it may be difficult to explain why is it that insertion of the same palindrome in a given plasmid exhibits, at least, 100 fold difference in its stability, depending on its insertion locus (Shafferman et al. 1983). Even more intriguing is the telestability phenomenon of the palindrom in pAS807 which requires more than 300bp of the palindrome proximal sequences on both sides of the palindrome in order for it to be excised out (Shafferman et al. 1983). Work in progress in our laboratory seems to indicate that in vivo, certain topological constrains may operate to produce cruciformic structures, not only via replication, but in the supercoiled state of the plasmid DNA molecules.

ACKNOWLEDGEMENT

This research was funded by the National Foundation of Cancer Research.

REFERENCES

Behnke K, Malke H, Hartmann M, Walter F (1979). Post-transfor-
    mational rearrangement of an in vitro reconstructed group –
    A Streptococcal erythromycin resistance plasmid. Plasmid 2:
    605–616.
Benham CJ (1982). Stable cruciform formation at inverted re-
    peat sequences in supercoiled DNA. Biopolymers 21: 679–696.
Bolivar F, Betlach MC, Heyneker HL, Shine J, Rodriguez RL,
    Boyer HW (1977). Origin of replication of pBR345 plasmid
    DNA. Proc. Natl. Acad. Sci. U.S.A. 74: 5265–5269.
Brutlag D, Fry K, Nelson T, Hung P (1977). Synthesis of hybrid
    bacterial plasmids containing highly repeated satellite DNA.
    Cell 10: 509–519.
Challberg MD, Englund PT (1979). The effect of template secon-
    dary structure on Vaccinia DNA polymerase. J. Biol. Chem.
    254: 7820–7826.
Cold Spring Harbor Sym. Quant. Biol. (1980). Moveable genetic
    eléments. 43: Vol. 1 and 2.
Collins J (1980). The instability of palindromic DNA. Cold
    Spring Harbor Symp. Quant. Biol. 45: 409–416.
Collins J, Volckaert G, Nevers P (1982). Precise and nearly-
    precise excision of the symmetrical inverted repeats of
    Tn5: common features of recA-independent deletion events in
    E. coli. Gene 19: 139–146.
Courey AJ, Wang JC (1983). Cruficorm formation in a negatively
    supercoiled DNA may be kinetically forbidden under physio-
    logical conditions. Cell 33: 817–829.
Cozzarelli NR (1980). DNA gyrase and the supercoiling of DNA.
    Science 207: 953–960.
Enger C, Berg DE (1981). Excision of transposon Tn5 is de-
    pendent on the inverted repeats but not on the transposase
    function of Tn5. Proc. Natl. Acad. Sci. U.S.A. 78:459–463.
Farabaugh PJ, Schmeissner U, Hofer M, Miller JH (1978). Genetic
    studies of the lac repressor. VII. On the molecular nature
    of spontaneous hotspots in the lacI gene of E. coli. J. Mol.
    Biol. 126: 847–863.
Foster TJ, Lunblad V, Hanley-Way S, Halling SM, Kleckner N (1981).
    Three Tn10-associated excision events: relationship to trans-
    position and role of direct and inverted repeats. Cell 23:
    215–227.
Gellert M, O'Dea MH, Mizuuchi K (1983). Slow cruciform trans-
    ition in palindromic DNA. Proc. Natl. Acad. Sci. U.S.A.
    80: 5545–5549.

Gellert M (1981) DNA topoisomerases. Ann. Rev. Biochem. 50: 879–910.

Gierer A (1966). Model for DNA and protein interaction and the function of the operator. Nature 212: 1480–1481.

Gupta SC, Weith HL, Somerville RL (1983). Biological limitations on the length of highly repetitive DNA sequences that may be stably maintained within plasmid replicons in Escherichia coli. Biotechnology 1: 602–609.

Hsieh T, Wang J (1975). Thermodynamic properties of superhelical DNA. Biochemistry 14: 527–535.

Kelley WS, Grindley DF (1976). Mapping of the polA locus of Escherichia coli K12: Orientation of the amino- and carboxy-termini of the cistron. Molec. gen. Genet. 147: 307–319.

Kolter R, Helinski DR (1979). Regulation of initiation of DNA replication. Ann. Rev. Genet. 13: 355–391.

Kolter R, Helinski DR (1978). Construction of plasmid R6K derivatives in vitro: Characterization of the R6K replication region. Plasmid 1: 571–580.

Kornberg A (1982). DNA replication. San-Francisco: WH Freeman & Co.

Larsen A, Weintraub H (1982). An altered DNA conformation detected by S1 nuclease occurs at specific regions in active chick globin chromatin. Cell 29: 609–622.

Lilley DMJ (1980). The inverted repeat as a recognizable structural feature in supercoiled DNA molecules. Proc. Natl. Acad. Sci. USA. 77:6468–6472.

Maniatis T, Ptashne M, Backman K, Kleid D, Flashman S, Jeffrey A, Maurer R (1975). Recognition sequences of repressor and polymerase in operators of bacteriophage lambda. Cell 5: 109–113.

Mizuuchi K, Mizuuchi M, Gellert M (1982). Cruciform structures in palindromic DNA are favored by DNA supercoiling. J. Mol. Biol. 156: 229–243.

Panayatatos N, Wells RD (1981). Cruciform structures in supercoiled DNA. Nature 289: 466–470.

Platt JR (1955). Possible separation of intertwined nucleic acid chains by transfer-twist. Proc. Natl. Acad. Sci. U.S.A. 41: 181–183.

Rosenberg M, Gurt D (1979). Regulatory sequences involved in the promotion and termination of RNA transcription. Ann. Rev. Genet. 13: 319–353.

Saedler JR, Betz JL, Tecklenburg M, Goeddel DV, Yansura DG, Caruthers MH (1978). Cloning of chemically synthesised lactose operators. II. EcoRI-linkered operators. Gene 3: 211-232.

Scildkraut CL, Richardson CC, Kornberg A (1964). Enzymic synthesis of deoxyribonucleic acid. XVII. Some unusual physical properties of the product primed by native DNA templates. J. Mol. Biol. 9: 24-45.

Shafferman A, Kolter R, Stalker D, Helinski DR (1982). Plasmid R6K DNA replication, III. Regulatory properties of the π initiation protein. J. Mol. Biol. 161: 57-76.

Shafferman A, Helinski D (1983). Structural properties of the β origin of replication of plasmid R6K. J. Biol. Chem. 258: 4083-4090.

Shafferman A, Flashner Y, Hertman I (1983). Genetic instability of an artificial palindrome DNA sequence. J. Biomolecular Str. Dyn. 1: 729-742.

Sherman AL, Gefter ML (1976). Studies on the mechanism of enzymatic DNA elongation by E. coli DNA polymerase II. J. Mol. Biol. 103: 61-76.

Sinden RR, Broyles SS, Pettijohn DE (1983). Perfect palindromic lac operator DNA sequence exists as a stable cruciform structure in supercoiled DNA in vitro but not in vivo. Proc. Natl. Acad. Sci. U.S.A. 80: 1797-1801.

Singleton CK, Wells RD (1982). Relationship between super-helical density and cruciform formation in plasmid pVH51. J. Biol. Chem. 257: 6292-6295.

Tomizawa J, Sakakibara Y, Kakefuda T (1975). Replication of colicin E1 DNA added to cell extracts. Proc. Natl. Acad. Sci. U.S.A. 72: 1050-1056.

Vologodskii AV, Frank-Kamenetskii MD (1982). Theoretical study of cruciform states in supercoiled DNAs. FEBS Lett. 143: 257-260.

Weisbrod S (1982). Active chromatin. Nature 297: 289-295.

Molecular Basis of Cancer, Part A: Macromolecular
Structure, Carcinogens, and Oncogenes, pages 37–46

VARIATION OF DOUBLE-HELIX STABILITY ALONG DNA MOLECULAR
THREAD AND ITS BIOLOGICAL IMPLICATIONS: HOMOSTABILIZING
PROPENSITY OF GENE DOUBLE-HELIX

Akiyoshi Wada and Akira Suyama

Department of Physics, Faculty of Science
The University of Tokyo, Bunkyo-ku, Tokyo
Japan

INTRODUCTION

If we look at a DNA molecule along its long double
helical molecular thread, its chemical structure is
immediately recognizable as an array of well-known purine
and pyrimidine bases, A, G, T, and C, making A-T and G-C
pairs.   In contrast to this clear chemical structural
pattern, biological or genetic structures such as codons,
promoters, terminators, the origin of DNA replication,
splicing regions, and protein-coding regions are invisible
from a geometrical structural viewpoint.   They are
perceptible only through the direct physical interaction of
functional biological macromolecules, such as RNA polymerase,
the proteins related to DNA replication, transfer RNAs and
so on (for a review, see von Hippel, McGhee 1972 ; Champoux
1978 ; Wells et al. 1980).   The size of the unit in the
biological structure of DNA ranges from 3 bases in the case
of codons to several hundreds or thousands in the case of
genes.   Some of the rules of the transformation which
connect the chemical structure and the biological ones (i.e.
biological signals transmitted by base sequences) have now
been disclosed; they are in the library of the codon table
and consensus sequences.
A third type of structure, which is also not directly
perceptible from the geometrical structure of DNA, is the
distribution of physical properties along the double strand.
The aim of this report is to present evidence showing that
the pattern of heterogeneous distribution of physical
stability of the double helix along a DNA chain has a
remarkable positional correlation with its genetic map.   The

correlation not only is recognizable intuitively but also proves quantitatively to be a real one, as revealed by the quite high value of its statistical confidence level (see also our previous reports: Suyama, Wada 1983 ; Wada, Suyama 1983, 1984).

We are interested in the existence of a physico-genetic correlation in DNA, and stress its biological importance, for the following reason. Living organisms are believed to have accumulated advantageous characteristics found in the living mechanism as genetic information. In other words, as a result of natural selection, these advantages have been incorporated into the genetic structure by a newly added DNA fragment or an altered base sequence in the course of evolution. As already described, the process connecting the base sequence and genetic functions is a physical one of molecular interaction, which is governed by the structures of and the interaction energy between the DNA and interacting functional molecules. Thus, a change in the physical properties of functional sites of DNA, which is produced by a change in base sequence due to a mutation or a recombination, affects the molecular interaction, and will eventually result in changing the economy of biological function. This improved function should be fed back and ultimately fixed to the base sequence by the mechanism of natural selection.

Fig.1
Triangular correlation among three aspects of DNA. Other physical properties besides the double helical stability may be included in the physical aspect.

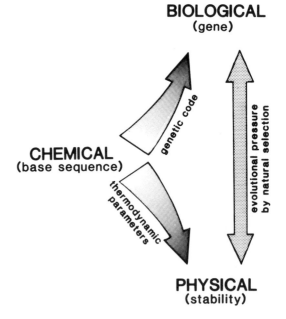

Syllogistically, the three types of DNA structure, which belong to the different categories specified above, establish a cyclic sequence of cause and effect. The relationships are schematically drawn in Fig.1 along with the factors that connect the different structures. The significant implication in this scheme is that the correlation between chemical and biological structure is not necessarily always direct. The redundancy in the translation rule between them (i.e. the wobble in the codon table) leaves some margin for base substitution without an affect on proteins' amino acid sequences and functions (i.e. synonymous translation). In other words, the DNA base sequence that is the best for cell systems may be determined primarily for the best protein function and, at the same time, for presenting the best conditions for DNA-functional protein interaction, within the redundancy of wobbled codons. Thus full understanding of the molecular genetic mechanism of DNA may not be established without comprehension of its structure in terms of physical properties.

PHYSICAL STABILITY MAP: PRINCIPLES AND PROCEDURE OF CALCULATION

A change of bases alters many kinds of physical properties, some of which are local and some non-local. For instance, base substitution will alter the distribution of hydrophobicity and hydrogen-bonding ability along the major or minor grooves of the double helix, and the electrostatic molecular potential surface as well. The effects of these changes are relatively localized at the site of an altered base. On the other hand, the physical stability of the double helix is affected over a stretch of several tens to several hundreds of bases by one base-pair substitution (Wada et al. 1980). There are two reasons why we have chosen in the present study to analyse the double-helix stability distribution among many physical properties. 1) The opening capability of the double helix, and thus its local stability, may be a factor which controls the DNA-functional protein binding. 2) The cooperative length of the stability (the length of a cooperatively melting region which will be described below) is comparable with the length of genes. Therefore, a physico-genetic coupling may take place in this dimension.

Cooperatively Melting Region

A DNA double strand consists of a series of virtual blocks with different double helix stability, whose length ranges from a hundred to several thousand base pairs

(Vizard, Ansevin 1976 ; Gotoh et al. 1976 ; Tachibana et al. 1978 ; Wada et al. 1980). The pattern of stability distribution is determined by the effect of the base sequence on the cooperative nature of the double helical structure, so that it is unique to a given base sequence. Broadly speaking, the stable region is a region rich in G-C pairs, which are more stable than A-T pairs. In this regard, the stability map may not be much different from the map of local G+C content. However, a complex feature is brought into the stability of the double helix by its cooperative nature due to base-base stacking and by long-range interactions which originate in the electrostatic interaction and in the entropy effect arising from the motional freedom of internal loops. These cooperative and long-range factors cannot be attributed to each nucleotide residue separately, so that the stability map appears greatly different from the map of local G+C content. These long-range effects provide a smoother stability distribution than that expected from the local G+C content and gives more definite divisions, i.e. cooperatively melting region (CMR), in DNA (Wada et al. 1980; Tachibana et al. 1978).

The evidence of the cooperative melting of DNA is observable either by plotting a differential thermal melting curve (Wada et al. 1980 and references therein) or by electron microscope (Funnel and Inman 1979). The former has a higher temperature-resolution but lacks the ability to directly locate unfolded regions, which can be done by the latter method. However, although electron microscopy is a unique way of directly observing CMR, the environmental condition of DNA, e.g. temperature or ionic strength, is obscure because of the necessity of drying samples for observation.

The present authors have used an indirect but more universal procedure to locate CMR for the stability mapping of DNA. The state of a double helix, that is, whether a particular site is in the helix state or coil state, is calculated by the statistical mechanical theory of the helix-coil transition taking the base sequence explicitly. Information required for the calculation is the base sequence and thermodynamic parameters that characterize the contribution of the base pairs and the internal freedom of motion (i.e. the entropy of the nucleotide chain) to the stability of the double helix (Ueno et al. 1978). The values of molecular thermodynamic parameters are universal for all DNA and have been determined by comparing experimentally observed differential thermal melting curves of several DNAs of known base sequence with theoretically calculated curves. The values of the parameters used in this report are for the solvent of 0.1 x SSC and are the same as those proposed by Gotoh (1983) except for the value of the cooperativity parameter : $\sigma = 6 \times 10^{-6}$.

Once the universal parameters have been determined, stability maps can be delineated by computer work, without making experimental observations, for any DNA of which the whole base sequence is given. Therefore, stability distribution maps of a few million bases in total which have been stored in the DNA data bank can now be the subject of the analyses.

All the calculations are made by the algorithm of Fixman and Freire (1977). The details of the calculation and the way the calculated differential melting curve agrees well with the experimentally obtained one is described in separate articles (Ueno et al. 1978; Gotoh, Tagashira 1981; Gotoh 1983; Suyama, Wada in preparation).

The stability distribution is plotted along the axis of base numbers, 1 to n, from 5' to 3' terminus. Stability of the i-th base pair is expressed in terms of the temperature Tm, giving it a probability of 50% helix.

Generality of Thermal Stability Map.

The stability map thus obtained is that for thermal perturbation. In this regard, it might be thought that stability maps in such a non-physiological condition will not provide any biologically significant information. This is not true because the thermal stability has a more comprehensive meaning: It represents the local resistivity of a double helix against the force to open it. As a matter of fact, the DNA unfolding produced by ligand binding, e.g. single-strand binding protein, which occurs in a normal physiological condition and is believed to play an important role in the processes of DNA replication, transcription, and recombination, is found to be quite similar to the mode of thermal melting. We have demonstrated, in a theoretical study, that calculated ligand-induced melting profiles of DNA (degree of unfolding vs. ligand concentration curve) reveal fine structures, and when the binding cooperativity is large, the profile becomes similar to the thermal melting profile (Tachibana, Wada 1982). Furthermore, in this high-cooperative binding case, cooperatively melting regions are found to be identical in their relative stabilities and in the positions of their boundaries whether the melting is ligand-induced or thermally induced. With the variation of ligand concentration inside a cell, therefore, it is expected that the unfolding of the double strand takes place in the same way as the unfolding by thermal perturbation.

RESULTS AND DISCUSSION

   We have calculated double-helix stability distributions
in the following DNAs : DNAs of T7 phage; human, bovine,
mouse, yeast, and A. nidulans mitochondrions; humanα -globin
gene cluster (ζ-,$\psi\zeta$-,$\psi\alpha$1-,α2-, andα1-globin genes); goat
βx- and βz-globin pseudogenes; avian, moloney mouse, and
feline sarcoma virus oncogenes; human T24 bladder carcinoma
oncogene; plasmids pCl94, pEl94 and pTl81 from Staphylococcus
aureus; and plasmid pEl94 from B. subtilis.
   The base sequences used are based on sequence data in
the Los Alamos Sequence Library.
   Fig. 2 shows a typical result of the stability map of
the DNA of phage T7. Fig. 3 shows a set of maps of globin
genes which are reproduced from our previous report (Wada,
Suyama 1983). In these plots we can find immediately that
the   genes   have   fairly   uniform   stabilities   while   the
intervening regions or introns have a remarkable tendency to
have fluctuating stability.   The stability fluctuation is
also found to be clustered around the boundary of these
genetic divisions.
   The cases exhibited above, and others, demonstrate that
the double-helix stability distribution showing a correlated
pattern with the distribution of genetic divisions is a
general characteristic of a variety of DNAs.   The principal
feature of the stability maps of the 21 DNA species examined
in this study, together with the results of the previous
studies on DNAs of phages ϕx174, G4, fd (Suyama and Wada
1983) and λ (Wada and Suyama 1984) ; of tumor viruses SV40,
BKV, and polyoma (Suyama and Wada 1983); and of seven globin
genes (Wada and Suyama 1983) may be summarized as follows.
1. A protein coding region has homostabilizing propensity
around   a   defined   stability   which   is   specific   to   each
individual gene (Wada et al. 1976 ; Wada, Suyama 1984).
2. There is a statistically significant   correlation (level
of   significance : α =0.01~0.001)   between   boundaries   of
cooperatively melting regions and boundaries of protein
coding   regions;   that   is,   the   double-helix   stability
fluctuates at gene boundaries (Suyama, Wada 1983).
3. Introns are found to be relatively unstable and to have
fluctuating stability.   In a stability map they are often
shown as a basin with a bumpy bottom (Wada, Suyama 1983).
4. Non-protein coding regions are regions of large stability
fluctuation.   The coincidence is statistically confident at
the level of significanceα=0.01 (Wada, Suyama 1984).
5. In spite of the homostable nature of protein coding
regions on the average, they have fluctuating stability near
their termini (Wada, Suyama 1984).

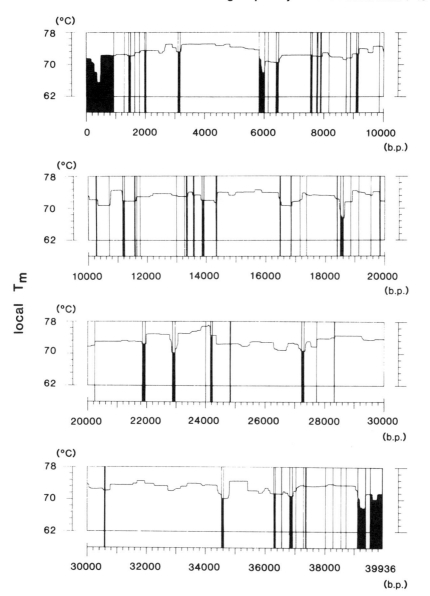

Fig. 2   Double-helix stability map of T7 phage DNA.
Molecular thermodynamic parameters used in the calculation
are for the solvent condition of 0.1 x SSC.   Gene boundaries
are indicated by vertical lines and non-coding regions by
shadowing.

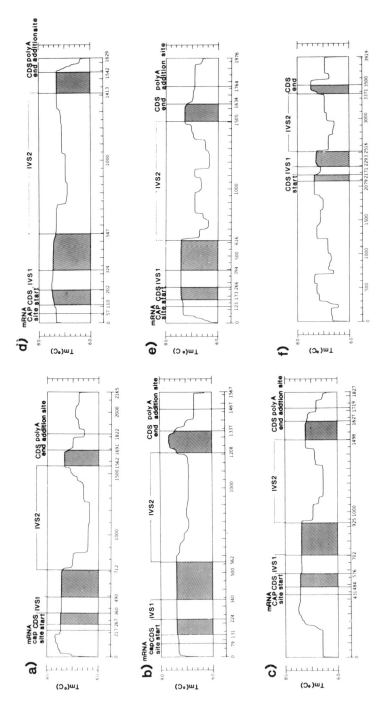

Fig. 3 Stability maps of DNAs of globin genes and flanking regions compared with their genetic maps. Exons are indicated by shadowing.

a) human β-globin   b) mouse β-globin   c) rabbit β₁-globin(typeI allele)
d) human fetal γ-globin A   e) human δ-globin   f) human embryonic ε-globin

6. The DNAs of pseudogenes and oncogenes show the same pattern of stability distribution; no difference was found from other DNAs examinined in our studies.

The physico-genetic correlation which is found in the varieties of DNAs mentioned above seems to be related in some sense to the nature of base distribution (i.e. the chemical structure) in DNA (Tong, Battersby 1979 ; Wada, Suyama 1984).

As for the specific feature of the chemical structure, Sueoka (1962) has pointed out that a DNA has a homogeneous distribution of local G+C content. For fairly long DNAs of bacterial and higher organisms, in other words, even though their average G+C contents varies from 25 to 75%, the distribution of the local base composition in individual DNAs is found to be rather narrow, not deviating much from binomial distribution (see Ueno et al. 1978 ; Wada et al. 1980). Sueoka (1962) and Freese (1962) interpreted this evidence as due to a species-specific balance in the equilibrium of the GC $\rightleftarrows$ AT transversion. Recently Gojobori et al. (1982) demonstrated, by the analysis of patterns of nucleotide substitution in pseudogenes and functional genes, that pseudogenes have a tendency to be rich in A and T bases. It is well known that nucleotide base substitution is much more frequent in the DNA regions with no functional constraints than in functional genes (Kimura 1980 ; Miyata, Yasunaga 1981; Hayashida, Miyata 1983 ; Li et al. 1981 ; Gojobori et al. 1982). The non-functional region is also known to provide recombination sites because of the absence of functional constraints. These factors in base substitution and recombination might be considered to be the origins of the less stable and fluctuating nature of intervening non-functional regions.

Tong and Battersby (1979) have demonstrated that denaturation maps (stability distribution maps in our terminology) correlate somewhat with the boundary where sharp changes in local A+T contents take place. This finding is supported by a more detailed statistical analysis by us (Wada, Suyama 1984).

There is no doubt that some functional constraints have provided the characteristic features in the physical and chemical maps of DNA as described above. It is hard, however, to say which of the physical and chemical effects is the cause and which is the result. Even though the question is somewhat similar to the famous puzzle of "which came first, the chicken or the egg," we now tend to believe that convenience in a physical process, such as the smoothness of the "zippering" of the DNA double strand, comes first. If the reverse were true, it would seem to be quite improbable for base sequences, which have been selected just for the economy of a biological function (for instance, by limiting the types of t-RNA), to just happen to have a regular characteristic in the stability distribution.

This work was supported by a grant-in-aid from the Ministry of Education, Science and Culture, Japan.

References

Champoux JJ (1978) Annu Rev Biochem 47:449.

Freese E, (1962) J Theo Biol 3:82.

Fixman M, Freire JJ (1977) Biopolymers 16:2693.

Funnel BE, Inman RB (1979) J Mol Biol 131:331.

Gojobori T, Li W-H, Graur D (1982) J Mol Evol 18:360.

Gotoh O, Husimi Y, Yabuki S, Wada A (1976) Biopolymers 15:655.

Gotoh O, Tagashira Y (1981) Biopolymers 16:2693.

Gotoh O (1983) Adv Biophys 16:1.

Hayashida H, Miyata T (1983) Proc Natl Acad Sci 80:2671.

Kimura M (1980) J Mol Evol 16:111.

Li W-H, Gojobori T, Nei M (1981) Nature 292:237.

Miyata T, Yasunaga T (1981) Proc Natl Acad Sci 78:450.

Sueoka N (1961) J Mol Biol 3:31.

Suyama A, Wada A (1983) J Theor Biol 105:133.

Tachibana H, Wada A, Gotoh O, Takanami M (1978) Biochim Biophys Acta 517:319

Tachibana H, Wada A (1982) Biopolymers 21:1873.

Tong BY, Battersby SJ (1979) Nucl Acid Res 6:1073.

Ueno S, Tachibana H, Husimi Y, Wada A (1978) J Biochem 84:917.

Vizard DL, Ansevin AT (1976) Biochemistry 15:741.

Von Hippel PH, McGhee JD (1972) Annu Rev Biochem 41:231.

Wada A, Tachibana H, Gotoh O, Takanami M (1976) Nature 263:439.

Wada A, Yabuki S, Husimi Y (1980) CRC Crit Rev Biochem 9:87.

Wada A, Suyama A (1983) J Phys Soc Japan 52:4417.

Wada A, Suyama A (1984) Abstract "International Symposium of Static and Dynamic Structures of Nucleic Acids, Proteins and Membranes" April 23-28, 1984, Rome.

Wells RD, Goodman TC, Hillen W, Horn GT, Klein RD, larsen JE, Muller VR, Nevendorf SK, Panayotatos N, Stirdivant SM (1980) Prog Nucl Acid Res Mol Biol 24:167.

Molecular Basis of Cancer, Part A: Macromolecular
Structure, Carcinogens, and Oncogenes, pages 47–53
© 1985 Alan R. Liss, Inc.

BIOLOGICAL AND CHEMICAL PROPERTIES OF LEFT HANDED Z-DNA

Robert D. Wells

Department of Biochemistry
University of Alabama in Birmingham
Birmingham, Alabama 35294

INTRODUCTION

Studies with DNA polymers which were initiated in
approximately 1966 provided the first evidence that
different DNA sequences have different conformations and
properties. In the past five years, investigations on the
structure of DNA have generated renewed interest due to the
demonstration of left handed helices in oligonucleotides,
DNA polymers, restriction fragments, and recombinant
plasmids.

A variety of recombinant plasmids have been
constructed in this laboratory which contain different
lengths of several types of sequences which can adopt left
handed Z structures. (dC-dG) inserts which are 58, 32, 26,
and 10 bp in length have been inserted into pBR322 in a
flanking orientation around the E. coli lac operator.
Furthermore, we have cloned sequences with repeating T and
G residues (C and A in the complimentary strand), as well
as mixtures of these types of sequences. All of these
sequences adopt left handed structures.

A major interest which derives from these studies is
the demonstration of a stable junction between the right
handed B and left handed Z structures.

Substantial information has been learned in the past
five years from this and other laboratories on structural
questions related to left handed Z DNA. A major thrust for

the future will be the evaluation of the biological
properties of this and other unusual forms of DNA.

Studies which were performed on restriction fragments
include circular dichroism, laser Raman spectroscopy, and
^{31}P-NMR (Wells, Brennan, Chapman, Goodman, Hart, Hillen,
Kellogg, Kilpatrick, Klein, Klysik, Lambert, Larson,
Miglietta, Neuendorf, O'Connor, Singleton, Stirdivant,
Veneziale, Wartell, Zacharias 1983). In the case of large
recombinant plasmids, left handed structures have been
demonstrated by supercoil relaxation studies (in both one
and two dimensions), S_1 and BAL31 nuclease sensitivity of
the junctions between right handed and left handed
structures, and antibody binding determinations (reviewed
in Wells, Brennan, Chapman, Goodman, Hart, Hillen, Kellogg,
Kilpatrick, Klein, Klysik, Lambert, Larson, Miglietta,
Neuendorf, O'Connor, Singleton, Stirdivant, Veneziale,
Wartell, Zacharias 1983).

The purpose of this review is to describe work from
this laboratory. Work from other laboratories has been
identified in the contributions listed in references.

MICROHETEROGENEITY

Left handed Z-DNA can neighbor right handed regions in
close proximity on the same chain (Wells, Brennan, Chapman,
Goodman, Hart, Hillen, Kellogg, Kilpatrick, Klein, Klysik,
Lambert, Larson, Miglietta, Neuendorf, O'Connor, Singleton,
Stirdivant, Veneziale, Wartell, Zacharias 1983; Klysik,
Stirdivant, Larson, Hart, Wells 1981; Klysik, Stirdivant
Wells 1982; Stirdivant, Klysik, Wells 1982; Wells,
Miglietta, Klysik, Larson, Stirdivant, Zacharias 1982;
Wartell, Klysik, Hillen, Wells 1982; Singleton, Klysik,
Stirdivant, Wells 1982; Zacharias, Larson, Klysik,
Stirdivant, Wells 1982; Klysik, Stirdivant, Singleton,
Zacharias, Wells 1983; Singleton, Kilpatrick, Wells 1984;
Singleton, Klysik, Wells 1983; Kilpatrick, Klysik,
Singleton, Zarling, Jovin, Hanau, Erlanger, Wells 1984;
Kilpatrick, Wei, Gray, Wells 1983). A large number of
prior studies on natural DNAs as well as DNA polymers had
demonstrated the presence of unusual conformations (such as
A or C forms). However, prior to the types of studies
which are described herein, it was not possible to show the
presence of more than one helical form of DNA in the same

molecule. Since a variety of determinations have shown the presence of left handed helices within molecules which are otherwise right handed, the concept of DNA microheterogeneity seems firmly established.

SUPERCOILING INDUCES LEFT HANDEDNESS

Negative supercoiling (at levels found in vivo) is sufficient to convert the (dC-dG) regions (58, 32, 26 and 10 bp in length) in recombinant plasmids into a left handed structure under physiological ionic conditions. Thus, it is likely that left handed DNA exists in vivo (Singleton, Klysik, Stirdivant, Wells 1982; Zacharias, Larson, Klysik, Stirdivant, Wells 1982; Klysik, Stirdivant, Singleton, Zacharias, Wells 1983; Singleton, Kilpatrick, Wells 1984; Singleton, Klysik, Wells 1983; Kilpatrick, Klysik, Singleton, Zarling, Jovin, Hanau, Erlanger, Wells 1984; Kilpatrick, Wei, Gray, Wells 1983).

One possible role for left-handed DNA is to modulate the extent of supercoiling and thereby affect biological processes such as transcription at a distant location on a topologically constrained segment of DNA. It is known that a number of promoters are effected by supercoiling. Some promoters are enhanced, some are turned down and others are unaffected. A small change in the primary helix at one location on a topologically constrained DNA can affect the overall structure at a distant location. In addition, it is possible that left handed structures will serve as energy sinks with relationship to supercoiling.

B-Z JUNCTIONS

Single-strand specific nucleases (S_1 and BAL31) recognize and cleave aberrant structural features at the B-Z junctions (Singleton, Klysik, Stirdivant, Wells 1982; Singleton, Kilpatrick, Wells 1984; Singleton, Klysik, Wells 1983; Kilpatrick, Klysik, Singleton, Zarling, Jovin, Hanau, Erlanger, Wells 1984; Kilpatrick, Wei, Gray, Wells 1983). These junctions exhibit both sequence and superhelical-dependent conformational flexibility (Singleton, Klysik, Wells 1983; Kilpatrick, Klysik, Singleton, Zarling, Jovin, Hanau, Erlanger, Wells 1984).

One of the major outstanding questions regarding left handed DNA concerns the structure and properties of junctions. It is possible that these unusual structural features serve as entry points for DNA recombination.

OTHER LEFT HANDED STRUCTURES

(dC-dG) sequences may exist in a family of left handed conformations. Spectroscopically identifiable conformational intermediates exist between the B and Z structures (Zacharias, Larson, Klysik, Stirdivant, Wells 1982). In addition to spectroscopic studies, x-ray analysis of small oligonucleotides has revealed variants of the Z conformation. Furthermore, antibody binding studies in the laboratories of Stollar and of Jovin are consistent with the notion of more than one type of left handed conformation.

CONDITIONS INDUCING Z-DNA

A variety of divalent metal ions (at μM concentrations) and dehydrating conditions are effective in causing the R to L transition (Zacharias, Larson, Klysik, Stirdivant, Wells 1982; Zacharias, Martin, Wells 1983). Other workers referenced in Zacharias, Larson, Klysik, Stirdivant, Wells 1982 have shown the importance of heat in effecting the B to Z transition.

ENERGETICS

The free energy cost of a junction region is approximately 5 kcal/mol of junction (Klysik, Stirdivant, Singleton, Zacharias, Wells 1983; Singleton, Klysik, Wells 1983). The free energy difference between between a B and a Z GC base pair is 0.44 kcal/mole for the unmethylated GC tract in a plasmid and 0.21 kcal/mole GC base pair for the methylated state (Klysik, Stirdivant, Singleton, Zacharias, Wells 1983).

LEFT HANDED $(dT-dG)_n \cdot (dC-dA)_n$

$(dT-dG)_n \cdot (dC-dA)_n$ adopts a left handed Z conformation in a recombinant plasmid (Kilpatrick, Klysik,

Singleton, Zarling, Jovin, Hanau, Erlanger, Wells 1984).
Also, when the DNA polymer with this sequence is first
modified by acetylaminofluorene (AAF), the DNA adopts a
left handed structure in concentrated salt solution (Wells,
Miglietta, Klysik, Larson, Stirdivant, Zacharias 1982).

This sequence appears to be ubiquitous in eucaryotic
cells. We subcloned this sequence from the 3' side of the
mouse kappa immunoglobin gene which contained a region of
64 bp of the repeating T and G sequence. The biological
role of these ubiquitous sequences are unknown but may be
related to their capability of forming unusual structures.

METHYLATION

Methylation of cytosine in a (dC-dG) region stabilizes
the left handed Z structure in fragments and plasmids
(Klysik, Stirdivant, Singleton, Zacharias, Wells 1983).
The observed free energy contributions of the B-Z junction
and cytosine methylation suggests that two junctions offset
the favorable effect of methylation on the Z conformation
in (dC-dG)$_n$ sequences (29 bp in length).

Methylation is believed to play an important role in
regulation of gene expression in eucaryotic cells. The
energetics of the B to Z transition with methylated
plasmids is consistent with methylation serving as a
triggering mechanism for conformational changes.

Studies on methylation of recombinant plasmids are
also important as they provide probes for conformational
changes (see below).

IVS2 SEQUENCES: RECOMBINATION

The large intervening sequences of three human fetal
globin genes containing tracts of alternating purine-
pyrimidine sequences (40-60 bp in length) adopt left handed
Z helices under the influence of supercoiling (Kilpatrick,
Klysik, Singleton, Zarling, Jovin, Hanau, Erlanger, Wells
1984). These sequences are involved in genetic
recombination and intergenic exchange (gene conversion).
Other studies indicated a possible role for sequences with
left handed structure potential in recombination in E. coli
(Klysik, Stirdivant, Wells 1982).

METHYLASE AS A PROBE FOR LEFT HANDED DNA

We have recently demonstrated that the Hha I methylase and restriction endonuclease can serve as probes for DNA conformational changes (B to Z) in (dC-dG) sequences (Zacharias, Larson, Kilpatrick, Wells submitted for publication). Recombinant plasmids containing (dC-dG) tracts have been analyzed for their capability to serve as substrates for the Hha I methylase when the alternating G and C tract is in a right handed structure or a left handed structure as modulated by supercoiling. Our results demonstrate that the (dC-dG) tract is completely resistant to methylation when the supercoil density is sufficiently high to generate a left handed region. The presence of a large number of other Hha I sites in right handed structures within the pBR322 vector provides an important positive control. Kinetic evaluations have been performed using radioactive SAM and we have mapped the sites of incorporation of labelled methyl groups into different segments of the recombinant plasmids. These determinations have been performed with populations of topoisomers at different supercoiled densities as well as with individual topoisomers which have been analyzed by two dimensional gel electrophoresis.

Completely analogous conclusions can be drawn regarding the capability of the Hha I restriction endonuclease to cleave right handed DNA but not left handed Z-DNA.

These results are significant from enzyme mechanistic and biological standpoints as well as for establishing a sensitive probe for left handed helices.

ACKNOWLEDGEMENTS

These studies were supported by grants from the NIH (GM21839) and the NSF (PCM-8002622).

REFERENCES

References are focused on work from this laboratory; this article is not intended to serve as a general review of left handed DNA, however, more than 500 references to

the work of other laboratories are cited in the
contributions listed below.

Kilpatrick MW, Wei CF, Gray HB, Wells RD (1983). Nucleic
  Acids Research 11:3811-3822.
Kilpatrick MW, Klysik J, Singleton CK, Zarling D, Jovin TM,
  Hanau LH, Erlanger BF, Wells RD (1984). J Biol Chem
  259:7268-7274.
Klysik J, Stirdivant SM, Larson JE, Hart PA, Wells RD
  (1981). Nature 290:672-677.
Klysik J, Stirdivant SM, Wells RD (1982). J Biol Chem
  257:10152-10158.
Klysik J, Stirdivant SM, Singleton CK, Zacharias W,
  Wells RD (1983). J Mol Biol 168:51-71.
Singleton CK, Klysik J, Stirdivant SM, Wells RD (1982).
  Nature 299:312-316.
Singleton CK, Klysik J, Wells RD (1983). Proc Natl Acad
  Sci 80:2447-2451.
Singleton CK, Kilpatrick MW, Wells RD (1984). J Biol Chem
  259:1963-1967.
Stirdivant SM, Klysik J, Wells RD (1982). J Biol Chem
  257:10159-10165.
Wartell RM, Klysik J, Hillen W, Wells RD (1982). Proc Natl
  Acad Sci 79:2549-2553.
Wells RD, Miglietta JJ, Klysik J, Larson JE, Stirdivant SM,
  Zacharias W (1982). J Biol Chem 257:10166-10171.
Wells RD, Brennan R, Chapman KA, Goodman TC, Hart PA,
  Hillen W, Kellogg DR, Kilpatrick MW, Klein RD, Klysik J,
  Lambert PF, Larson JE, Miglietta JJ, Neuendorf SK,
  O'Connor T, Singleton CK, Stirdivant SM, Veneziale CM,
  Wartell RM, Zacharias W (1983). Cold Spring Harbor
  Symposium 47:77-84.
Zacharias W, Larson JE, Klysik J, Stirdivant SM, Wells RD
  (1982). J Biol Chem 257:2775-2782.
Zacharias W, Martin JC, Wells RD (1983). Biochemistry
  22:2398-2405.

Molecular Basis of Cancer, Part A: Macromolecular
Structure, Carcinogens, and Oncogenes, pages 55–69
© 1985 Alan R. Liss, Inc.

ELECTROSTATICS AND SPECIFICITY IN NUCLEIC ACID REACTIONS

Bernard Pullman

Institut de Biologie Physico-Chimique
Fondation Edmond de Rothschild
13, rue Pierre et Marie Curie – 75005 Paris – FRANCE

1. INTRODUCTION

The determination of the factors and mechanisms which
govern the specificity of intermolecular interactions is one of the
main problems of modern molecular biology. For a long time it was
considered essentially in relation to proteins, where it was realized
that although the reactions take place at a local "active site" their
mechanism and turnover rate are under the dependence of the
overall structure of the macromolecule.

In recent years the problem has acquired great importance in
relation to the nucleic acids and this for two reasons. One of them is
the accumulation of evidence that the nucleic acids are the main or
the most significant target for reactions with a large number of
exogenous compounds including carcinogens, mutagens, antibiotics, antitumor drugs, antiviral drugs etc.

The second is the discovery, or at least the full realization of
the significance, of the polymorphism and microheterogeneity of
DNA, a realization which was particularly stimulated by the specta-
cular discovery of Z-DNA by Rich and collaborators (Wang et al,
1979, 1980) and the demonstration of the probable biological
significance of this variety of DNA.

There is not much doubt that for a long period specificity of
interaction was considered as being due essentially to geometrical
factors : accessibility, adaptability, complementarity between the
ligands and the target macromolecule (the "key and lock" or "hand
and glove" concepts). Today the problem has broadened and few
modern biophysicists would still pretend, I believe or at least I hope

so, that these geometrical factors are the only ones involved. Evidence is accumulating which shows that what broadly may be referred to as electronic factors play also a very important role in specificity. This situation means that specificity, although it frequently takes up the appearance of a local phenomenon, may in fact be determined in a quite important if not decisive way be distant influences springing from the overall global structure of the reacting species. It is this aspect of the specificity problem that I would like to present to you here in connection with some features of the reactivity of the nucleic acids, in particular DNA, related to chemical carcinogenesis or therapy.

2.   MOLECULAR ELECTROSTATIC POTENTIAL IN DNA AND ITS CONSTITUENTS

In order to determine the possible role of the overall electronic structure of a macromolecule on the specificity of its local interactions with external ligands, it is essential to choose an appropriate electronic property of the polymer which is liable to translate the effect of its distant parts on the region of space involved. Such a suitable characteristic seems to be available in the form of the molecular electrostatic potential generated by the charge distribution of the polymeric species. This potential is defined, at point P, as (Scrocco and Tomasi 1973, 1978) :

$$ V \ (P) \ = \ \sum_{\alpha} \ \frac{Z_{\alpha}}{\left| r_{-\alpha P} \right|} \ - \ \int \ \frac{\rho(i)}{\left| r_{-iP} \right|} \ d\tau_i $$

where Z_{α} is the charge of nucleus α, distant by $r_{\alpha P}$ from point P and $\rho(i)$ is the electronic distribution whose volume element $d\tau_i$ is at a distance of r_{iP}. Its long range effect is due to its relatively light dependence upon distance.

The methods of evaluating the potentials in biomolecules and biopolymers have been described in (Pullman, A. and Pullman, B., 1981 ; Pullman, B., Lavery, Pullman, A., 1982) and will not be repeated here. May we just recall that for simple biomolecules, of limited dimensions, such as the fundamental constituents of the nucleic acids (phosphates, sugars, purine and pyrimidine bases) they are computed from the electronic distributions of these subunits, obtained from ab initio SCF computations. The potentials of the macromolecules are constructed by the superposition of the potentials of all the subunits forming the nucleic acid, appropriately positioned in space. In order to facilitate the calculation of the macromolecular electrostatic properties, the electronic distribution of each subunit is replaced by a multicenter, multipole expansion which is capable of reproducing the exact electrostatic properties of the subunit down to a short distance from its constituent atoms.

Before investigating the problem of how such, at first sight a relatively non-discriminatory property, as the electrostatic potential may contribute to the specificity of interactions, a more simple question may be considered of whether the electrostatic properties can be shown altogether to contribute significantly to the reactivity of the nucleic acids. The answer to this question is yes and can be reached for exemple by studying the evolution of the potential minima associated with the reactive sites of the purine and pyrimidine bases of the nucleic acids in the series free bases, nucleosides, nucleotides, single helices and finally double helices, comparing it with the parallel evolution to the accessibilities to these sites and, finally, with their known appropriate reactivities.

Such studies have been carried out (Pullman A., Pullman B., 1981) and they invariably show that :

1) There is a general constant, progressive increase in the absolute value (depth) of the potential minima associated with the reactive sites of the purine and pyrimidine bases when we follow the series of the indicated substrates in order of increasing complexity. The increase is particularly striking when we compare the values at the extremes of the sequence, between the isolated bases and the bases in DNA.

2) In distinction to the situation concerning the electro-static potential there is, on the contrary and not surprisingly, a general decrease of the accessibilities of the sites involved, when going over from the isolated bases to the bases in DNA (Lavery, Pullman, A., Pullman, B., 1981)

3) There is thus an antagonism between the evolution of the molecular electrostatic potential at the reactive centers of the bases and their accessibility when the bases are incorporated into more complex structures, in particular into the double helix.

4) Experimental data referring to a large number of electrophilic reagents indicate that they react much better with DNA than with its constituents. Particularly interesting from that point of view are the chemical

carcinogens (Pullman, A. and Pullman, B., 1980 ; Pullman, B. and Pullman, A., 1980). It is well established today that the active forms of the great majority of them (the so-called proximate or ultimate carcinogens) are electrophilic agents, generally positive ions. This is true both for carcinogens considered as being active per se (a number of relatively simple alkylating agents) and those which necessitate a metabolic activation (aromatic hydrocarbons, aromatic amines, aflatoxin B_1 etc...). Now practically, all these substances (as also a certain number of antitumor drugs) react much better with double stranded DNA than with its consituents or any simpler systems. Because of the reduced target accessibility in DNA, it seems logical to attribute this increase in reactivity to the effect of the increased electrostatic potential. In fact, this proposition introduces a unifying principle for an important aspect of the interaction of carcinogens with one of their probable major receptor.

3. INTERACTION OF NON-INTERCALATING ANTITUMOUR LIGANDS WITH THE GROOVES OF DNA

The fact that the sites of action of the electrophilic carcinogens, referred to in the previous section, are the nucleophilic centers on the purine and pyrimidine bases, relates to another significant demonstration made in our laboratory (Pullman, A., Pullman, B., 1981), namely that the deepest electrostatic potentials are concentrated in the grooves of DNA. This fundamental result may seem surprising at first sight because when the potentials of the constituent units of the nucleic acids (purine and pyrimidine bases, sugars, phosphates) are investigated separately the deepest one is that of the monoionic phosphate. The concentration of the deepest potentials of DNA in their grooves is, however, the natural result of their long-range superposition.

This strong concentration of deep potentials in the grooves of DNA seems to be of particular significance for the much investigated recently problem of the tendancy of a large number of non intercalating drugs to bind to the grooves of DNA. (see e. g. Zimmer, 1975 ; 1984 ; Braithwaite, Baguley, 1980 ; Baguley, 1982).

Outstanding examples of such preferential binding are represented by netropsin, distamycin A (Dist-3), Dist-2, SN 18071

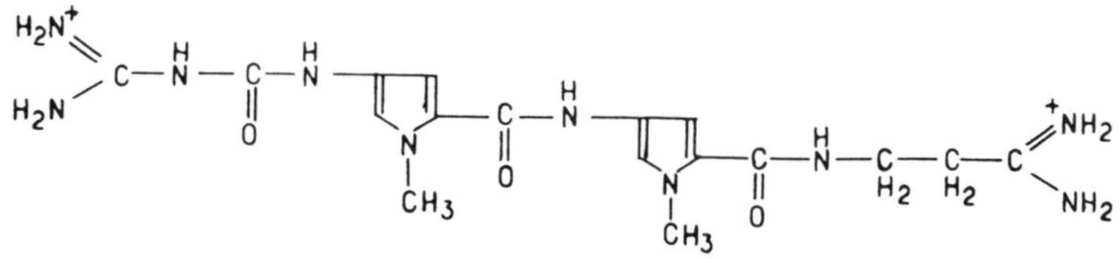

Netropsin

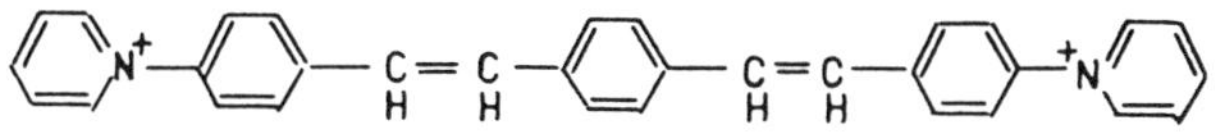

SN 18071

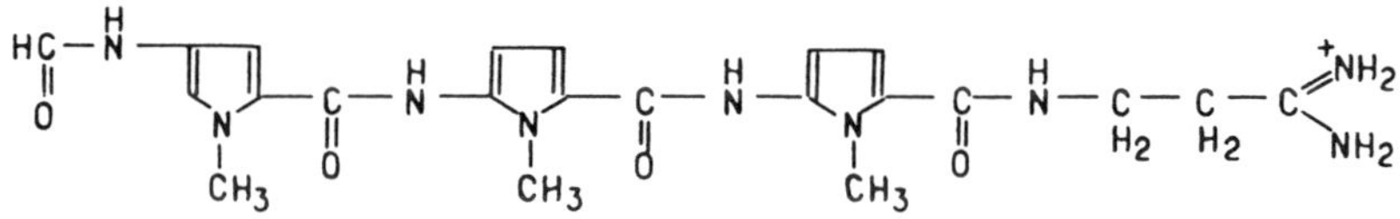

Distamycin A (Dist 3)

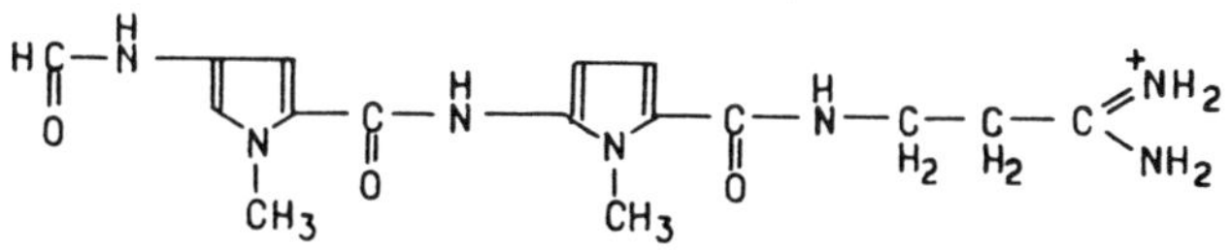

Distamycin 2

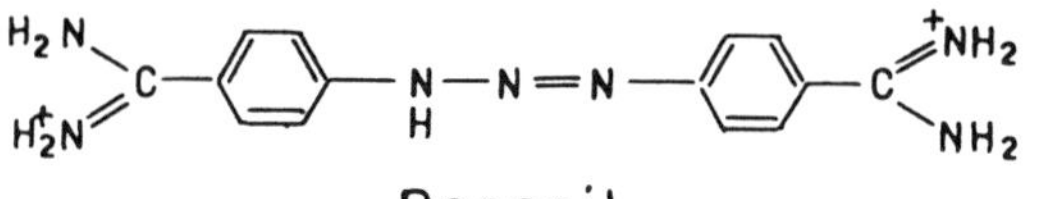

Berenil

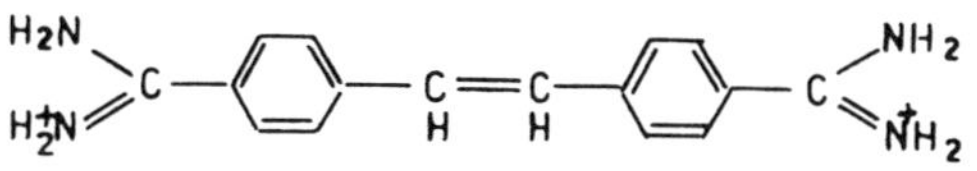

Stilbamidine

FIGURE 1. Examples of non intercalating ligands binding preferentially or exclusively to the minor groove of A–T sequences of DNA.

berenil and stilbamidine (Fig. 1). The biological importance of these compounds stems in particular from the fact that they are antibiotics with antitumor activity. All of them (and many other related molecules) bind in a highly specific way to the minor groove of A–T rich sequences of B–DNA. The most extensively investigated compounds in this series are netropsin and distamycin A and because of the apparent structural features of these molecules, a widely accepted model for their interaction with nucleic acids (Gursky et al., 1977 ; Berman et al., 1979 ; Patel, 1982) postulates that the drugs, having their concave side (Berman et al., 1979), carrying their peptidic hydrogen donors oriented towards DNA, interacts with the minor groove through hydrogen bonds, essentially with the 02 atoms of thymine and N3 atoms of adenine. The charged end groups are considered to be also involved in the interaction in a less clearly specified way.

That the situation is more complicated than this simple picture suggests and that, in particular, the precise role of the formal charges and the hydrogen bonds for the energy and the specificity of the bonding has to be reconsidered become evident from some perplexing findings. Thus, although the charged ends of the drugs appear to be important for the binding, a netropsin derivative with both ends removed, although showing a decrease in binding efficiency, still complexes to poly(dA).poly(dT) (Zimmer, 1975). The ability to form hydrogen bonds may thus seem to be essential, but in fact it is not, as can be seen from the fact that the bisquarternary ammonium heterocycle, SN 18071, which cannot form such bonds (fig. 1), binds also to DNA and shows a similar AT minor groove specificity (Braithwaite and Baguley, 1980 ; Baguley, 1982).

The situation becomes still more puzzling when more quantitative aspects of the binding are considered. Truly not much data are available in this respect, but at least some information about the relative affinity of the ligands for the A–T minor groove can be obtained from the so-called C_{50} values, defined as micromolar drug concentrations required to halve the observed fluorescence due to DNA-bound ethidium (Baguley, 1982). The results indicate that the just mentioned SN 18071 compound, although devoid of hydrogen bonding possibilities shows a greater AT affinity (C_{50} = 0.20) than does netropsin (C_{50} = 0.55). On the other hand distamycin A, having more hydrogen bonding possibilities than netropsin but carrying only one positive charge shows the greatest affinity (C_{50} = 0.07). Berenil and stilbamidine with two positive charges but no hydrogen bond possibilities in their central chain have the lowest affinities : C_{50} = 0.9 and 1.8, respectively. (The central NH bond in berenil is on the convexe side of the molecule and is not engaged in H-bonding with DNA (Gresh and Pullman, 1984b).

This situation shows that the determination of the factors involved in the binding and selectivity is not a straightforward adventure. We have originally suggested (Pullman and Pullman, 1981) that altogether this preferential binding to the A-T minor groove of B-DNA could be related to the presence of a very negative surface potential in this receptor zone. It became, however, soon obvious that a more detailed analysis was necessary.

We have carried it out recently and it involves two fundamental steps.

In the first step, we have performed explicit comparative calculations of the complexing energy of the six above listed compounds with model poly(dA) . poly(dT) and poly(dG) . poly(dC) duplexes, in B-DNA conformation (with the phosphates screened by Na^+ ions), taking into account the electrostatic and Lennard-Jones type components and allowing for the conformational adaptability of the drugs (Zakrzewska, Lavery and Pullman, 1983). The conformation of the polynucleotide system was maintained rigid, an approximation justified by the NMR results of Patel and Canuel (1977) which show that the base pairing and stacking interactions remain nearly unperturbed by netropsin binding and that the only significant conformational changes occur in the glycosidic torsion angles, the alteration of which has following (Marky, Patel and Breslauer, 1981) little if any effect on the enthalpy of binding.

The results obtained are summarized in Table I, in details for netropsin and SN 18071 and only for the essential binding sites for the others. They show that in all cases the strongest complex is formed in the minor groove of the AT sequences. It is the most favoured one by both the electrostatic and Lennard-Jones energy terms. This last term may be considered as a measure of the quality of steric fit between the ligand and the macromolecule because of its strong distance dependence which causes it to become favourable only for very close interactions, but also to rapidly become extremely repulsive if any close contacts are produced. Its significant value signifies a good fit.

The overall results clearly demonstrate that whatever the significance of hydrogen bonds for the stability of the complex, the formation of these bonds is not necessary neither for binding nor for the preference for the minor groove of the AT sequences of B-DNA.

TABLE 1. Interaction energies for the formation of DNA–ligand complexes (kcal/mole)

Ligand	DNA conformation	DNA sequence	DNA groove	Interaction energy Electrostatic	Lennard–Jones	Ligand conformational energy	Total
Netropsin	B	AT	Min.	-203.5	-42.3	7.6	-238.2
		AT	Maj.	-104.4	-19.5	15.3	-108.7
		GC	Min.	-155.3	-34.1	8.2	-181.2
		GC	Maj.	-138.0	-15.6	17.2	-136.4
SN 18071	B	AT	Min.	-86.4	-31.1	9.8	-107.7
		AT	Maj.	-49.8	-21.3	9.8	-61.3
		GC	Min.	-72.2	-25.8	9.8	-88.2
		GC	Maj.	-65.6	-21.3	9.8	-77.1
Distamycin 3	B	AT	Min.	-95.9	-48.8	15.3	-129.4
		GC	Min.	-77.8	-42.4	18.0	-102.2
Distamycin 2	B	AT	Min.	-94.1	-36.7	16.6	-114.2
		GC	Min.	-75.6	-30.9	18.5	-88.0
Berenil	B	AT	Min.	-174.3	-25.2	15.3	-184.3
Stilbamidine	B	AT	Min.	-143.5	-26.5	5.2	-164.8
Netropsin	A	AT	Min.	-74.4	-15.6	15.4	-77.6
		AT	Maj.	-40.2	-22.3	13.9	-48.7
		GC	Min.	-60.5	-14.0	16.0	-58.6
		GC	Maj.	-53.1	-25.4	13.9	-64.6

It seems that if a relatively good steric fit can be obtained in the minor groove the ligand will be sufficiently stabilized there by the favourable potentials generated by the AT sequences.

This, however, does not terminate the problem. It may be seen from Table 1 that the order of the binding energies obtained is :

netropsin > berenil > stilbamidine > distamycin A > SN 18071

which is altogether in strong contradiction with the order indicated by the C_{50} values.

It may also be remarked that the values of the binding energies obtained are very high, of the order of 1-2 hundreds kcal/mole. The experimental values may be expected to be much smaller. In fact, a recent determination of the enthalpy of binding of netropsin indicates a value of -9.2 kcal/mole (Marky, Blumenfeld, Breslauer, 1983).

This situation brings us to the second stage of our study. It seems obvious that the previous results carried out for binding in vacuum are far away from the real interaction which occurs in water. It seems natural to assume that although they obviously correctly indicate the nature of the specificity which seems thus to be an intrinsic property of the systems studied, they need to be significantly refined in order to describe similarly the quantitative aspects of the energetics of binding. A preliminary investigation in this direction, carried out for netropsin and SN 18071 (B. Pullman, 1984), indicated that in fact the taking into account of the dehydration energies of these ligands, before their complexation with DNA, should help appreciably to bring the theoretical results in line with the experimental order of reactivity : the energy necessary to dehydrate netropsin was shown to be sufficiently greater than that necessary for dehydrating SN 18071 to compensate for the reverse contribution of the ligand–DNA interaction energies (For a similar example in the series of bisguanylhydrazones see Gresh, Pullman 1984).

We have presently refined this procedure (Zakrzewska, Lavery, Pullman, 1984) by taking into account in a much more extended way the overall contribution of the solvation to the energy balance of the interaction. The methodology involves first a discrete representation of water molecules which are directly bound to the entities in interaction. This part of the procedure is based on a spherical, point dipole model of water and is limited to the evaluation of the electrostatic interaction energy. The hydration shells are energy optimized with respect to both water–solute and water–water interactions for the complexes and for the isolated DNA oligomers and the ligands. The effect of the bulk solvent is then added by a cavity treatment, following the procedure of Halicioglu and Sinanoglu (1969). (For more details see Zakrzewska, Lavery and Pullman, 1984).

The binding energy of the complex in solution E_W is then equated to :

$$E_W = E_V + \Delta H + \Delta C$$

where E_V is the interaction energy in vacuum.

$$\Delta H = H_{comp} - (H_{DNA} + H_{lig})$$

with H_{comp}, H_{DNA} and H_{lig}, respectively, the hydration energies of the complex, of DNA and of the ligand and where :

$$\Delta C = C_{comp} - (C_{DNA} + C_{lig})$$

with C_{comp}, C_{DNA} and C_{lig}, respectively, the cavity energies of the complex, of DNA and of the ligand.

The principal results of this evaluation of the interaction, energies in water are summed up in table 2, in details for netropsin and SN 18071 and only for the main binding sites for the others. (For information about the individual values involved in ΔH and ΔC see Zakrzewska, Lavery, Pullman, 1984).

The main conclusions are the following :

1) The hydration energy change upon complexation, ΔH, is always positive, corresponding to the considerable loss of hydration sites when DNA and the ligand are brought together.

2) The cavity energy change upon complexation, ΔC, is always negative, since the complex has a smaller surface area than the sum of the isolated species.

3) ΔC contributes thus to the enhancement of the binding energy while ΔH has a reverse effect.

TABLE 2. Solvent corrected DNA-ligand binding energies

Ligand	Conformation	sequence	groove	E_v	ΔH	ΔC	E_w
Netropsin	B	AT	Min.	-238.2	+380.7	-159.2	- 16.7
		AT	Maj.	-108.7	+322.2	- 98.5	+115.0
		GC	Min.	-181.2	+408.7	-147.5	+ 80.0
		GC	Maj.	-136.4	+336.2	- 80.5	+119.3
SN 18071	B	AT	Min.	-107.7	+214.6	-127.0	- 20.1
		AT	Maj.	- 61.3	+193.0	- 89.0	+ 42.7
		GC	Min.	- 88.2	+188.4	- 96.4	+ 3.8
		GC	Maj.	- 77.1	+147.8	- 65.1	+ 5.6
Distamycin 3	B	AT	Min.	-129.4	+265.5	-163.7	- 27.6
		GC	Min.	-102.2	+233.3	-139.3	- 8.2
Distamycin 2	B	AT	Min.	-114.2	+212.4	-125.7	- 27.5
		GC	Min.	- 88.0	+218.7	- 97.8	+ 32.9
Berenil	B	AT	Min.	-184.3	+270.5	- 95.0	- 8.8
Stilbamidine	B	AT	Min.	-164.8	+249.0	- 89.2	- 5.0
Netropsin	A	AT	Min.	- 77.6	+248.9	- 71.3	+103.0
		AT	Maj.	- 48.7	+327.7	-136.4	+142.6
		GC	Min.	- 58.6	+152.1	- 64.6	+ 28.9
		GC	Maj.	- 64.6	+307.8	-143.6	+ 99.6

4) The resulting E_W corresponds always to a preference for binding to the minor groove of AT sequences.

5) The relative affinity of the ligands in these interactions now becomes :

distamycin A > SN 18071 > netropsin > berenil > stilbamidine.

This order corresponds exactly, and truly surprisingly, to the experimental order indicated by the C_{50} values. Surprisingly, because E_W is obtained as a small difference between contributions represented by great numbers and because of the approximations involved in the evaluation of all of them. Obtaining a correct order for five compounds is more than could really be expected, but at the same time constitutes a confirmation for the overall soundness of the procedure.

6) The absolute values of E_W are strongly reduced with respect to the values of the interaction in vacuum and are now much more in line with the experimental results. Indeed, for netropsin the computed value of − 16.7 kcal/mole is at least in the range of magnitude of the experimental binding enthalpy (−9.2 kcal/mole, as quoted before).

These conclusions may be complemented by two more related to two other results contained in table 2.

The first one pertains to the possible binding of these ligands, at least some of them, to some extent, to the G−C sequences of B−DNA. This problem has gained recently interest with the discovery by some authors that while distamycin 2 does not bind to GC sequences, distamycin 3 (distamycin A) does so slightly (Zimmer, 1984). This problem was investigated by us and the results are included in table 2. The theoretical results agree fairly well with the experimental observations : while the two distamycins have a rather similar affinity for the A−T sequences, their E_W for the interaction with the G−C sequences is positive (repulsive) for distamycin 2, but negative (attractive), although only a little, for distamycin 3.

The second remark concerns the specificity of binding of the non intercalating ligands mentioned here to B−DNA. They quite generally do not bind to A−DNA. The problem was investigated on the example of netropsin and the corresponding results in table 2 show that E_W for the interaction of this ligand with A–DNA is always positive, it means repulsive.

CONCLUSION

The present study shows that no simple property of ligands, in particular as visualized in their chemical formulas, is liable to allow an easy prediction of their binding specificities and still less energetics. The preference for the minor groove of A–T sequences appears to be an intrinsic property of the ligands studied, present already in vacuum, where it is basically independent of hydrogen bonding possibilities. It is confirmed in solution. The order of the binding affinities can, however, only be obtained after the solvation effects have been included in the computations. In this respect it must be borne in mind that a compound capable of a strong hydrogen bonding to a substrate will also manifest a similar tendancy to bind water. Its affinity for binding to DNA will imply a delicate balance between these two tendancies, whose result is difficult to be predicted without carrying out explicit computations.

Altogether, it appears that our approximate treatment is able to account for many of the major problems related to the specificity of interaction of these important different antitumor antibiotics with DNA. Because of limitations in space and time and the very nature of this lecture, I insisted more on the results than on the methodology. However satisfied we may appear to be with it, I can assure you that we are perfectly aware that it can and needs to be refined in many ways. In fact, we are engaged in a number of such refinements, as also in the extention of these studies to a wider group of DNA binding ligands, including intercalators. Many basic processes and events in life involve and depend on such inter-actions. Because of the involvement of the ligands concerned in many harmful but also in many chemotherapeutic processes, the elucidation of the intimate mechanisms of these interactions may thus be of particular importance for the progress not only of molecular biology but also of molecular pharmacology.

One possible contribution in this last direction may be obtained by investigating the consequences of the binding reactions on the biochemical behaviour of so perturbed DNA. As an example of possibilities in this field we may quote our recent study on the effect of netropsin binding on the electrostatic potential of DNA (Zakrzewska and Pullman, 1983). The results indicate that the binding produces an important weakening of the potential, not only in the minor groove, where netropsin is located, but also in the major groove, spreading moreover far beyond the interaction zone.

This situation enables to predict a modulation (decrease) of the reactivity of the so perturbed DNA towards electrophilic reaagents, in particular carcinogens. Experimental results observed upon binding of the closely related distamycin A confirm this presumption (Rajalakshani, Rao, Sarma, 1978).

ACKNOWLEDGMENT

This work was supported by the National Foundation for Cancer Research (Bethesda, U.S.A.) to which the author wishes to express his profound gratitude.

REFERENCES

Baguley BC (1982) Molecular and Cellular Biochemistry 43:167.

Berman HM, Neidle S, Zimmer Ch, Thrum H (1979) Biochem Biophys Acta 561:124.

Braithwaite AW, Baguley BC (1980) Biochemistry 19:1101.

Gresh N, Pullman B (1984a) Theoret Chim Acta 64:383.

Gresh N, Pullman B (1984b) Molecular Pharmacology, in press.

Gursky GV, Tumanyan VG, Zasedatelev AS, Zhuze AL, Groknovsky SL, Gottikh BP (1977) Nucleic Acid-Protein recognition, Ed HJ Vogel, Academic Press p 189.

Halicioglu T, Sinanoglu O (1969) Ann NY Acad Sci 158:308-317.

Lavery R, Pullman A, Pullman B (1981) Intern J Quantum Chem 20:49.

Marky LA, Blumenfeld KS, Breslauer KJ (1983) Nucl Acids Res 11:2857.

Marky LA, Patel DJ, Breslauer KJ (1981) Biochemistry 20:1427.

Patel DJ (1982) Proc Natl Acad Sci USA 79:6424.

Patel DJ, Canuel LL (1979) Proc Natl Acad Sci USA 74:5207.

Pullman B (1984) in Specificity in Biological Interaction. International Symposium at the Pontifical Academy of Sciences (Chagas C, Pullman B Eds) Vatican Press, in press.

Pullman A, Pullman B (1980) Intern J Quantum Chem, Quantum Biol Symp 7:245.

Pullman A, Pullman B (1981) Quart Rev Biophys 14:289.

Pullman B, Pullman A (1980) in Carcinogenesis : Fundamental Aspects and Environmental Effects (Pullman B, Ts'o POP, Gelboin H Eds) Reidel Publishing Co, Dordrecht, Hollande, p 55.

Pullman B, Pullman A (1981) Studia Biophys 86:95.

Pullman B, Lavery R, Pullman A (1982) Eur J Biochem 124:229.

Rajalakshani S, Rao PM, Sarma DSR (1978) Biochemistry 17:4515.

Scrocco E, Tomasi J (1973) Topics Current Chem 42:95.

Scrocco E, Tomasi J (1978) Adv Quantum Chem 11:115.
Wang AH-J, Quigley GJ, Kolpak FJ, Crawford JL, van Boom JH, van der Marel G, Rich A (1979) Nature 282:680.
Wang AH-J, Quigley GJ, Kolpak FJ, van der Marel G, van Boom JH, Rich A (1980) Science 211:171.
Zakrzewska K, Lavery R, Pullman B (1983) Nucl Acids Res 11:8825.
Zakrzewska K, Lavery R, Pullman B (1984) Nucl Acids Res, in press.
Zakrzewska K, Pullman B (1983) Nucl Acids Res 11:8841.
Zimmer C (1975) Progress Nucleic Acids Res and Mol Biol 15:285.
Zimmer C (1984) in Specificity in Biological Interactions. International Symposium at the Pontifical Academy of Sciences (Chagas C, Pullman B Eds) Vatican Press, in press.

Molecular Basis of Cancer, Part A: Macromolecular
Structure, Carcinogens, and Oncogenes, pages 71–86
© 1985 Alan R. Liss, Inc.

STERIC AND ELECTRONIC FACTORS IN THE REACTIVITY OF YEAST
tRNA^{Phe}

Alberte Pullman

Institut de Biologie Physico-Chimique,
Laboratoire de Biochimie Théorique
13 rue Pierre et Marie Curie – 75005 Paris, FRANCE

Introduction

The various functions of transfer ribonucleic acids in the
cellular machinery make a detailed understanding of their reactivity
an important objective. Since the high resolution by X-ray techniques of the structure of one such macromolecule, yeast tRNA^{Phe},
the elucidation of this reactivity in terms of structural characteristics
of the polymer became feasible and a rather substantial effort in this
direction has been carried out in our laboratory.

The problem is particularly challenging because of the
dimensions (2513 atoms) and great complexity of this biopolymer
which makes it, in fact, the most complicated system studied so far
by quantum-mechanical methods. Because of its highly convoluted
structure, it is moreover obvious that its overall macromolecular
conformation will play a very great role in the reactivity of its
different atoms or zones.

During our studies on the relation structure–activity in this
nucleic acid, use has been made of four concepts, demonstrated in
our laboratory to be crucial in the elucidation of the biochemical
reactivity of nucleic acids in general. These concepts are :

1) <u>The accessibility to reactive sites</u>

Originally developed by Lee and Richards (1971 ; Richards
1977), this approach consists of rolling a spherical probe over the
van der Waals surface of a macromolecule and determining, for a
given atom, the positions of the probe which do not lead to its
intersection with the van der Waals spheres of any of the other

atoms of the macromolecule. In this framework, the accessibility of the atom concerned can be expressed either as a "contact surface area" (CSA) which is the accessible area on the surface of the van der Waals sphere (radius r_i) of the target atom in the macro-molecule or as a "surface accessible area" (SAA) which is the corresponding accessible area on the surface of a sphere of radius equal to that of the target atom plus that of the probe ($r_i + r_a$), that is, the area covered by the locus of the center of the attacking sphere for the accessible positions of the probe. We have, on the one hand, extended this technique to the explicit treatment of polyatomic species (Lavery, Pullman A., Pullman B., 1981), and, on the other hand, indicated under what conditions one could model such species by a sphere with an appropriately chosen radius (Lavery, Pullman A., 1984).

2) The molecular electrostatic potential (MEP), defined at point P by :

$$(MEP) = \sum_\alpha \frac{Z_\alpha}{|\underline{r}_{\alpha P}|} - \int \frac{\rho(i)}{|\underline{r}_{iP}|} d\tau_i$$

where Z_α is the charge of nucleus α, distant by $r_{\alpha P}$ from point P and $\rho(i)$ is the electronic distribution whose volume element $d\tau_i$ is at a distance r_{iP}. (Scrocco, Tomasi 1978 ; Pullman A., Pullman B. 1981)

This index represents thus the electrostatic potential created in the neighbouring space by the nuclear charges and the electronic distribution of the system. Its significance in reactivity stems from the fact that, in difference to such local entities as electronic charges or populations, it is an expression of the global molecular or macromolecular reality closely related to what a reactant, in particular an ionic one, "feels" upon approaching the substrate.

3) The molecular electrostatic field (MEF), defined at point P by :

$$(MEF) = \sum_\alpha \frac{Z_\alpha \, \underline{r}_{\alpha P}}{|\underline{r}_{\alpha P}|^3} - \int \frac{\rho(i) \, \underline{r}_{iP}}{|\underline{r}_{iP}|^3} d\tau_i$$

where the different symbols have the same meaning as in the definition of the potential (Lavery, Pullman A., Pullman B., 1982, 1983 ; Lavery, Pullman B., 1982). Although the field is simply minus the derivative of the potential with respect to distance its distribution in macromolecular systems may present a drastically different shape from that of the potential (see e.g. Pullman A., Pullman B., Lavery 1983 ; Pullman B. 1983). Moreover, conceptually, it is particularly suitable for the studies of the interactions of the nucleic acids with neutral "dipolar" molecules, of which water is the most outstanding representative.

Because of the polyanionic nature of the nucleic acids, the electrostatic component of their interaction energy with an attacking species is generally dominating and often exerts a strong influence in favouring a particular reactive site. The combined knowledge of the potential and the field is thus able to provide important information on the main features of the interaction of the nucleic acids with a large variety of species.

    4) <u>ASIF (Accessible Surface Integrated Field)</u> (Lavery, Pullman A., 1984).

The three previous indices define the essential steric and electrostatic properties liable to play a role in the biochemical reactivity of tRNA ^{Phe}. It is, however, obvious that when dealt with independently, the information produced by these two types of indices may not be sufficient. In particular, there need not be for a particular reaction at a given position in the nucleic acid a convergence between the indication drawn from its accessibility, on the one hand, and the potential or field, on the other.

Attempts at a simultaneous consideration of these two factors have been made by us (Pullman B., Lavery, Pullman A. 1982 ; Pullman B., Pullman A., Lavery 1983) in the form of two-dimensional potential/accessibility graphics for many sites in yeast tRNA ^{Phe}. However, it seemed desirable to achieve a closer combination of the two properties by generating a single index which contains both aspects.

This has been achieved by the ASIF index, obtained by a numerical integration of the field over the SAA on the target atom of the macromolecule, generated by the center of the probe modelling the attacking species. In order to make a distinction between atoms which are attractive or repulsive towards electrophiles we replace the net field at each point by its projection on the radius vector ($\vec{r}$) joining the center of the attacked atom of the macromolecule to the center of the attacking sphere, so that the index is given by :

$$\int_S \vec{F} \cdot \vec{r}_u \cdot ds$$

where S is the SAA defined earlier and $\vec{r}_u$ is a unit vector along the direction $\vec{r}$.

With this definition, if the electrostatic field is more or less aligned with the radius vector and pointing outwards from the attacked atom concerned, this atom will be repulsive towards positively charged electrophiles and the resulting integral will be positive. If, conversely, the field is again more or less aligned with the radius vector but points towards the attacked atom this atom will be attractive for positively charged electrophiles and the resulting integral will be negative. Finally, if the field is more or less perpendicular to the radius vector the resulting integral will be small, corresponding to an atom which is unlikely to react since the ambient field will slide a charged attacking species towards a neighbouring atom which is a stronger field source. The values of ASIF will be expressed in units of volt. angstrom.

It may be remarked that the ASIF index represents, in fact, the flux of the electrostatic field through the accessible surface described and hence may be expressed in units of electronic charge. The factor of conversion between volt. angstrom and electronic charge is 5.5266×10^{-3}.

METHOD

The methods of evaluating the potentials and the fields in biomolecules and biopolymers have been described previously (Pullman A., Pullman B. 1981 ; Lavery, Pullman A., Pullman B. 1982) and will not be repeated here. May we recall that for simple biomolecules, of limited dimensions, such as the fundamental constituents of the nucleic acids (phosphates, sugars, purine and pyrimidine bases) they are computed from the electronic distributions of these subunits, obtained from ab initio SCF computations. The potential and the field of the macromolecules are constructed by the superposition of the potentials and fields of all the subunits forming the nucleic acid, appropriately positioned in space. In order to facilitate the calculation of the macromolecular electrostatic properties, the electronic distribution of each subunit is replaced by a multicenter, multipole expansion which is capable of reproducing the exact electrostatic properties of the subunit down to a short distance (2 Å) from its constituent atoms.

Numerous representations are available for describing the molecular potentials and fields. Among the most significant ones are :

a) Point potentials or fields
b) Plane potentials or fields (isopotential or field intensity maps, whose minima or maxima represent, respectively, the main site potentials or fields at reactive centers in the chosen plane.
c) Surface envelope potentials or fields : potentials or fields on envelopes formed by the intersection of spheres centered on each atom of DNA with radii equal to the van der Waals radius of the atoms concerned, multiplied, if desired, by a factor F ; they are generally presented in the form of their projection on a two-dimensional "window". For technical details on this representation see (Lavery, Pullman B. 1981).

For technical details on computing ASIF see (Lavery, Pullman A. 1984).

As input data for the structure of tRNA^{Phe} we have used the X-ray crystallographic results on the orthorhombic form (Fussman et al 1978), in the form of a refined coordinate system provided by Dr. S. H. Kim.

RESULTS AND DISCUSSION

The development of our research on the steric and electronic factors in the reactivity of tRNA^{Phe} involved a number of stages of which the principal may be summed up as follows.

1) The evaluation of the electrostatic molecular potential generated by the 76 phosphate groups of the macromolecule, placed in their crystallographic coordinates and presumed to provide the major part of this potential (Lavery, Pullman A., Pullman B. 1980a ; Lavery, Oliveira, Pullman B. 1980). For this sake isopotential maps were evaluated in nine planes cutting through the nucleic acid, at a separation of 4 $\overset{\circ}{A}$ from each other. The general features of the results obtained enabled to localize the main potential wells, whose position was considered in relation to the binding of Mg^{2+} ions. The results indicated also that the deepest potentials of tRNA^{Phe} were appreciably deeper than those which could be obtained with a double helical B−DNA composed of the same number of phosphates.

2) The evaluation of the electrostatic potential and of the accessibility associated with each of the 76 phosphates of the macromolecule (Lavery, Pullman A., Pullman B. 1980b). The

results, represented schematically in fig. 1, show that there is frequently an opposition between these two properties in the sense that, for instance, strong potentials occur in regions of low accessibility and weak potentials in zones of high accessibility. At the time of the production of these results, no experimental data were avaibable which could enable us to estimate the respective roles of these two factors in the biochemical reactivity of the phosphates. Since then, appropriate data have become available. They will be presented later in this discussion.

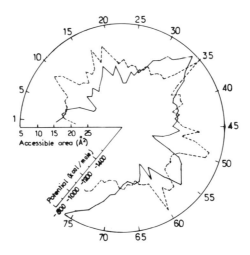

Fig. 1. Phosphate potential (——) and accessibilities (---) in tRNA^{Phe}.

3) The evaluation of the electrostatic potential and of the steric accessibility of the reactive sites associated with the purine and pyrimidine bases of the macromolecule (Lavery, Pullman A. , Pullman B. , Oliveira, 1980). The results illustrated in table 1 for the guanines, point to the extreme diversity of situations, announcing great differences in possible reactivities of these bases, according to their positioning in the macromolecule. Two dimensional plots of potential versus accessibility for a number of important reactive atoms of tRNA^{Phe} were used for a preliminary evaluation of their reactivity towards reagents known to attack these atoms.

4) The evaluation of the effect of counterion binding (Mg^{2+} and Na^+) on the electrostatic potential and steric accessibility of the

TABLE 1. Guanine : Site potentials and atom accessibilities.

Residue	Site potentials (kcal/mole)						Atom accessibilities (Å²)					
	N1	N2	N3	N7	C8	O6	N1	N2	N3	N7	C8	O6
1	-978	-949	-979	-1116	-1060	-1055	0.0	0.09	1.21	5.33	2.11	2.34
3	-1068	-1028	-1044	-1189	-1109	-1170	0.0	0.14	0.09	4.36	0.79	2.02
4	-1091	-1068	-1086	-1206	-1125	-1196	0.0	0.09	0.60	2.60	0.53	0.97
15	-1195	-1138	-1156	-1302	-1189	-1302	0.0	0.0	0.60	3.38	1.0	3.31
18	-973	-1033	-1043	-986	-931	-983	0.0	0.0	0.37	4.13	0.53	3.55
19	-859	-870	-928	-908	-887	-861	0.93	1.76	1.95	5.47	1.0	7.35
20	-1016	-1104	-1031	-952	-955	-1005	1.02	1.81	1.39	5.75	2.27	5.17
22	-1147	-1121	-1149	-	-1126	-1126	0.0	0.0	0.0	-	0.0	0.0
24	-1098	-1071	-1119	-1223	-1141	-1183	0.0	0.32	0.97	1.71	0.0	0.28
30	-965	-930	-968	-1047	-966	-1021	0.0	1.90	0.0	3.11	0.11	1.90
34	-668	-660	-713	-767	-744	-717	0.88	0.0	1.21	5.05	2.06	7.31
42	-1059	-1026	-1041	-1169	-1093	-1145	0.0	0.0	0.56	4.03	0.74	2.71
43	-1077	-1040	-1062	-1201	-1108	-1183	0.0	0.05	0.19	4.22	0.74	2.42
45	-1130	-1146	-1181	-1225	-1129	-1229	0.0	0.0	0.0	3.75	1.05	6.30
51	-1096	-1056	-1079	-1257	-1132	-1230	0.0	0.09	0.42	3.29	0.58	1.74
53	-1073	-1034	-1055	-1172	-1047	-1176	0.0	0.0	0.0	3.57	0.79	2.46
57	-931	-957	-987	-926	-892	-949	0.0	0.09	0.42	0.0	0.0	3.55
65	-1160	-1131	-1144	-1248	-1161	-1241	0.0	0.05	0.19	4.17	0.69	2.26
71	-1010	-991	-987	-1089	-983	-1085	0.0	0.0	0.28	2.04	0.21	1.09
10	-1078	-1060	-1067	-1182	-1133	-1105	0.0	0.0	0.74	0.0	0.79	0.0
26	-1093	-1112	-1100	-1187	-1075	-1186	0.0	0.09	0.37	0.51	0.0	2.91
46	-1133	-1166	-1237	-	-1072	-1152	0.0	0.0	0.0	-	0.95	0.28

reactive sites in tRNA^{Phe} (Lavery, Corbin, Pullman A. 1981).

5) The evaluation of the electrostatic molecular potential on the surface envelope of the macromolecule (Lavery, Pullman A. , Corbin 1981), carried out within the technique developed in our laboratory by Lavery and Pullman B. (1981). The results have been shown to be significant for the binding of Mg^{++} ions and of spermine to this acid.

6) The evaluation of the electrostatic field on the surface envelope of tRNA^{Phe} and a comparison with the corresponding distribution of the potential (Lavery and Pullman A. , 1983). It was shown that the two distributions are very different (as they also are in DNA) and further, that the binding of counterions has very different effects on them.

7) Finally, our most recent work in this field was devoted to the utilization of our new theoretical index of biochemical reactivity ASIF, combining the steric and the electrostatic factors, for the exploration of a series of different reactions of tRNA^{Phe} (Lavery and Pullman A. , 1984). This extension has substantially increased the possibility of structure-reactivity correlations in tRNA^{Phe}.

We propose now to select from these numerous and long investigations some of the most striking examples pertaining to the significance of the theoretical computations for the understanding of the factors governing the reactivity of tRNA^{Phe} towards represen- tative biochemical reagents.

A subject of special interest in connection with this macro- molecule and which seems somewhat to dominate the debates on the factors responsible for its biochemical reactivity is the respec- tive role of the steric and electronic (electrostatic) factors in this behaviour. Because of the very convoluted structure of tRNA^{Phe} it is obvious a priori that the steric factors, that is essentially the accessibility to the attacked targets, must play a very significant role in the reactivity, certainly superior to that played in the much more regular B-DNA. The problem is, how important a role and how much of a playground is left to other factors.

The computations provide an answer to this question which seems to be dual depending on the nature of the target, whether on the phosphates or on the bases.

Thus, recently, the reactivity of the phosphates in yeast tRNA^{Phe} has been assayed with ethylnitrosourea by Ebel and coworkers (Vlassov, Giégé, Ebel, 1980, 1981). This reactant alkylates the anionic oxygens of the phosphodiester bonds. In the unfolded macromolecule all phosphates are reactive. In contrast, in the folded form phosphates in different sites react differently. In particular the reactivity of phosphate 9, 10, 11, 19, 49, 58 and 60 is strongly reduced and that of phosphates 23 and 24 is partially so. The technique utilized in this study did not permit to determine the reactivity of the terminal phosphates, 7–10 residues apart from each end of the molecule. The reactivity of phosphate 35 could not be determined precisely either but a decrease in its reactivity is announced.

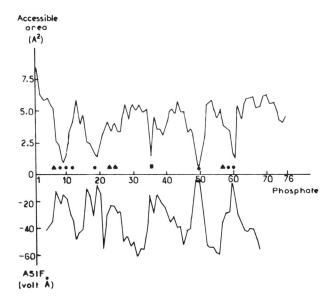

Fig. 2. Accessibility of phosphate groups of tRNA^{Phe} for a probe sphere of 2.2 $\overset{o}{A}$ (upper part), the related ASIF (lower part) and reactivity of phosphates towards ethylnitrosourea :

● least reactive phosphates
▲ phosphates of reduced activity

The upper part of fig. 2 relates these experimental findings to the accessibilities of the anionic oxygens of the different phosphates (Pullman A., 1981). The correlation is very striking, the reduced reactivity being closely associated with highly reduced accessibility. This conclusion is further corroborated if one tries to relate the experimental reactivities to the electrostatic potentials of the phosphates (Pullman, A., 1981). Not only is no correlation observed but in many cases the unreactive phosphates are those which have the deepest potentials. This, at first sight surprising, situation is in fact easily understandable inasmuch as in this highly convoluted macromolecule the sites of deepest phosphate potential are also those of their greatest crowding and thus also of their greatest inaccessibility (see fig. 1). Therefore, while in the unfolded acid all phosphates react with ethylnitrosourea, indicating thus their intrinsically high affinity for this reagent, it is the steric inaccessibility of some of these sites in the folded structure which prevents their reaction, in spite of the high value of the associated potential.

On the other hand, if we consider the ASIF index (lower part of fig. 2) its correlation with the experimental results is practically identical to that obtained by the sole consideration of accessibilities. This closeness of the results for the two indices is not surprising in this case as the anionic nature of the phosphate groups means that each residue is a source of very strong local electrostatic field. Hence, its inclusion does not influence noticeably the order of results obtained from accessibilities.

A much more diversified and sometimes quite different situation is found for the reactive sites of the purine and pyrimidine bases of tRNA^{Phe}. (Lavery, Pullman, A., 1984). A number of reactions of these bases with a number of reagents have been investigated experimentally. They always occur on selected bases, in a range of relative reactivities. Contrary to the proposition of some authors (Alden, Kim 1979, 1980) estimating that they can all be satisfactorily accounted for by the sole accessibilities of the target atoms, it was shown (Lavery, Pullman 1984) that if this is sometimes the case, it is certainly not always so and that in a number of cases a very significant improvement in the structure-reactivity relation is obtained with the ASIF index.

We may illustrate this situation on three examples.

Fig. 3 presents the comparison of the experimental and theoretical results on the reactivity of the N3 atom of cytosines of tRNA^{Phe} towards dimethylsulfate (reactive species CH_3^+). The theoretical results relate in this figure (as in the two following ones) to both the surface accessible area (SAA) and ASIF of the target atom. It can be seen that only two cytosines N°74 and 75 are

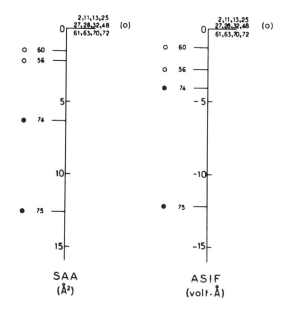

Fig. 3. Accessibility (left) and ASIF (right) for N3 of cytosine in tRNA^{Phe} and reactivity towards dimethylsulphate . In this figure and in figures 4 and 5 the numbers refer to the nucleotide positions in yeast tRNA and the symbols indicate the experimental reactivities : (●) reactive, (◓) partially reactive and (O) unreactive.

reactive. They are both the most accessible and have the greatest (in absolute value) ASIF. In this case the taking into account of ASIF does not improve the conclusions drawn from the sole consideration of accessibility.

The situation is different in fig. 4 and 5. Fig. 4 presents the comparison of the experimental and theoretical results on the reactivity of the N1 atoms of adenines of tRNA^{Phe} with monoperphtalic acid (active species OH^{+}). Four bases are known to be reactive (numbers 35, 36, 38 and 76). The accessibility index exhibits an inversion in the ordering, placing the unreactive adenine 73 at a higher (absolute) value than the reactive bases 35 and 38. ASIF, on the other hand, brings things into order, grouping together the four reactive bases at the bottom of the scale.

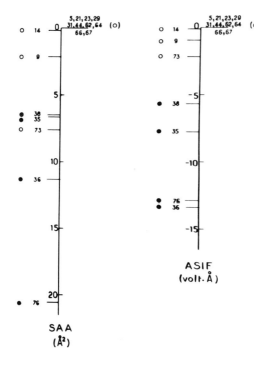

Fig. 4. Accessibility and ASIF for N1 of adenine in tRNA^{Phe}. Symbols represent reactivity towards monoperphthalic acid.

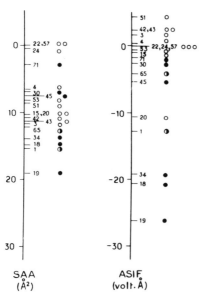

Fig. 5. Accessibility and ASIF for N7 of guanine in tRNA^{Phe}. Symbols represent reactivity towards dimethylsulphate.

Fig. 5 represents a still more persuasive case. It relates to the results of the reaction of guanines of tRNA^{Phe} with dimethylsulphate, which methylates their N7 position.

It can be seen from fig. 5 that six guanines (numbers 18, 19, 30, 34, 45 and 71) are fully methylated and that two are partially reactive (numbers 1 and 65). The left-hand scale shows that the accessibility of these bases does not account well at all for the experimental results.

In contrast, when electrostatic effects and accessibilities are both taken into account, by using the ASIF index, a much better correlation is achieved. With the sole exception of guanine 20, all the reactive and partially reactive residues are now grouped together at more negative ASIF values. This improvement shows that the inclusion of electrostatic effects is vital in this case for obtaining a satisfactory correlation with reactivity.

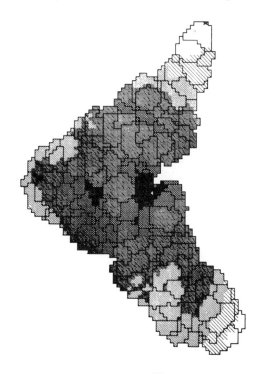

Fig. 6. The surface potential of tRNA^{Phe} viewed through the "windows" A and C of fig. 7. The darker, the shadow, the deeper, the potential.

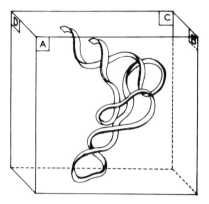

Fig. 7. The orientation of tRNA^{Phe} with respect to the "windows" used to view its surface envelope.

Finally, I would like to indicate an example pertaining to the utilisation and utility of the surface envelope representation of the potential, which enables to have a view of its regional distribution. Fig. 6 represents the two dimensional representation (following the techniques of Lavery and Pullman, A., 1981), of the surface envelope potential of tRNA^{Phe} viewed from the C direction (Fig. 7)). In this figure, the darker the shading, the deeper the potential. It is immediately obvious from the figure that there is a big potential well localized in a zone corresponding to the "P10 loop" of this compound. Now, a recent study by Sundaralingam and coworkers (Liebman, Rubin, Sundaralingam 1977) on the crystal structure of ethidium bromide–tRNA^{Phe} molecular complex demonstrates that the drug binds specifically and is lodged in a cavity at the very mouth of this "P10 loop", it means in the zone of deepest potential. The binding is stabilized by hydrogen bonds between the ethidium amino groups and the anionic oxygens of phosphates 8 and 15 and by stacking of the ethidium ring over U8 and, partially, G15. Nevertheless, the significance of the deep potential is substantiated by Sundaralingam's own observation that although similar conformations of the polynucleotide fold are observed in the anticodon and pseudouridine hairpin loops, no ethidium binding is observed in these regions. It may be interesting to add that a reinterpretation by Sundaralingam of the NMR data relating to the same complex in solution, (which have originally been intepreted by some authors as involving intercalation between the base pairs U6–A67 and U7–A66 of the amino acid stem), indicates that the interactions in solution are, in fact, similar to those in the crystal. A similar conclusion was also reached recently (Nielsen, 1981) through studies using the limited nuclease digestion method.

This work was supported by the National Foundation for Cancer Research (Bethesda U. S. A.) to which the author would like to express her gratitude.

Addendum : After this paper has been prepared, we have learned (Pascale Romby, Thèse 3ème Cycle, 1983, Univ. Louis Pasteur, Strasbourg) that Guanine 20, which appears as an exception in figure 7, is in fact reactive towards dimethylsulfate on its N7.

Alden CJ, Kim SH (1979). J. Mol. Biol. 132:411.

Alden CJ, Kim SH (1980). In Nucleic Acid Geometry and Dynamics ed. RH Sarma, Pergamon Press p 399.

Liebman M, Rubin J, Sundaralingan M (1977). Proc. Natl. Acad. Sci. U.S. 74:4821.

Lee B, Richards FM (1971). J. Mol. Biol. 55:379.

Lavery R, Corbin S, Pullman A (1981). Int. J. Quantum Chem. Quantum Biol. Symp. 8:171.

Lavery R, Oliveira M, Pullman B (1980). J. Comput. Chem. 1:301.

Lavery R, Pullman A (1983). In New Horizons of Quantum Chemistry (Lowdin PO and Pullman B eds) Reidel Publishing Co. p 439.

Lavery R, Pullman A (1984). Biophys. Chem. in press.

Lavery R, Pullman B (1981). Int. J. Quant. Chem. 20:259.

Lavery R, Pullman B (1982). Nucl. Acid Res. 10:4383.

Lavery R, Pullman A, Corbin S (1981). In Biomolecular Stereo-dynamics (R.H. Sarma ed) Adenine Press N.Y. 1:185.

Lavery R, Pullman A, Pullman B (1980a). Nucleic Acid Res. 8:1061.

Lavery R, Pullman A, Pullman B (1980b). Theoret. Chem. Acta 57:233.

Lavery R, Pullman A, Pullman B, Oliveira M (1980). Nucleic Acid Res. 8:5095.

Lavery R, Pullman A, Pullman B (1981). Int. J. Quant. Chem. 20:49.

Lavery R, Pullman A, Pullman B (1982). Theoret. Chim. Acta 62:93.

Lavery R, Pullman A, Pullman B (1983). Biophysical Chem. 17:75.

Nielsen PE (1981). Biochim. Biophys. Acta 655:89.

Pullman A (1981). In Steric Effects in Biomolecules, (Naray-Szabo

Ed.). Hungarian Academy of Sciences, Budapest p 247.

Pullman A, Pullman B (1981). Quart. Rev. Biophys. 14:289.

Pullman A, Pullman B, Lavery R (1983). In Nucleic Acids – The Vectors of Life (B. Pullman and J. Jortner Eds) Reidel Publishing Co. p 75.

Pullman B (1983). J. Biomolecular Structure and Dynamics 1:773.

Pullman B, Lavery R, Pullman A (1982). Eur. J. Biochem. 124:229.

Pullman B, Pullman A, Lavery R (1983). In Structure, Dynamics, Interactions and Evolution of Biological Macromolecules (C. Hélène Ed) Reidel Publishing Co. p 23.

Richards FM (1977). Ann. Rev. Biophys. Bioeng. 6:151.

Scrocco E, Tomasi J (1978). Advances in Quantum Chomistry 11:116.

Sussman JL, Holbrook SR, Warrant RW, Church GM, Kim SH (1978). J. Mol. Biol. 123:607.

Vlassov VV, Giege R, Ebel JP (1980). FEBS Letters 120:12.

Vlassov VV, Giege R, Ebel JP (1981). Eur. J. Biochem. 119:51.

**Molecular Basis of Cancer, Part A: Macromolecular
Structure, Carcinogens, and Oncogenes, pages 87–98**
© **1985 Alan R. Liss, Inc.**

MOLECULAR MECHANISM OF CATALYSIS BY RNA

Karen Haydock and Leland C. Allen

Department of Chemistry
Princeton University
Princeton, N.J. 08544

It is now known that RNA can perform both autocatalytic
and enzymatic reactions, acting either on itself or on other
RNA substrates. The best characterized examples occur in the
Tetrahymena 26 S pre-rRNA "ribozyme" (Zaug et al. 1983, 1984)
and the M1 RNA of E. coli RNase P (Guerrier-Takada et al.
1983, 1984). Our objective is to understand how these reactions occur and to establish the chemical and structural
requirements for catalysis by RNA. Using analogy to known
enzymatic and non-enzymatic reactions, comparison of the different RNA catalysts, model building, and computer graphics,
we have proposed the reaction mechanisms and modeled the
active sites and modes of enzyme/substrate recognition at the
secondary and tertiary structure level.

All of the presently known RNA catalysts carry out
phosphoryl transfer or hydrolysis reactions at P-O bonds of
RNA. P-O3' bonds are cleaved and ligated (or hydrolyzed) in
the ribozyme and in RNase P. There are other cases where RNA
may catalyze hydrolysis at P-O5' bonds with a 2',3'-cyclic
phosphate intermediate, the same type of reaction which is
catalyzed by the protein enzyme RNase A (Dugas & Penney,
1981). The non-enzymatic cleavage of RNA by heavy metals has
been well characterized (i.e. the cleavage of tRNA by Pb(II)
at P-O5' bonds with a 2',3'-cyclic intermediate (Rubin &
Sundaralingam, 1983; Brown et al., 1983)).

In all known phosphoryl transfer reactions it is
generally believed that a nucleophile makes an S_N2 attack in-
line with the P-O bond to be broken, producing a trigonal

bipyramid transition state. For high specificity and rate enhancement, a base is needed to deprotonate the incoming nucleophile and an acid is needed to protonate the leaving group. In protein enzymes, various amino acid residues can fulfill these roles. Cationic amino acids or metal ions make the phosphate more susceptible by increasing the charge on the phosphorous atom and inducing P-O bond polarization. A metal may also activate the nucleophile or increase the acid strength of the leaving group, either by direct coordination, or interaction through a ligand such as a water molecule (Cooperman, 1976).

The basis of catalysis in nucleic acids is likely to be similar to that in proteins and thus we propose that RNA catalyzes a P-O3' bond cleavage/ligation reaction as shown below.

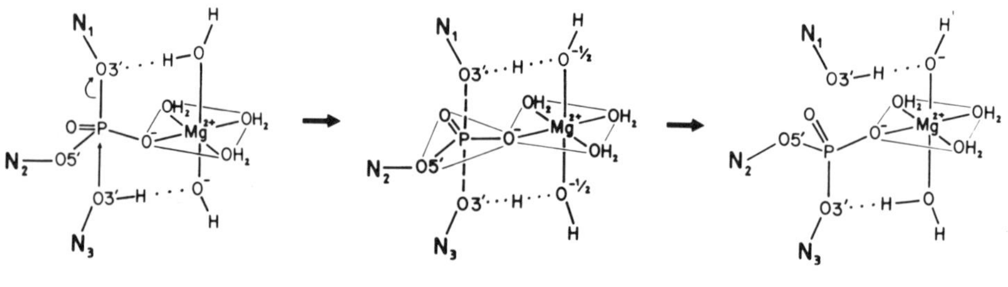

transition state

N_1 and N_2 are nucleosides and N_3 is either a nucleoside (for phosphoryl transfer or a proton (for hydrolysis). Deprotonation of the nucleophile and protonation of the leaving group are carried out by a hydroxyl ion and a water molecule which are both coordinated to an Mg^{2+} ion.

RIBOZYME MECHANISM

The 413 nucleotide intron of the Tetrahymena pre-rRNA is self-spliced out of the exon in three steps (Zaug et al., 1983, 1984). First the left splice junction is cleaved and a guanosine cofactor is linked to the 5'-end of the intron. In the second step the right splice junction is cleaved and the two ends of the exon are ligated. The excised intron is cyclized in the third step, with the release of a 15 nucleotide oligomer from the 5'-end of the intron. Each of these steps is a phosphoryl transfer reaction in which the O3'-hydroxyl

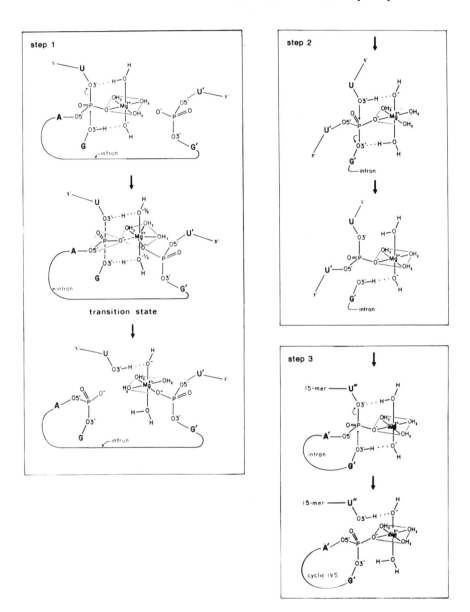

Fig. 1. Mechanism of the self-splicing ribozyme (described
in text). The 5'-exon ends with U; the intron begins with A,
includes U"pA', and ends with G'; and the 3'-exon begins with U'.

of a nucleoside (N_3) attacks a P-03' bond between nucleosides N_1 and N_2:

$$(N_1)03'-P(N_2) + (N_3)03'-H \rightarrow (N_3)03'-P(N_2) + (N_1)03'-H$$

In both the first and third steps N_3 is G, N_1 is U, and N_2 is A. According to our proposed mechanism (Haydock & Allen, 1984) the three steps of the ribozyme reaction proceed as shown in Figure 1, using a Mg-water complex for acid/base catalysis.

Knowing that the splicing reaction requires a guanosine cofactor, that A, U, C and 7-methylguanosine are all inactive as cofactors, and also noting the similarities between steps 1 and 3, we hypothesized that in both steps the guanine may be specifically recognized by hydrogen bonding to either the uracil or the adenine of the (U)03'-P(A) which it is attacking. After examining all possible hydrogen bonding schemes between G and (U)03'-P(A) which are geometrically feasible when the 03' of G is making an in-line attack on the P-03' bond, we found only one possible scheme. As shown in Figure 2(a), guanine makes a hydrogen bond from its N2-H1 to 02 of uracil. Both components of this scheme are in their normal A RNA conformations, except guanine is rotated 180° about its glycosidic torsion angle into the syn position and the C3'-03' torsion angle in th ribose of U has been rotated by -90°.

Very recently, Bass and Cech (1984) have reported testing the activities of the modified guanosine analogues shown in Table 1, and proposed that four hydrogen bonds are made from unspecified sites on the ribozyme to H1-N2, H2-N2, H-N1, and 06. We agree it is possible that additional hydrogen bonds are made to all these sites, although not from the U or A, as noted above. However, recognition of all these sites may not be necessary to explain the data.

According to our model it is easy to understand why the analogues on the right side of Table 1 are completely inactive. The reasons for the observed degrees of reduced activity by the analogues on the left may be quite complex. However, the partial activity of inosine can be explained by its ability to form a linear hydrogen bond from N1-H to 02 of uracil (see Figure 2). The reduced activities of 2-aminopurine and N1-methylguanosine can be accounted for by

Table 1. Activities of guanosine cofactor analogues as determined by Bass and Cech (1984).

guanosine
(100%)

REDUCED ACTIVITY	INACTIVE
2-aminopurine (50%)	purine ribonucleoside
6-thioguanosine	isoguanosine
1-methylguanosine (very low)	adenosine
N2-methylguanosine	xanthosine
inosine (50%)	N2,N2-dimethyl-guanosine

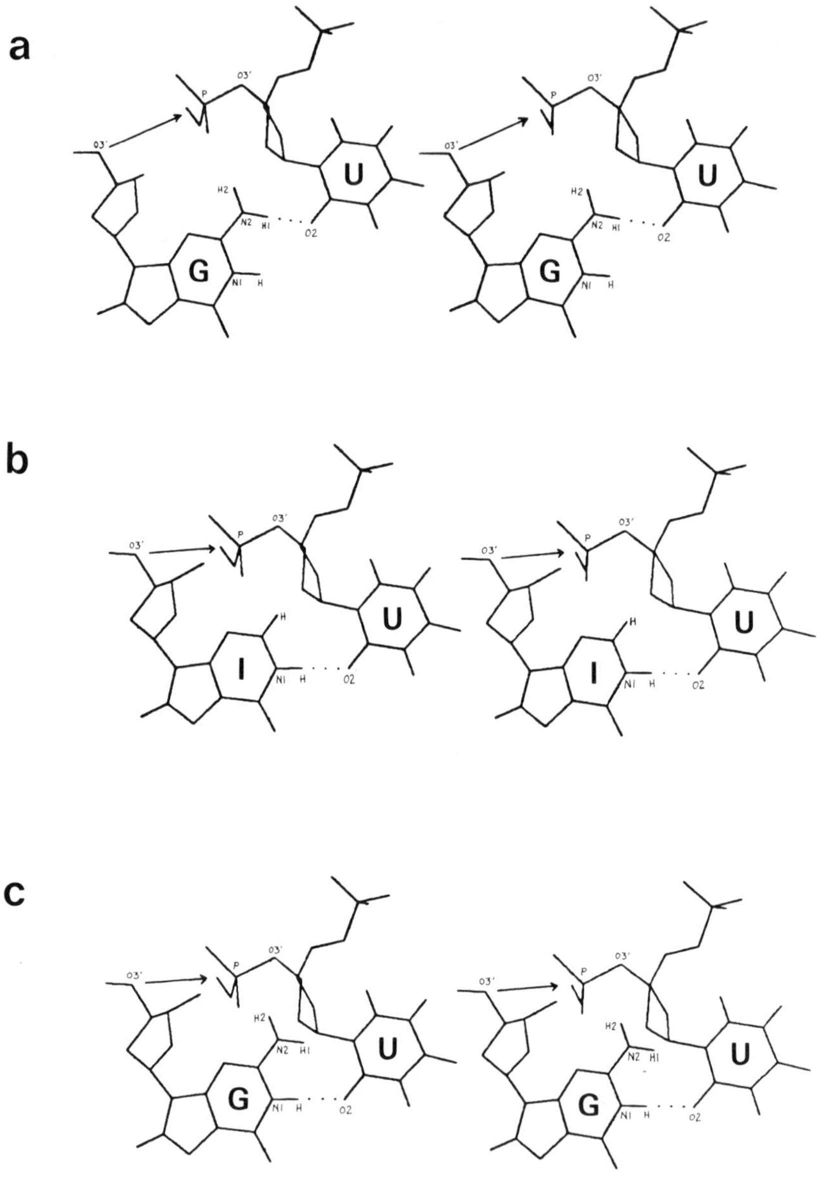

Fig. 2. Stereo views of cofactor recognition: (a) G···U; (b) I···U; (c) unallowed G···U, due to interference of N_2 amino group.

a non-linear (weak) hydrogen bond from guanine's N1-H to O2
of uracil, in addition to the (G)N2-H1•••O2(U) hydrogen bond.
On the other hand, if four hydrogen bonds are made to the
sites proposed by Bass and Cech, it is hard to explain why
N2-methylguanosine is partially active. Also, one might
expect 1-methylguanosine to be completely inactive if a
linear hydrogen bond is normally made to H-N1. In addition,
xanothosine in the Bass and Cech base recognition scheme
might be expected to be partially active if it could make two
out of four hydrogen bonds.

Our prediction that U is specifically recognized in
steps 1 and 3 appears to be holding up to further new experimental results. Zaug et al. (1984) have recently found an
alternative cyclization site at the (U)O3'-P(U) which is four
nucleotides downstream from the usual (U)O3'-P(A) site. Thus
the common feature of step 1 and these two cyclization reactions is that in each case a G attacks the phosphate on the
3'-side of a U. Recognition of both G and U can be suc-
cinctly explained by our minimum assumption model.

A third set of new results by Cech and coworkers
(personal communication) is that the cyclization reaction can
be reversed with the addition of certain di- and tri-
nucleotides (substituting for the 15-mer on the 5'side of the
cyclization site). The minimum length of the oligonucleotide
is a dinucleotide (all mononucleotides are inactive), and the
reaction depends on the oligonucleotide base sequence.
Therefore, recognition of the 5'-side must extend beyond the U
which is adjacent to the cleavage site. Since the oligonucleotide UU appears to be just as active as CC (but less
active than UUU) it is unlikely that these bases are being
recognized by making normal base pairs to some adenine or
guanine residues. (A G•C base pair should be more favorable
than G•U.) It is more likely that these bases are recognized
by hydrogen bonds such as the one we have proposed to O2 of
U, since both C and U have an O2 keto group.

We have built a Kendrew skeletal model of the active
site region of the ribozyme in which the critical components
for all three steps are in position for the reaction,
according to the schematic diagram (Fig. 3). Thus, we propose that the ribozyme reaction occurs as follows: (Step 1):
The cofactor G recognizes a specific site on the ribozyme by
hydrogen bonding to the uracil of UpA and to the Mg-water

complex. The Mg—water complex is bound specifically to the
phosphate of UpA and to other bases through its equatorial
ligands. The (U)03'-P(A) bond is broken and a (G)03'-P(A)
bond is formed. (Step 2): The (U)03' attacks the phosphate
of G'pU', which is already in position for this attack due
to the secondary and tertiary structure of the ribozyme (of
which the hairpin structure at the 5'-end of the intron is a
part) and the recognition of G' by U" (Fig. 3(b)). This
results in the cleavage of the (G')03'-P(U') bond and the
formation of a (U)03'-P(U') bond (exon ligation). (Step 3):
Cyclization reaction. Analogous to Step 1, G' recognizes
its specific site by hydrogen bonding to the uracil of U"pA'
and to the Mg—water complex (which is bound to U"pA'). (The
existence of the hairpin structure at the 5' end of the
intron is irrelevant at this stage.) The (G')03' attacks the
(U")03'-P(A') bond, which breaks as a (G')03'-P(A') bond
forms, producing the 15—mer and the cyclic IVS. As an
alternative to Step 3, the minor reaction producing a
19—mer and a shorter cyclic IVS can occur when G' hydrogen
bonds to U_{19} rather than U_{15}. This can occur because the
two ends of the linear IVS must be somewhat floppy (and
their conformation pH dependent) after removal from the
exon.

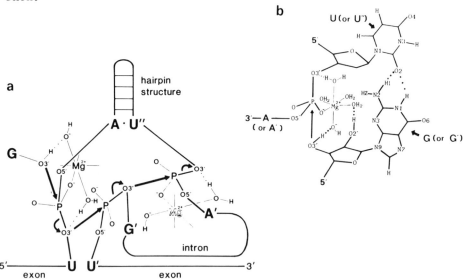

Fig. 3. The ribozyme reaction: (a) Schematic diagram of the
active site geometry. (b) G···U and G'···U" hydrogen bonds.

RNASE P MECHANISM

     RNase P is an RNA-protein enzyme which catalyzes the
hydrolysis of an oligonucleotide from the 5'-end of pre-tRNA.
Altman and coworkers (Guerrier-Takada et al. 1983, 1984a)
have shown that the M1 RNA component by itself is capable of
catalyzing this reaction. The protein appears to be playing
a structural role which can also be satisfied by polyamines
or structural Mg ions. By analogy to the ribozyme mechanism,
we have proposed (Guerrier-Takada et al, 1984b) that the
M1 RNA active site contains a Mg-water complex which acts
according to the same mechanism as the ribozyme, except the
nucleophile is a water molecule rather than a nucleoside.

     Each step in the reaction is shown in Figure 4. The
secondary and tertiary structure of the enzyme forms an
active site pocket in which the Mg^{2+} is coordinated to a
phosphate of the M1 RNA, four water molecules, and one
sequestered hydroxyl ion (Fig. 4(a)). We note that either
the three equatorial water molecules hydrogen bond to other
sites on the M1 RNA or the Mg is instead directly coordinated
to sites on the bases or ribose oxygens. The M1 RNA binds to
the pre-tRNA substrate as shown in Figure 4(b), making contacts with recognition sites on the tRNA. This brings the
phosphate containing the P-O3' bond which is to be hydrolyzed
into the active site where its negatively charged oxygen
becomes coordinated to the Mg as the enzymes phosphate becomes uncoordinated. A water molecule which is hydrogen bonded
to the Mg-bound hydroxyl ion makes an in-line S_N2 attack on
the P-O3' bond (Fig. 4(c)). The phosphate forms a trigonal
bipyramid transition state (Fig. 4(d)) as the axial hydroxyl
and water become protonated and deprotonated and the M1 RNA
phosphate becomes recoordinated to the Mg(Fig. 4(e)). The
tRNA is then released, but a strong anionic hydrogen bond
keeps the oligonucleotide in the active site as solvent water
molecules enter (Fig. 4(f)). Proton transfer through the
water chain results in deprotonation and protonation of the
axial water and hydroxyl ligands, allowing the oligonucleotide to dissociate and the enzyme to return to its original state (Fig. 4(g)).

P-O5' BOND CLEAVAGE REACTION

     In distinction to the ribozyme and M1 RNA catalyzed
P-O3' bond cleavage/ligation reactions, the enzyme RNase A

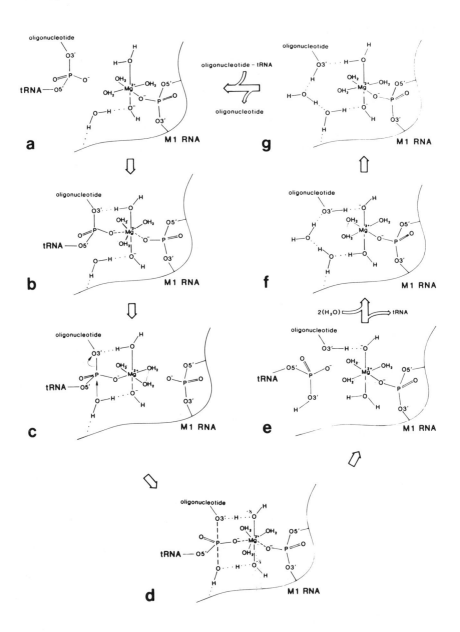

Fig. 4. Mechanism of M1 RNA catalyzed pre-tRNA hydolysis
(described in text).

catalyzes the hydrolysis of P-05' bonds. This reaction is accomplished in two steps. First, the 02' hydroxyl makes an in-line attack on the P-05' bond, forming a 2',3'-cyclic phosphate intermediate. In the second step a water molecule replaces the 05' leaving group and hydrolyzes the P-02' bond, resulting in a terminal 3'-phosphate.

We have examined the possibility that this type of reaction could also be catalyzed by RNA rather than protein. We propose that the amino acid residues which are involved in catalysis by RNase A (e.g. histidine and lysine) could be replaced by a Mg-water complex in an RNA-enzyme (or in an autocatalytic RNA). As shown in Figure 5, the mechanism could proceed as follows. First, the Mg-coordinated hydroxyl ion deprotonates the 02'-hydroxyl as the P-02' bond forms and the P-05' bond breaks, with a trigonal bipyramid transition state. The axial Mg-bound water molecule simultaneously protonates the 05' leaving group. The 2',3'-cyclic phosphate intermediate is hydrolyzed when the nucleoside N-05'-H is replaced by a water molecule in the reverse reaction.

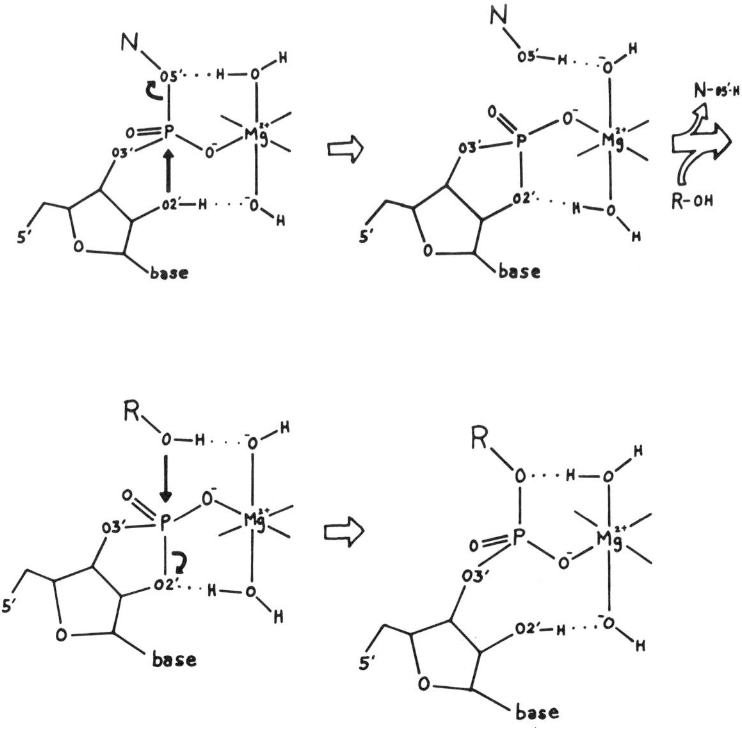

Fig. 5. P-05' cleavage with cyclic intermediate.

Since the nucleophiles in both steps make in-line attacks on the P-O bonds, the entering water molecule must occupy the same position as the 05' leaving group. This requirement for geometrical repositioning suggests that RNA cannot be hydrolyzed at a P-05' bond in one step. Furthermore, it may not be possible for any single enzyme to catalyze a nucleotidyl transfer reaction involving P-05' bond cleavage and ligation (where R in Fig. 5 is a nucleoside rather than a proton) because water would enter the active site before the 05' leaving group could be replaed by an 05'-nucleophile. Once hydrolysis has occured, ATP would then be required for a nucleotidyl addition reaction. Thus, splicing RNA at P-05' bonds appears to require a more complex mechanism than P-03' bond splicing.

Bass BL, Cech TR (1984). Biological catalysis by RNA. Nature (in press).

Brown RS. Hingerty BE, Dewan JC, Klug A (1983). Pb(II) catalyzed cleavage of the sugar-phosphate backbone of yeast tRNA^{Phe}. Nature 303:543.

Cooperman BS (1976). The role of divalent metal ions in phosphoryl and nucleotidyl transfer. In Sigel, H (ed.) "Metal Ions in Biological Systems", Vol. 5, New York: Dekker, p. 79.

Dugas H, Penney C (1981). "Bioorganic Chemistry", New York: Springer-Verlag.

Guerrier-Takada C, Gardiner K, Marsh T, Pace N, Altman S (1983). The RNA moiety of ribonuclease P is the catalytic subunit of the enzyme. Cell 35:849

Guerrier-Takada C, Altman S (1984a). Catalytic activity of an RNA molecule prepared by transcription in vitro. Science 224:574.

Guerrier-Takada C, Baer M, Lawrence N, Haydock K, Allen L, Altman S (1984b). Manuscript in preparation.

Haydock K, Allen LC (1984). Mechanism of self-splicing rRNA. Proc Natl Acad Sci USA (in press).

Rubin JR, Sundaralingam M (1983). Lead ion binding and RNA chain hydrolysis in phenylalahine tRNA. J Biomol Struct Dyn 1: 639.

Zaug AJ, Grabowski PJ, Cech TR (1983). Autocatalytic cyclization of an excised intervening sequence RNA is a cleavage-ligation reaction. Nature 301:578.

Zaug AJ, Kent JR, Cech TR (1984). A labile phosphodiester bond at the ligation junction in a circular intervening sequence RNA. Science 224:574.

**Molecular Basis of Cancer, Part A: Macromolecular
Structure, Carcinogens, and Oncogenes, pages 99–108**
© **1985 Alan R. Liss, Inc.**

PHYSICAL CHARACTERIZATION OF A NUCLEIC ACID JUNCTION

[+][#]Nadrian C. Seeman, [%]Marcos F. Maestre, [*]Rong-Ine
Ma, and [*]Neville R. Kallenbach
[#]Department of Biological Sciences, SUNY Albany,
Albany, NY 12222, [*]Department of Biology,
University of Pennsylvania, Philadelphia, PA 19104
and [%]Biology and Medicine Division, Lawrence
Berkeley Lab 70-A, Berkeley, CA 94220

[+]Recipient of an NIH Research Career Development Award

ABSTRACT
     Normally unstable transient states of DNA, in which the
linear duplex branches to form junctions with three or more
arms, can be studied at the oligonucleotide level if their
sequences are carefully selected. We have designed a series
of oligonucleotide complexes with sequences that are restricted to prevent any major overlap among the arms, and
chosen to exhibit high equilibrium stabilities, as well.
The electrophoretic mobility of these complexes on polyacrylamide gels permits us to demonstrate formation of a
stable four-strand complex with 1:1:1:1 stoichiometry. We
review here the evidence for formation of a stable stoichio-
metric junction, and present new circular dichroism data
showing that the arms remain in B helix geometry within the
complex, and that no significant loss of structure occurs on
forming a junction.

INTRODUCTION
     DNA molecules exist predominantly in the form of linear
or circular extended double helices. Despite the success of
fiber diffraction analysis, base-paired duplexes involving
oligonucleotides of specific sequence, rather than polynucleotides, have provided the major source of detailed
structural and dynamic information concerning the state of
the bases and backbones in various forms of double helical
structure (reviewed in Sarma (1981)). While it is known
that triply and quadruply branched structures (junctions) of
DNA have a transient existence as intermediates in the
replication or recombination of DNA molecules (Dressler and
Potter, 1982), it has not been possible to investigate these
forms structurally at high resolution in short chain mole-

cules. This is because these naturally occurring intermediates are inherently unstable, due to internal sequence
symmetry, which permits their resolution to double helices,
via a rapid isomerization process called branch point migration. As shown in Figure 1, this process allows bases
across the junction to pair, thereby redistributing the
residues in each of the arms. Even if the direction of each
step is random, random-walk kinetics dictate that this
structure will eventually resolve to double helices
(Thompson, et al., 1976; Warner, et al., 1979; Meselson,
1972). Clearly, such unstable symmetric molecules are not
suitable to analysis at the oligonucleotide level.
Nevertheless, it is only in oligonucleotide systems that the
region of chain at the site of branching can provide a
significant component of the signal in any physical probe of
structure or dynamics.

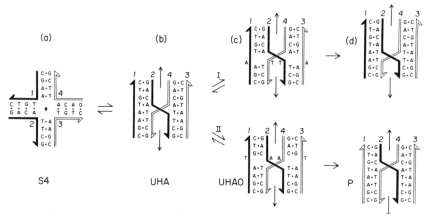

Fig. 1. Nucleic acid junctions and branch point migration.
(a) A four-fold symmetric (S4) junction backbone structure.
The similarly shaded backbones were initially paired to each
other; the lens-shaped object indicates the two-fold
sequence symmetry. (b) A Holliday (1964) structure with
unperturbed helix axes (UHA). Migration of the branch point
in either direction through an open structure (UHAO) is
indicated by reactions I and II in the transition to (c);
the migrated products (P) are indicated in (d). Repetition
of reaction I yields a return to the original pairing, while
iterating reaction II yields a new hybridization.

Transient branched symmetric DNA intermediates, such as
the cruciform structures proposed by Holliday (1964), Sigal
and Alberts (1972), and Gierer (1966) provide biologically
important examples of nucleic acid junctions. It has

recently been suggested that migration can be eliminated, thereby forming immobile (non-migratory) junctions from oligonucleotides (Seeman, 1981, 1982). The idea is that oligonucleotides can be constructed which will preferentially associate to form all of the arms of junctions via Watson-Crick base pairing, while the sequences of these molecules lack the symmetry necessary to permit branch point migration. At the same time, the overall sequence symmetry is minimized so that the pairing configuration corresponding to the desired junction architecture is the most probable one (Seeman, 1981, 1982; Seeman and Kallenbach, 1983).

The essential feature of the "sequence symmetry minimization" procedure is that no pairing which interferes with the designed architecture is permitted. Operationally, this is accomplished by assuming that a stretch of contiguous base pairs constitutes a single, favorable interacting unit; the longer the stretch, the more favorable. In order to achieve unique pairing, one must minimize the length of redundant stretches. An example of a specific immobile nucleic acid junction is illustrated in Figure 2. Each of the four hexadecamer strands shown in Figure 2 may be treated as a series of 13 overlapping tetramers. The architecture of the junction dictates 52 of these tetramers. In this junction, all the tetramers are unique, and redundancy is only seen at the level of trimers, for example the G.G.A sequences seen at the middle of the third and fourth strands. While it is desirable to limit redundancy to the level of dimers only, it was not possible to choose the 56

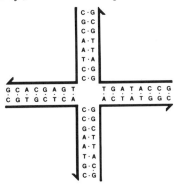

Fig. 2. An immobile nucleic acid junction composed of four hexadecanucleotides. Strand numbering is counterclockwise from the upper left. Note the lack of symmetry around the center, eliminating migration. These sequences were commercially synthesized by phosphotriester techniques.

required trimers from the 64 possible trimers. The process of generating suitable sequences is not trivial, and it is strongly dependent on the additional constraints imposed, as described below.

The discrete procedure for minimizing sequence symmetry must be supplemented by equilibrium stability calculations, in order to maximize the probability of achieving this junction architecture (Seeman and Kallenbach, 1983) with the redundant trimers chosen. Only competing Watson-Crick base pairs are considered in this procedure. Nevertheless, it is advisable to eliminate possible non-Watson-Crick interactions, as well: In the region near the junction, the double helical constraints are not strong, and non-Watson-Crick interactions might be more favorable than within double helical domains. This is done by including arbitrary constraints; for example, in the design of this junction, stretches of G's longer than two were forbidden. Furthermore, we routinely calculate a thermal transition profile for each of the sequences which passes the other criteria. It is very useful to know whether to expect a monophasic or polyphasic melting curve.

We present here gel electrophoretic data which indicate that the four hexadecameric molecules, whose sequences are shown in Figure 2, indeed form a tetrameric junction complex in solution. Therefore, we are able to present ultraviolet optical absorbance and circular dichroism data on this system. With these data, we have begun to characterize this unusual, but extremely interesting, nucleic acid system.

GEL ELECTROPHORESIS EXPERIMENTS

Direct evidence for the formation of a specific complex involving all four strands is obtained from inspection of polyacrylamide gel electrophoretic patterns. For uniformly charged oligonucleotide linear duplexes, electrophoretic mobility is an approximately inverse function of chain length (Fangman, 1978; Sealey and Southern, 1982). When the individual strands, two equimolar mixtures of pairs, and the tetrad corresponding to the complete junction, are subjected to electrophoresis, the radioautographic patterns shown in Figure 3 result.

In this experiment, the 5' terminus of each of the arms was labelled with $\gamma-^{32}$ATP (Amersham, 5000 Ci/mMol) using T4 polynucleotide kinase (BRL), in a reaction mixture containing 8 mM of each strand, 0.5 M Tris HCl, pH 7.6, 0.01 M

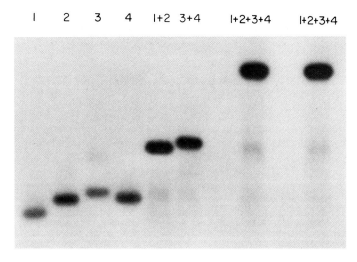

Fig. 3. Polyacrylamide gel electrophoresis of oligodeoxynucleotide strands and mixtures. The four single strands
are in the four left-most lanes, the pairs 1+2 and 3+4 are
in the next two lanes and the tetrameric complex in the next
two lanes.

$MgCl_2$, 5 mM dithiothreitol (Calbiochem) and 0.1 mM EDTA.
After 30 minutes at 37°C., the reaction mixes were extracted
once with phenol, the aqueous phase was removed, washed with
ether, and loaded onto a pre-equilibrated 3 ml column of
Sephadex G-50. Fractions containing the first peak with
absorbance at 254 nm were pooled following elution with a
buffer containing 0.5 mM Tris HCl, pH 8, 25 μM EDTA, lyo-
philized and 2 μg of each sample was electrophoresed on 20%
polyacrylamide at 10°C., as previously described
(Kallenbach, et al., 1983). The gel was taped to a sheet of
Kodak X-ray film, exposed for 24 hours at -70°C., to produce
the autoradiogram in Figure 3.

The single strands in the first four lanes migrate with
mobilities greater than the two pair-wise combinations shown
in the fifth and sixth lanes. Mixing these two pairs as
shown in the replicate experiments in the two right-hand
lanes yields a complex migrating much more slowly still,
incorporating all the label present in the 1+2 and 3+4
mixtures, within experimental error. Each of the bands
containing arms 1+2 and 3+4 and complex was then cut out
from the gel, and counted in a scintillation counter, with
the results shown in Table 1.

Table 1.
Radioactivity in the Paired Arms and Tetrameric Complex

Sample	D.P.M. x 10^{-3}
1+2	50
3+4	58
1+2+3+4 a	114
1+2+3+4 b	113

This experiment confirms the mobility studies previously reported, because (1) the mixtures of four strands
migrate as a single band of distinct mobility, and (2) the
strands 1+2 and 3+4 quantitatively react to yield complex
within the accuracy of these data. Higher unclosed complexes do not represent a significant fraction of the
material present. Further evidence of the 1:1:1:1
stoichiometry from a Job plot-type analysis has been
reported previously (Kallenbach, et al., 1983).

ULTRAVIOLET ABSORBANCE EXPERIMENTS
    The stability of the different complexes of strands 1 to
4 can be assessed by thermal denaturation studies. Base
paired nucleic acid duplexes are hypochromic (absorb less),
relative to single strands or a mixture of their constituent
mononucleotides, at wavelengths near 260 nm (e.g.,
Freifelder, 1976). Figure 4 shows the thermal transition
profiles of individual strand 3 and an equimolar mixture of
strands 1+2, compared with that of the quaternary complex at
half the total strand concentration. The fact that the
hyperchromism in the junction is twice as great as in the
same concentration of pairs strongly suggests that the complex is closed with four arms nearly intact. The increase
in junction stability (seen in the higher melting temperature, T_m) further strengthens this argument. Contrary to
estimates made by several workers in the field, no major
fraction of open base-pairs has to exist at the junction, and
the structure is not intrinsically an unstable one.

CIRCULAR DICHROISM MEASUREMENTS
    One of the first questions to ask about the junction is
to what extent the structure of the DNA in the arms is perturbed in the complex. Circular dichroism (CD) in the ultraviolet provides an extremely sensitive probe of geometrical
relationships among the bases in ordered nucleic acid
duplexes. The positive CD band near 275 nm has been shown to
be sensitive to variations in base tilt, twist, displacement
from the helix axis and step height (Johnson, et al., 1981).

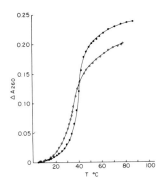

Fig. 4. Thermal transition profiles of the quaternary complex (25 µM total strands), an equimolar mixture of strands 1+2 (49 µM total strands) and individual strand 3 (98 M total strand) at 260 nm. The UV absorbance of the samples was measured at each of a series of temperatures (T), and the results expressed as $\Delta A_{260} = \Delta A_{260}(T)/\Delta A_{260}$ (10°)-1. Fragment 3 alone exhibits a typical non-cooperative transition characteristic of nucleic acids in the absence of base pairing. Note that the concentration of 4-fold complex is 6.25 µM, while that of the paired arm is 24.5 µM. Hence the hyperchromicity in the junction is actually more than four times that of a single arm.

Figure 5 compares the ultraviolet CD spectrum of the equimolar junction complex with the spectrum derived from averaging the spectra of each of the pairing dimers: 1+2, 2+3, 3+4, and 1+4. The molar ellipticity of the junction in the positive band near 275 nm is observed to exceed that in the paired arms at all temperatures below the T_m of the junction. Thus, there is no evidence for significant loss of helical structure in the complex. The wavelengths corresponding to the two positive bands and the negative band at 250 nm in both spectra are characteristic of B-DNA.

The behavior of the CD spectrum as a function of temperature is shown in Figure 6. The presence of isoelliptic points at 298 nm and 267 nm is consistent with an overall transition in which the junction dissociates directly to disordered strands, with no substantial population of any intermediates intervening in the reaction. This is consistent with the higher T_m of the junction seen in the absorbance transition data.

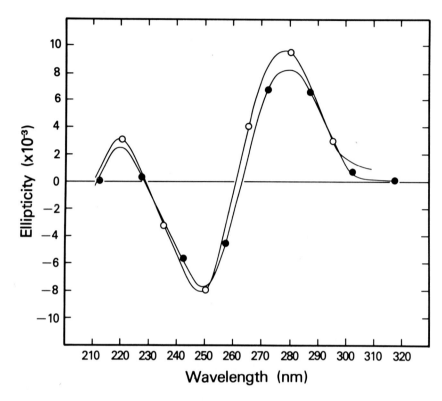

Fig. 5. Circular dichroism spectra for the junction and its constituent pairs. The open circles correspond to the junction, 1+2+3+4, while the filled circles are the average of the four pairs of arms, 1+2, 2+3, 3+4, 4+1.

We conclude also that the additional asymmetry imposed by constraining four arms to form a junction does not lead to a detectable characteristic CD signal, at least in the present case. Shorter stable junctions (Kallenbach, et al., 1983a) can be investigated to increase the relative signal from the center region.

DISCUSSION
The above experiments show that it is possible to de-sign and synthesize immobile nucleic acid junctions by sequence symmetry minimization (Seeman, 1981, 1982), together with appropriate equilibrium stability calculations (Seeman and Kallenbach, 1983). The stability and stoichiom-etry of the 1:1:1:1 tetrameric complex have been shown. The

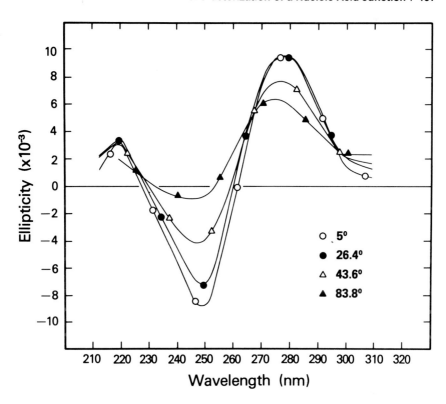

Fig. 6. Melting of the junction monitored by circular dichroism spectroscopy.

current level of characterization does not permit us to conclude that the junction is completely immobile, despite the
presence of non-complementary sequences flanking the junction. Further experimentation and comparison with semi-
mobile junctions are needed to firmly establish that a
limited amount of non-Watson-Crick mobility is not taking
place in the vicinity of the junction.

This demonstration opens up a number of new experimental possibilities, which should shed light on the molecular
details of the biologically important symmetric analogs of
these complexes. Further physico-chemical and structural
characterization of immobile junctions will be presented in
subsequent reports. A number of direct biological applications of these model complexes are evident, and these experiments are also in progress. Several chemical aspects of

non-linear branched nucleic acid structures have been postulated (Seeman, 1981, 1982; Seeman and Robinson, 1981), and
these hypotheses are open to experimental verification for
the first time.

ACKNOWLEDGMENTS
     This work has been supported by Grants GM-29554,
ES-00117, AI-08247 and CA-24101 from the National Institutes
of Health, Contract #W-7405-ENG-48 from the Division of
Environmental Research and Development of the Department of
Energy.

REFERENCES

Dressler D, Potter H (1982). Ann Rev Biochem 51:727.
Fangman WL (1978). Nuc Acid Res 5:653.
Freifelder DM (1976) In Physical Biochemistry, W.H.
  Freeman, San Francisco, p 377.
Gierer A (1966). Nature 212:1460.
Holliday R (1964). Genet Res 5:282.
Johnson BB, Dahl KS, Tinoco I, Jr, Ivanov VI, Zhurkin VB
  (1981) Biochemistry 20:73.
Kallenbach NR, Ma R-I, Seeman NC (1983). Nature 305:829.
Kallenbach NR, Ma R-I, Wand AJ, Veeneman GH, van Boom JH,
Seeman NC (1983a). Biomolecular Structure and Dynamics
  1:159.
Meselson M (1972). J Mol Biol 72:795.
Rodbard D, Chrambach A (1971). Anal Biochem 40:95.
Sarma RH (ed) (1981). In Biomolecular Stereodynamics,
  Adenine Press, New York, Vol 1, p 1.
Sealey PG, Southern EM (1982). In Rickwood D, Hames BD
  (eds): Gel Electrophoresis of Nucleic Acids, IRL Press,
  Oxford, p 39.
Seeman NC (1981). In Sarma RH (ed): Biomolecular
  Stereodynamics, Adenine Press, New York, p 269.
Seeman NC (1982). J Theor Biol 99:237.
Seeman NC, Kallenbach NR (1983) Biophys J 44:201.
Seeman NC, Robinson, BH (1981) In Sarma RH (ed):
  Biomolecular Stereodynamics, Adenine Press, New York, Vol
  1, p 279.
Sigal N, Alberts B (1972). J Mol Biol 71:789.
Thompson BJ, Camien MN, Warner RC (1976). Proc Nat Acad Sci
  (USA) 73:2299.
Van Holde KE (1971). In Physical Biochemistry,
  Prentice-Hall, Englewood Cliffs, p 168.
Warner RC, Fishel R, Wheeler R (1979). Cold Spring Harbor
  Symp Quant Biol 43:957.

Molecular Basis of Cancer, Part A: Macromolecular
Structure, Carcinogens, and Oncogenes, pages 109–121
© 1985 Alan R. Liss, Inc.

THEORETICAL STUDIES OF PERTURBED NUCLEIC ACID STRUCTURES

Wilma K. Olson, Nancy L. Marky, Annankoil R.
Srinivasan, Khang D. Do, and Janet Cicariello
Rutgers University
Department of Chemistry
New Brunswick, New Jersey 08903

INTRODUCTION

The interactions of the nucleic acids with
small molecules frequently involve perturbations of
the double helical structure. The intercalative
associations of planar drugs and dyes with the
heterocyclic bases, for example, increase the
spacing between adjacent chain units and unwind the
intervening sugar–phosphate backbone (Neidle, 1981;
Krugh, 1981; Taylor & Olson, 1983). More dramatic
are the covalent interactions of the nucleic acids
with carcinogenic agents such as
acetylaminofluorene. The primary adduct formed by
its chemical complexation at the C(8) position of
guanine apparently involves major structural
variations that expose the purine to its local
chemical environment and permit conformational
interconversions about its glycosyl linkage (Nelson
et al, 1971; Fuchs & Daune, 1972; Chang et al,
1974). Such conformational changes are sterically
forbidden by the close stacking of adjacent bases
in the standard right–handed A– and B–DNA double
helices. The C(8) of guanine, however, is exposed
in the left–handed Z–DNA duplex (Sage & Leng, 1980;
Santella et al, 1982), but the likelihood and ease
of an A– or B– to Z–DNA conformational transition
is poorly understood (Olson et al, 1982).

This work examines the likelihood of
perturbing standard A– and B–DNA helices into
three-dimensional spatial arrangements capable of
binding bulky carcinogenic agents. The probability

of forming bulges with mispaired or exposed bases is estimated using an elaborated form of Jacobson-Stockmayer cyclization theory (Jacobson & Stockmayer, 1950). Some of the likely conformational routes that link an intact duplex to a bulged form are presented. The bases in such structures are found to rotate as freely about their glycosyl linkages as they would in an isolated nucleoside. Interestingly, some of the conformational patterns associated with bulge formation are also found to be a natural consequence of the deformation of the DNA duplex along a supercoiled trajectory.

CHAIN STATISTICS

The relative ease of deforming the DNA duplex into a bulged form with bases misaligned or positioned on the surface of the structure can be estimated from the distribution of conformations assumed by a theoretically equivalent single-stranded chain. As illustrated in Figure 1, the bulge can be represented by a sequence of vectors-- here the P-to-C5' and C5'-to-P virtual bond vectors previously developed to treat polynucleotide extension and orientation (Olson & Flory, 1972b; Yevich & Olson, 1979; Marky & Olson, 1982)--that proceed down one of the chains, across the base-paired end of the bulge, and back up the complementary strand. The end-to-end vector $\underset{\sim}{r}$ joining the chain termini is required to meet specific vectorial criteria associated with base pair formation, and the terminal vectors of the chain sequence are expected to align in an orientation (given by the scalar product $\gamma = \underset{\sim}{v}_1 \cdot \underset{\sim}{v}_n / |\underset{\sim}{v}_1| |\underset{\sim}{v}_n|$) that assures the desired base pair formation. In an A-DNA helix the required end-to-end vector and angular orientation defined relative to a Cartesian coordinate reference frame placed in the standard fashion (Olson & Flory, 1972a) along the first virtual bond of the chain fragment are $\underset{\sim}{r}_0 = (+7.1\text{Å}, -6.2\text{Å}, -15.2\text{Å})$ and $\gamma_0 = 0.28$. These constraints are very similar to those associated with RNA hairpin loop formation (Marky & Olson, 1982). Indeed, the duplex bulge is simply an internally constrained hairpin structure. Except for the rigid link that joins the complementary

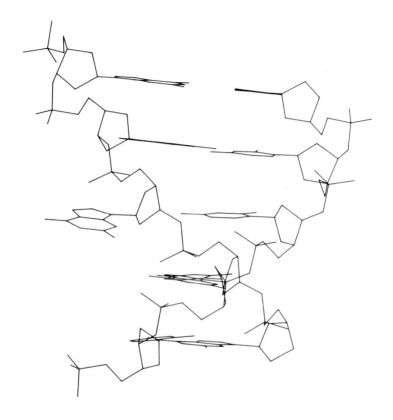

Figure 1: Schematic illustrating the virtual bond
scheme (dashed lines) used in the
statistical mechanical treatment of
duplex bulge formation

strands in the middle of the chain, the intervening
bonds are free to adopt any combination of states
so long as they satisfy the chain closure
constraints. Accordingly, the duplex can either
bend or preserve the helical direction at the bulge
site. For simplicity, in the data presented below,
one of the complementary strands is assigned A-DNA
helical geometry so that the duplex remains linear.

The extent to which the closure constraints are met in such a system is given by the product of two correlated probabilities

$$Q(\underset{\sim}{r}_0, \gamma_0) = \left[W(\underset{\sim}{r}_0) \delta \underset{\sim}{r} \right] \left[2\Gamma_{\underset{\sim}{r}}(\gamma_0) \delta \gamma \right] \tag{1}$$

$W(\underset{\sim}{r}_0) \delta \underset{\sim}{r}$ is the probability of the end-to-end vector falling within δr of the ideal closure position $\underset{\sim}{r}_0$ while $2\Gamma_{\underset{\sim}{r}}(\gamma_0)$ is the probability that the first and last virtual bonds of the chain sequence assume an orientation within $\delta\gamma$ of γ_0 with $\underset{\sim}{r}$ already fixed at $\underset{\sim}{r}_0$. The former probability can be estimated by the leading terms of a Hermite series expansion (Flory & Yoon, 1974) of the average tensor moments of the end-to-end vector $<\underset{\sim}{r}^x P>$, while the latter is obtained from a Legendre polynomial expansion (Flory et al, 1976) of the scalar moments $<\gamma^k r^2 P>$. The chain moments are determined by the conformational character of the nucleotide repeating unit (Yevich & Olson, 1979).

The probabilities reported in Figure 2 are functions of the amount of bending permitted in the C5'-C4' (ψ) and the P-O5' (ω) torsions that immediately precede and follow the central base in the leading strand of a bulged A-DNA duplex. The two rotations are allowed to flip from their preferred gauche$^+$ (60 ±60° with respect to a 0°=cis reference) and gauche$^-$ (-60±60°) states to trans arrangements (180° ±60°). Such variations are well known to distort the A-DNA backbone with local bending and to disrupt adjacent base stacking (Srinivasan & Olson, 1980). Surprisingly, the bends have little influence on the computed values of $Q(\underset{\sim}{r}_0, \gamma_0)$. The likelihood of end-to-end closure is essentially the same for an unperturbed duplex (subject only to minor torsional fluctuations of the standard helical geometry) and a duplex with any degree of bending in the two torsional variables. The two bends, however, must be equally favored. In chains containing only the ψ bend, the computed likelihood of bulge formation is reduced by an order of magnitude over the above cases. When the bending is exclusively in ω, the probabilities are diminished by two to three orders of magnitude.

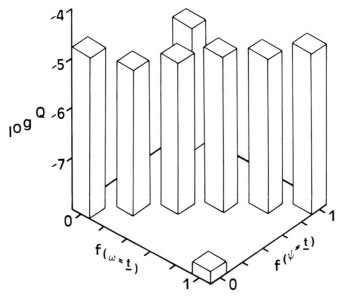

Figure 2: Computed probability of chain closure in a single-base bulged duplex as a function of bending in the C5'-C4' (ψ) and P-05' (ω) torsions.

LOCAL CONFORMATIONAL ANALYSIS

This somewhat bizarre prediction is readily understood from Figure 3 where a bulge created by simultaneous variations about the bonds of interest is illustrated. Because the pair of bonds is roughly parallel to one another, their correlated variations (in the opposite rotational sense) preserve the direction of the helical backbone (Olson, 1981). At the same time the intervening base flips to the outside of the duplex, forming an angle of roughly 90° with respect to the planes of the bases in the hydrogen-bonded interior. The exposed base is also free to rotate about its glycosyl torsion in this unencumbered position. Indeed, as illustrated by the computed variation in van der Waals' potential energy in Figure 4, the exposed base in the bulge rotates as freely about its glycosyl linkage as it would in an isolated nucleoside. The base used in the example is an adenine which, like guanine, can flip between an <u>anti</u> arrangement ($\chi = 30 \pm 30°$) where it is oriented

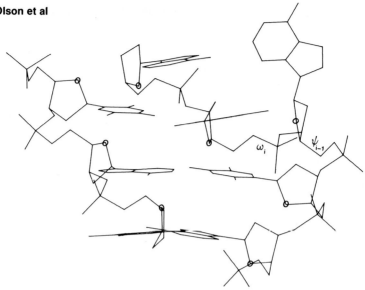

Figure 3: Bulged   B-DNA   duplex   generated   by
           correlated variations in ψ_{i-1} and ω_i.
           The O1' atoms of the sugar rings are
           noted by circles.

away from the sugar phosphate to a <u>syn</u> conformation
($\chi = 210 \pm 30°$) where the six-membered ring is directed
above the sugar and the C(8) atom is positioned for
easy interaction with a bulky carcinogen.

        The bulge structure illustrated in Figure 3 is
of further interest in that the exposed sugar ring
is flipped with respect to the direction of the
remaining sugars in the structure (i.e., the oxygen
atom in the exposed sugar points downward while the
oxygens on the remaining sugars of the same strand
point upward).   Such an alternation of ring
direction is a characteristic feature of the Z-DNA
helix, suggesting a likely mechanism involved in
the B- to Z-DNA helical transition. A route like
this also preserves the direction of the
polynucleotide backbone, unlike a previously
suggested B-Z path (Olson et al, 1982) that creates
sharp bends in the DNA backbone. Finally, it is
recognized that the specific structure illustrated
here involves base mispairing at its terminal end.
The residues on either side of the exposed base are

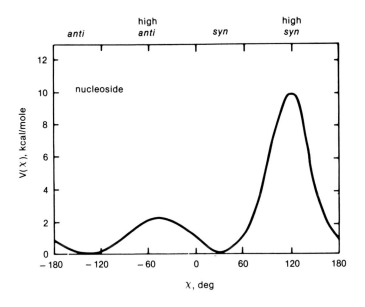

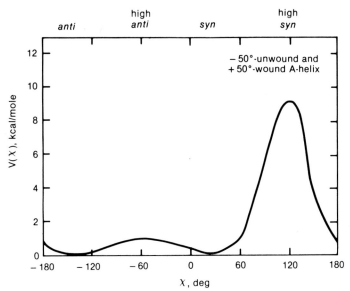

Figure 4: The computed variations in van der Waals energy as a function of the glycosyl torsion in (a) free adenosine and (b) a bulged residue of A-type poly dA.

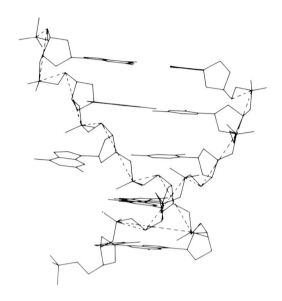

Figure 5: Bulged duplex generated by correlated
overwinding and unwinding of the B-DNA
duplex.

brought to normal stacking distances by the
correlated $\psi_{i-1}\omega_i$ variation. Indeed, the 6.8Å
separation of alternate base planes can only be
preserved by perturbing the duplex to a form which
orients the C5'-C4' and P-O5' bonds more nearly
parallel to the vertical axis.

A second type of bulge arising from the
correlated variations of successive O3'-P (ω')
torsions is illustrated in Figure 5. Like the
$\psi_{i-1}\omega_i$ angle pair discussed above, the ω' torsions
are parallel to one another. Because these
torsions are also parallel to the duplex axis,
their variation translates into local winding and
unwinding of adjacent base planes. The bases are
exposed on the helical surface if the overwinding
precedes the underwinding motion (Olson, 1982).
The intervening sugar is not inverted in such a
process, which is characteristic of the transitions
between right- and left-handed helices of the same
morphological sense, such as B-DNA and its closely
related left-handed analogs (Olson, 1976).

MACROSCOPIC CHAIN FOLDING

The horizontal twisting of base planes associated with the latter kind of bulge is a natural consequence of DNA supercoiling. The relative deviations of local twist (with respect to a regular linear duplex) are reported as a function of chain sequence for a representative toroidal structure in Figure 6. The supercoil of interest (illustrated in stereo at the base pair level in Figure 7) is obtained by smoothly deforming a tenfold right-handed helix along a closed circular superhelical (e.g., toroidal) trajectory. The radius of the superhelix (2.7Å) and the radius of the closed circle (43.2Å) are chosen to preserve, as closely as possible, the preferred 3.5Å vertical spacing of adjacent bases. In this particular example, the mean vertical distance between base planes is found to range from 3.3 to 3.7Å.

Although the presumed superhelical density (4 left-handed turns per 80 residues) is an order of magnitude greater than that observed in natural DNA's (Bauer, 1978), the model is useful in understanding the influence of higher order coiling upon secondary structure. The local twist (measured by the angle between the C1'···C1' long axes of successive base planes) is seen in Figure 6 to decrease throughout the chain. The majority of residues are found to unwind by 6-8° from the 36° reference angle. A sizable minority (10%), however, are found to unwind roughly 90° to a local left-handed backbone geometry. As a consequence of these events and as expected from topological arguments (Fuller, 1971; Crick, 1976), the duplex is seen (Figure 7) to intertwine four fewer times than it would in a relaxed closed circular trajectory of the same chain length.

The severe 90° unwinding sites in Figure 7 are potential nucleation points for the left-handed helix that might be induced by further supercoiling of the DNA. In the present example, the residues involved in the sudden turns are much more exposed to the local environment than the remaining chain units. In contrast to the exposed base models presented above, the base pairs are seen to bulge

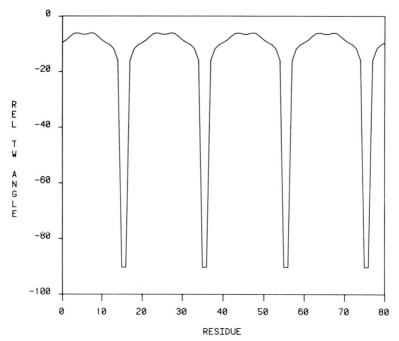

Figure 6: Variation of local base-base twist in an
80-residue closed circular toroidal
trajectory of B-DNA.

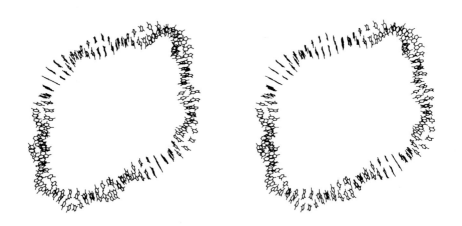

Figure 7: Stereo representation at the base pair
level of the toroidal trajectory
described in Figure 6.

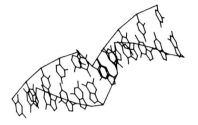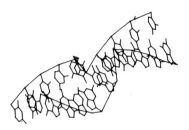

Figure 8:   Close-up stereo view illustrating the
            unwinding of complementary strands in
            the toroidal trajectory of Figure 6.

as units at specific points along the superhelical
trajectory, the most exposed sites occurring in
residues between the points of maximum and minimum
local twist (e.g., residues 15-16, 35-36, 55-56,
75-76 in Figures 6 and 7). A stereo close-up of
the bulged base pairs is provided for further
inspection in Figure 8. For clarification,
consecutive C1' atoms have been connected by
virtual bonds, the values ranging from 3.8 to 6.3Å
along this segment of the duplex. In the regular
tenfold linear chain this distance is constant at
5.0Å.

ACKNOWLEDGMENT

      This research was supported by grants CA-25981
and GM-20861 from the U. S. Public Health Service
and an award from the Charles and Johanna Busch
Memorial Fund. Computer resources were generously
supplied by the Center for Computer and Information
Services of Rutgers University.

REFERENCES

Bauer WR (1978). Structure and reactions of closed duplex DNA. Ann Rev Biophys Bioeng 7:287.

Chang C-T, Miller SJ, Wetmur JG (1974). Physical studies of N-acetoxy-N-2-acetylaminofluorene-modified deoxyribonucleic acid. Biochemistry 13:2142.

Crick FHC (1976). Linking numbers and nucleosomes. Proc Natl Acad Sci, USA 73:2639.

Flory PJ, Yoon DY (1974). Moments and distribution functions for polymer chains of finite length. I. Theory. J Chem Phys 12:5358.

Flory PJ, Suter UW, Mutter M (1976). Macrocyclization equilibria. I. Theory. J Am Chem Soc 98:5733.

Fuchs R, Daune M (1972). Physical studies on deoxyribonucleic acid after covalent binding of a carcinogen. Biochemistry 11:2659.

Fuller FB (1971). The writhing number of a space curve. Proc Natl Acad Sci, USA 68:815.

Jacobson H, Stockmayer WH (1950). Intramolecular reaction in polycondensations. I. The theory of linear systems. J Chem Phys 18:1600.

Krugh TR (1981). Oligonucleotide and polynucleotide-drug complexes in solution as investigated by NMR. In Neidle S (ed): "Topics in Nucleic Acid Structure," New York, John Wiley & Sons, p. 197.

Marky NL, Olson WK (1982). Loop formation in polynucleotide chains. I. Theory of hairpin loop closure. Biopolymers 21:2329.

Neidle S (1981). Oligonucleotide and polynucleotide-drug complexes in the crystalline state. In Neidle S (ed): "Topics in Nucleic Acid Structure," New York, John Wiley & Sons, p. 177.

Nelson JH, Grunberger D, Cantor CR, Weinstein IB (1971). Modification of ribonucleic acid by chemical carcinogens. IV. Circular dichroism and proton magnetic resonance studies of oligonucleotides modified with N-2-acetylaminofluorene. J Mol Biol 62:331.

Olson WK (1976). The spatial configuration of ordered polynucleotide chains. I. Helix formation and base stacking. Biopolymers 15:859.

Olson WK (1981). Understanding the motions of DNA.

In Sarma RH (ed): "Biomolecular Stereodynamics, Volume I," New York: Adenine Press, p. 327.

Olson WK (1982). Theoretical studies of nucleic acid conformation: potential energies, chain statistics, and model building. In Neidle S (ed): "Topics in Nucleic Acid Structure, Part 2," London: The Macmillan Press Ltd., p. 1.

Olson WK, Flory PJ (1972a). Spatial configurations of polynucleotide chains. I. Steric interactions in polyribonucleotides: a virtual bond model. Biopolymers 11:1.

Olson WK, Flory PJ (1972b). Spatial configurations of polynucleotide chains. II. Conformational energies and the average dimensions of polyribonucleotides. Biopolymers 11:25.

Olson WK, Srinivasan AR, Marky NL, Balaji VN (1982). Theoretical probes of DNA conformation: Examining the B Z conformational transition. Cold Spring Harbor Symp Quant Biol 47:229.

Sage E & Leng M (1980). Conformation of poly (dG-dC) poly(dG-dC) modified by the carcinogens N-acetoxy-N-acetyl-2-aminofluorene and N-hydroxy-N-2-aminofluorene. Proc Natl Acad Sci, USA 77:4597.

Santella RM, Grunberger D, Weinstein IB (1982). Carcinogens can induce alternate conformations in nucleic acid structure. Cold Spring Harbor Symp Quant Biol 47:339.

Srinivasan AR & Olson WK (1980). Yeast tRNA[Phe] conformation wheels: a novel probe of the monoclinic and orthorhombic models. Nucleic Acids Res 8:2307.

Taylor ER, Olson WK (1983). Theoretical studies of nucleic acid interactions. I. Estimates of conformational mobility in intercalated chains. Biopolymers 22:2267.

Yevich R, Olson WK (1979). The spatial distributions of randomly coiling polynucleotides. Biopolymers 18:113.

**Molecular Basis of Cancer, Part A: Macromolecular
Structure, Carcinogens, and Oncogenes, pages 123–129**
© **1985 Alan R. Liss, Inc.**

ATOMIC MOTIONS IN PHENYLALANINE TRANSFER RNA PROBED BY
MOLECULAR DYNAMICS SIMULATIONS

M. Prabhakaran*, J. Andrew McCammon+, and Stephen C. Harvey*

*Department of Biochemistry
University of Alabama in Birmingham
Birmingham, AL   35294

+Department of Chemistry
University of Houston
Houston, TX   77004

INTRODUCTION

The functions of biological macromolecules are intimately tied to their structures, and the determination of
structure-function relationships is one of the principal
goals of biochemical and biophysical research at the molecular level. Since many functions of biological macromolecules are dynamic, it is desirable to develop dynamic
structural models.

A variety of methods are available for modeling intramolecular motions. The most detailed models are provided by
molecular dynamics simulations in which the positions of
every atom in the molecule are followed over the time scale
from fractions of a picosecond to tens or hundreds of picoseconds (1 psec = 10^{-12} sec). In this method, a static
molecular model (usually obtained by x-ray crystallography)
is animated by assigning random thermal velocities to all of
the atoms, and a computer is used to keep track of atomic
positions and velocities as they evolve under the influence
of interatomic forces due to deformations of the covalent
structure and due to collisions between atoms that are not
covalently bonded to one another. The molecular dynamics
algorithm has the advantage of producing a very detailed
picture of the motions, but current limitations on computer
speed restrict the studies to systems of relatively small

size (total molecular weights below about 30,000) and very short times (total times less than about 300 psec). Several articles explain the molecular dynamics method in detail and describe applications of the algorithm to the simulation of protein dynamics (McCammon et al. 1979; Karplus, McCammon 1981; Northrup et al. 1981; Brooks et al. 1983; Levitt 1982a; Levitt 1983; McCammon 1984).

The results from the protein simulations were cause for both hope and apprehension about the ability to simulate motions in nucleic acids. Hope, because the simulations gave average protein structures close to the crystallographic structures and motions that were in reasonable agreement with thermal factors from crystallography (Northrup et al. 1980; Levitt 1983b). Apprehension, for two reasons. First, agreement with experiment is best in the interior of the proteins, (Northrup et al. 1981), and nucleic acids have much larger surface-to-volume ratios than globular proteins. Second, the original protein simulations were done for models in vacuo; the inclusion of explicit solvent has been shown to improve the agreement with experiment considerably (van Gunsteren, Karplus 1981; Swaminathan et al. 1982; van Gunsteren et al. 1983), and solvent effects are known to be particularly important in structural studies of nucleic acids, since nucleic acids are polyelectrolytes (Eisenberg 1976).

The past two years have produced the first reports of molecular dynamics simulations on nucleic acids, both DNA (Levitt 1982b; Tidor et al. 1983) and transfer RNA (Prabhakaran et al. 1983; Harvey et al. 1984a). Earlier apprehensions have been partly justified, because the models are prone to dynamic degradation (Levitt 1982b), although these problems can be overcome by scaling the electrostatic charges and by a careful warmup and equilibration of the model (Levitt 1982b; Tidor et al. 1983; Prabhakaran et al. 1983; Harvey et al. 1984a).

In this paper we examine some of the aspects of the atomic motions in phenylalanine transfer RNA (tRNA[Phe]) as revealed by a 24 psec molecular dynamics simulation in vacuo. The details of the methods and the energy parameters are published elsewhere (Prabhakaran et al. 1983; Harvey et al. 1984a; Tung et al. 1984).

RESULTS AND DISCUSSION

The overall structure of tRNA^{Phe} is well preserved
throughout the simulation, with a root mean square (rms)
displacement of 1.34Å from the crystallographic structure
(Hingerty et al. 1978). This value compares favorably with
those reported for in vacuo protein simulations. No large
scale bending or flexing motions are observed, even though
they were a prominent feature of one DNA simulation (Levitt
1982b) and have been predicted for tRNA^{Phe} because of
experimental results (for a review see Rigler, Wintermeyer
1983) as well as theoretical studies (Harvey, McCammon 1981;
Tung et al. 1984). The absence of large scale motions indicates that the model has probably been equilibrated near the
global energy minimum.

The amplitudes of the rms deviations of the atomic positions correlate very well with the thermal factors from the
crystallographic study (which were kindly provided by Dr.
Brian Hingerty). There is also a high correlation between
the average atomic mobility of a given residue and the residue's solvent-accessible surface area, indicating that
simple packing considerations are the dominant factor in
determing the size of atomic motions (Harvey et al. 1984a).

To further characterize these motions, it is useful to
examine their anisotropy. This has been done by calculating
the mean square displacement matrix for each atom (Northrup
et al. 1981). This matrix, S^2, is a 3x3 matrix whose elements represent the covariances of the rms displacements
along three orthogonal coordinate axes,

$$S^2_{ij} = \langle \Delta r_i \, \Delta r_j \rangle$$

Since this matrix is symmetric, it can be diagonalized, and
the three elements of the diagonalized matrix are the mean
square amplitudes of the thermal ellipsoid for the atom. We
order those amplitudes and define f_2 to be the ratio between
the second largest and the largest mean square amplitude,
while f_3 is the ratio between the smallest and largest
amplitude (Northrup et al. 1981). For isotropic motion, the
thermal ellipsoid would be a sphere, with $f_2 = f_3 = 1$.
Smaller values of these ratios correspond to more anisotropic motions. Table 1 compares the average values of these

ratios for interior and exterior atoms in the tRNA simulation with the same ratios for ferrocytochrome c (Northrup et al. 1981).

Table 1: Average Anisotropy Ratios

tRNA^{Phe}	All atoms	Interior atoms	Exterior atoms
f_2	0.31	0.28	0.34
f_3	0.11	0.10	0.11
Ferrocytochrome c			
f_2	0.50	0.53	0.47
f_3	0.26	0.29	0.23

There are two outstanding features of the anisotropies that are shown in Table 1. First, the atomic motions of tRNA are much more anisotropic than those seen in the protein. Second, the motions of atoms in the interior of the tRNA are more anisotropic than those on the surface, in sharp contrast with the protein results. The difference between atoms in the interior and those on the outside is due to the very anisotropic force field that acts on atoms in bases (for which $f_2 = 0.30$) versus the relatively more isotropic forces acting, for example, on atoms in phosphate groups ($f_2 = 0.36$). A similar role of structural anisotropy on atomic motions is seen when we divide atoms into those that are part of residues in the double helical stems ($f_2 = 0.27$) and those that are part of other regions ($f_2 = 0.36$).

The anisotropies are also time dependent, so the size, shape, and orientation of the thermal ellipsoids depend on the time interval over which the mean square displacement matrix is calculated. A similar phenomenon has been reported for atomic motions in ferrocytochrome c (Morgan et al. 1983). This is most easily seen in moving pictures run at different speeds (Harvey et al. 1984b). On the sub-picosecond scale, the largest amplitude motions for atoms in double helical regions are along the helix axis, as rapid fluctuations in the glycosidic torsion angle cause each base to flutter and jitter in the narrow space between its neighbors. Lateral sliding of the bases only occurs over a time scale of several picoseconds, because this requires the collective motions of the base, the ribose, and part of the backbone. Since there are only weak forces opposing this lateral motion, it is of larger amplitude than the longitudinal motion, and it is thus the lateral motions which are the largest components of the thermal ellipsoids for base atoms on this longer time scale.

The simulation allows tRNA to sample several local minima in the conformational energy surface. This fact produces many examples of atomic motions that are very anharmonic. This behavior has also been shown to occur in protein dynamics (Mao et al. 1982), and a detailed report on this phenomenon will be presented elsewhere.

SUMMARY

A 24 psec molecular dynamics simulation of tRNA^{Phe} reveals a very stable model whose average structure is close to that of the crystallographic studies. The root mean square atomic motions correlate very well with the thermal factors from crystallography and are largely determined by packing forces. These motions are generally more anisotropic than those seen in a molecular dynamics simulation of a globular protein, and the anisotropic effects are also primarily a consequence of packing considerations. The development and examination of molecular dynamics models for macromolecules is an interesting basic research problem in biophysical chemistry, and it is now reasonably well advanced. The more exciting tasks of using these models to predict experimental properties and to examine biological function are just beginning.

ACKNOWLEDGEMENTS

Supported by grants from the National Science Foundation to SCH and JAM.

REFERENCES

Brooks BR, Bruccoleri RE, Olafson BD, States DJ, Swaminathan S, Karplus M (1983). CHARMM: A program for macromolecular energy minimization and dynamics calculations. J Comp Chem 4:187.

Eisenberg H (1976). "Biological Macromolecules and Polyelectrolytes in Solution." Oxford: Clarendon Press.

Harvey, SC, McCammon JA (1981). Intramolecular flexibility in phenylalanine transfer RNA. Nature 294:286.

Harvey SC, Prabhakaran M, Mao B, McCammon JA (1984a). Phenylalanine transfer RNA: Molecular dynamics simulation. Science 223:1189.

Harvey SC, Suddath FL, Prabhakaran M (1984b). Computer graphics and moving pictures in the analysis of molecular dynamics simulations. Biophs J 45:404a.

Hingerty R, Brown RS, Jack A (1978). Further refinement of the structure of yeast tRNA^{Phe}. J Mol Biol 124:523.

Karplus M, McCammon JA (1981). The internal dynamics of globular proteins. CRC Crit Revs Biochem 9:293.

Levitt M (1982a). Protein conformation, dynamics and folding by computer simulation. Ann Rev Biophys Bioeng 11:251.

Levitt M (1982b). Computer simulation of DNA double-helix dynamics. Cold Spring Harbor Symp Quant Biol 47:251.

Levitt M (1983a). Molecular dynamics of native protein. I. Computer simulation of trajectories. J Mol Biol 168:595.

Levitt M (1983b). Molecular dynamics of native protein. II. Analysis and nature of motion. J Mol Biol 168:621.

Mao B, Pear MR, McCammon JA, Northrup SH (1982). Molecular dynamics of ferrocytochrome c: Anharmonicity of atomic displacements. Biopolymers 21:1979.

McCammon JA, Wolynes PG, Karplus M (1979). Picosecond dynamics of tyrosine side chains in proteins. Biochemistry 18:927.

McCammon JA, (1984). Protein dynamics. Rep Prog Phys 47:1.

Morgan JD, McCammon JA, Northrup SH (1983). Molecular dynamics of ferrocytochrome c: Time dependence of the atomic displacements. Biopolymers 22:1579.

Northrup SH, Pear MR, McCammon JA, Karplus M, Takano T (1980) Internal mobility of ferrocytochrome c. Nature 287:659.

Northrup SH, Pear MR, Morgan JD, McCammon JA, Karplus M (1981). Molecular dynamics of ferrocytochrome c: Magnitude and anisotropy of atomic displacemnts. J Mol Biol 153:1087.

Prabhakaran M, Harvey SC, Mao B, McCammon JA (1983). Molecular dynamics of phenylalanine transfer RNA. J Biomolec Struct Dyns 1:357.

Rigler R, Wintermeyer W (1983). Dynamics of tRNA. Ann Rev Biophys Bioeng 12:475.

Swaminathan S, Ichiye T, van Gunsteren W, Karplus M (1982).
Time dependence of atomic fluctuations in proteins:
Analysis of local and collective motions in bovine
pancreatic trypsin inhibitor. Biochemistry 21:5230.
Tidor B, Irikura KK, Brooks BR, Karplus M (1983). Dynamics
of DNA oligomers. J Biomolec Struct Dyns 1:231.
Tung CS, McCammon JA, Harvey SC (1984). Large amplitude
bending motions in phenylalanine transfer RNA.
Biopolymers in press.
van Gunsteren WF, Karplus M (1982). Protein dynamics in
solution and in a crystalline enrionment: A molecular
dynamics study. Biochemistry 21:2259.
van Gunsteren WF, Berendsen HJC, Hermans J. Hol WGJ, Postma
JPM (1983). Computer simulation of the dynamics of
hydrated protein crystals and its comparison with x-ray
data. Proc Natl Acad Sci USA 80:4315.

Molecular Basis of Cancer, Part A: Macromolecular
Structure, Carcinogens, and Oncogenes, pages 131–140
© 1985 Alan R. Liss, Inc.

DNA TERTIARY STRUCTURE OF DISK-SHAPED TORUSES: AN in vitro
VIRAL DNA MODEL SYSTEM

Kenneth A. Marx, Ph.D. and George C. Ruben, *Ph.D.

Departments of Chemistry and Pathology*
Dartmouth College and Dartmouth Medical School
Hanover, NH   03755

CONDENSED DNA TORUSES, ds VIRUSES AND CANCER

   DNA can exist in a variety of tertiary states both in
vivo and in vitro. One of the more intriguing of these
tertiary conformations is the torus (donut shape), formed
in vitro by the collapse of DNA upon itself at a critical
concentration of trivalent cation such as naturally occurring
spermidine. Toroidal spermidine-DNA tertiary structure
organization is relevant to the in vivo DNA state since in
certain double stranded DNA bacteriophage such as λ
(Chattoraj et. al. 1978) and T2 (Klimenko et. al. 1967;
Richards et. al. 1973) and viruses like herpes simplex
(Furlong et. al. 1972) the genomes appear to be packaged
into torus-like structures in the infectious virions and
polyamines, including spermidine, are commonly found as
counterions (Ames and Dubin 1958). That polyamines may
help collapse and crosslink viral or bacteriophage DNA in
vivo is suggested by the observation that close to one-half
of the thymine residues in the bacteriophage φW-14 DNA are
replaced by the modified base, α-putrescinylthymidine, a
covalent polyamine dication modified base (Gerhard and
Warren 1982). The double stranded DNA containing herpes
virus group includes at least two members whose infections
in humans are associated with and may be causal agents of
neoplasias. These are the Epstein-Barr virus with Burkitt's
lymphoma (Miller 1981) and the herpes simplex-2 virus with
cervical carcinoma (McDougall et. al. 1981). It is clear
that an understanding of the organization of DNA packaged
in these pathogens would provide insight into the packaging
mechanism as well as possible unique chemotherapeutic targets

in the intact or assembling virion. For these reasons we
have investigated the properties and DNA organization of
in vitro spermidine-condensed DNA torus preparations treating
them as model systems for the condensed viral DNA genomes.

   In previous studies with a variety of DNAs we have shown
that the DNA tertiary structure transition that forms toruses
is reversible. Furthermore, it is sensitive to monovalent
and divalent ion competition in a manner suggesting that the
spermidine-DNA collapse interaction is largely electrostatic
(Marx and Reynolds 1983). Micrococcal nuclease is able to
digest the collapsed DNA structures producing an arithmetic
series of broad DNA bands upon gel electrophoresis. These
data have been rationalized by a regional micrococcal nuclease
cleavage model of DNA toruses organized by the continuous
circumferential winding of DNA (Marx and Reynolds 1982; Marx
and Reynolds 1983; Marx and Ruben 1984). The organization
of DNA toruses by circumferential DNA winding was confirmed
by our freeze-etch TEM (transmission electron microscopy)
studies of hydrated calf thymus DNA torus structure (Marx
and Ruben 1983) and the average measured torus circumference
which was found to be consistent with the micrococcal nuclease
monomer band size predicted by the cleavage model.

ΦX-174 dsDNA TORUS DIMENSIONS AND PACKAGING MODELS

   The freeze-etch preparation technique not only allows the
macromolecular specimen to remain hydrated and avoids any
possibility of surface forces disrupting the native macromolecular conformation but coupled with very low Pt-C metal
deposition during thin replica formation (60-80 Å thick) high
contrast of surface detail can be obtained (Marx and Ruben
1983; Marx and Ruben 1984 review; Ruben and Marx 1984). This
has prompted the present study using freeze-etch low Pt-C
metal (9 Å) replica TEM (Marx and Ruben 1983 experimental
details) to visualize torus shaped structures formed from
1 mM spermidine collapse of identical length (5386 bp) but
different topological state linear and nicked, circular
ΦX-174 RF II DNAs. One of the most accessible parameters of a
torus population is the circumference distribution since
toruses are invariably oriented nearly horizontal to the ice
in the freeze-etch experiment at the time of replica formation.
Therefore, both inner and outer circumference distributions
of toruses formed from 5386 bp nicked, circular and linear
(Figure 1) ΦX-174 RF II DNA were measured. Within each group

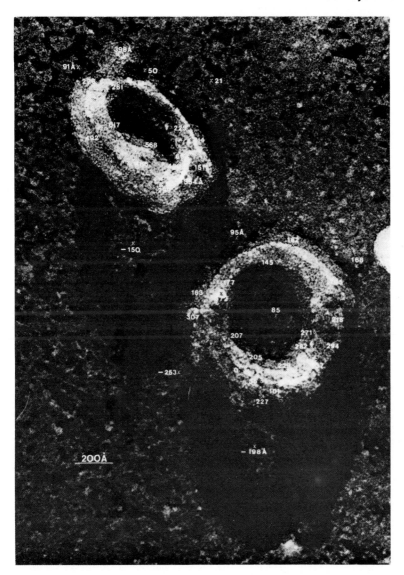

Fig. 1   Topography of two spermidine-condensed linear
φX-174 RF II DNA toruses.   The sterometer height measurements
were made on the stereomicrograph tilts in Fig. 3 panels a and
b.

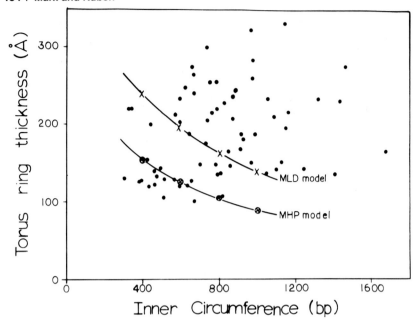

Fig. 2 Annulus measurement distribution vs. inner circumference (expressed as base pairs circumferentially wrapped B DNA) of 1 mM spermidine-condensed nicked, circular φX-174 RF II DNA toruses (n=63) from deep-etched replica TEM.

of toruses there is a highly significant correlation (0.94) between individual torus inner and outer circumference values (data not shown). The circular DNA population has a far more dispersed, almost polymodal distribution of torus circumferences than does the linear DNA torus population. This difference may be a consequence of the circular molecules' topological end constraint affecting the condensation mechanism or pathway.

Of great interest is another accessible parameter of a torus population—annulus (ring) thickness. We have tabulated this parameter for populations of both nicked, circular (n=63) in Figure 2 and linear (n=40) φX-174 toruses (data not shown). In both cases, there appears to be a compact grouping of toruses possessing smaller dimensions separated from a dispersed population possessing considerably larger dimensions. We surmised that the more compact torus population represented monomer DNA (5386 bp) packaging, whereas the larger

objects were packaging more than one DNA molecule (multimer).
Consistent with this interpretation are light scattering
measurements (Widom and Baldwin 1980; Post and Zimm 1982)
that demonstrate DNA aggregation under DNA collapse conditions
similar to ours. To develop a model that could account for
the distribution data and help us decide whether a monomer/
multimer explanation was justified we turned to a disk-shaped
torus organized by circumferential DNA winding. By extensive
tilting of replicas along the shadow direction we have been
able to directly view toruses on edge (Figures 3 and 4).
In all cases, toruses are flat disk-shaped objects rather
than being cylindrical shaped. Therefore, we calculated the
torus dimensions of monomer DNA (5386 bp B geometry: 29 Å
center-to-center helix spacing) packaged by a minimum
hexagonal packing model MHP:

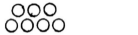

and a monomer limiting disk model MLD:

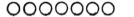 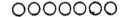

both shown here in cross-section perpendicular to the torus
annulus plane. The MHP model describes the monomer group of
torus measurements quite well (see Figure 2) and under these
solution conditions is greatly preferred energetically over
the extreme MLD model since the extent of helix-helix contact
is far greater. Therefore, these data and model studies
indicate that monomer DNA toruses can be discriminated from
multimers on the basis of simple annulus projection measurements and suggest that toruses are thin, disk-shaped objects
that closely resemble the MHP model of DNA organization.
This discrimination of monomer DNA disk-shaped toruses
allows us to reinterpret the circumference distribution data
above to identify a unimodal monomer population whose
dimensions are consistent with our published biochemical
study (Marx and Reynolds 1982).

STEREOMICROSCOPY REVEALS DNA TOPOLOGY IN TORUSES

   To help understand the 3-D microscopic details of DNA
writhe we have analyzed high-magnification stereomicrographs
of a few DNA toruses. Using a mirror stereoscope with
"floating" mark stereometer relative 3-D heights of surface

Table 1. Calculated Height Maximum Errors (95%) For Upper
Left Figure 1 Torus

H (Å)	N	*dH (Å)
458	10	13.2
354	11	10.5
568	13	29.6
486	11	10.4

*Calculated from the total differential of the parallax equation.

DNA double helices were mapped from paired stereomicrographs
of calf thymus DNA toruses (Marx and Ruben 1983; Marx and
Ruben 1984) and nicked, circular (data not shown) as well as
linear (Figure 1) φX-174 RF II DNA toruses. While largely
circumferential in orientation these DNA surface strands
reveal in most cases an irregular path that suggests a less
than crystalline hexagonal DNA packing and a non-unique DNA
collapse pathway. We have demonstrated that the measured
heights in Figure 1 are known with high precision (Ruben and
Marx 1984). In Table 1 two pairs of height values measured
from the upper left torus in Figure 1 are presented along
with their calculated 95% fractile errors. This degree of
precision is dependent upon error minimization by: making
a sufficient number of measurements (N) of each height point
(H), selection of the optimal reference point height (0 Å),
proper alignment of the stereomicrograph tilt axis preceding
measurement, careful printing of stereomicrographs to preserve
depth cue detail and calibration of the microscope so that
tilt error can be minimized (Ruben and Marx 1984). We feel
that individual height measurements accurate to 2-3% and
precisions of 5 Å are attainable.

As an independent assay of the relative accuracy of
stereometer height measurements we performed extensive
tilting (through 50-90°) of toruses along the metal shadow
direction axis (Figure 3). When the edge of the torus plane
is at an angle less than 75° to the shadow direction the
torus view tilted end-on (Figure 3f) can directly reveal the
vertical annulus thickness corroborating the less direct
Table 1 stereographic pair measurements. In Figure 4 the

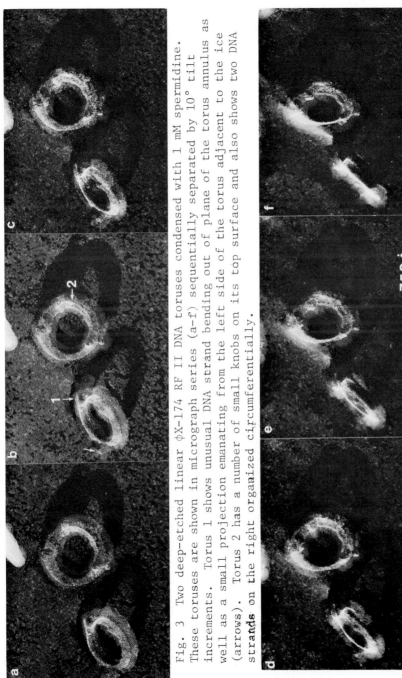

Fig. 3 Two deep-etched linear φX-174 RF II DNA toruses condensed with 1 mM spermidine. These toruses are shown in micrograph series (a–f) sequentially separated by 10° tilt increments. Torus 1 shows unusual DNA strand bending out of plane of the torus annulus as well as a small projection emanating from the left side of the torus adjacent to the ice (arrows). Torus 2 has a number of small knobs on its top surface and also shows two DNA strands on the right organized circumferentially.

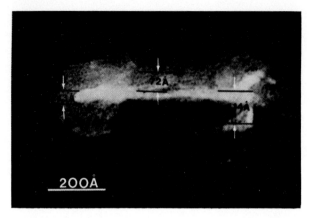

Fig. 4   The spermidine-condensed linear φX-174 DNA torus in
the upper left of Fig. 1 is tilted vertically so that it can
be viewed end-on (also Fig. 3f).   Features measured directly
as 72 Å and 114 Å correspond to the paired points in Table 1
and labelled positions in Fig. 1.

directly measured 72 Å and 114 Å torus surface point spacings
correspond to the real distances between the Table 1 paired
height points.   These have been calculated to be, respectively,
89 Å for the 568 Å, 486 Å points and 114 Å for the 458 Å,
354 Å points (see Ruben and Marx 1984), in good agreement
with the direct measurements.   The simple differences between
paired torus surface point heights in Table 1 do not correspond
to the directly measured Figure 4 spacings.   Besides
corroborating the stereometer measurements a tilt series has
the advantage of yielding more direct information on the
writhe of individual DNA strands and end-on views of a number
of toruses confirms our idea that DNA toruses on the average
possess disk-like shapes as embodied in the MHP model of
calculated monomer torus dimensions.

CONCLUSIONS

   Low Pt-C metal shadow freeze-etch TEM studies of
spermidine-condensed φX-174 RF II DNA toruses provide
additional direct evidence for the organization of these
structures by the continuous circumferential winding of DNA
(Marx and Reynolds 1982; Marx and Reynolds 1983; Marx and
Ruben 1983; Marx and Ruben 1984).   Circumference and annulus

thickness measurements of torus populations reveal two size classes. These are most easily explained as being comprised either of a single collapsed DNA molecule (monomer) or more than one collapsed DNA molecule (multimer). A minimum hexagonal packing (MHP) model for a torus organized from a single DNA molecule produces calculated dimensions that agree with the smaller measured dimension class of torus structures. That this class of toruses represents DNA monomer structures is further supported by stereomicroscopy of individual toruses where the specimen replica is tilted through large angles. Direct end-on views of putative monomer toruses confirm that these structures are basically disk-shaped and in fundamental agreement with the MHP model.

Careful stereometer measurements from paired stereomicrographs of toruses allows the 3-D mapping of individual DNA double helices in the condensed structures. Height measurements can be obtained with high precision, a 95% fractile error of 5-10 Å (Ruben and Marx 1984) and the heights are corroborated by direct measurement from end-on torus tilt views. The stereometer measurements reveal a less than crystalline hexagonal DNA packing of surface DNA strands suggesting microscopic variability in the organization of circumferentially wound DNA in individual toruses. Recent experiments on mapping nearest-neighbor DNA segments and DNA-capsid head contacts in bacteriophage λ have reached a somewhat similar conclusion (Widom & Baldwin 1983; Haas et. al. 1982). The low Pt-C metal, freeze-etch TEM techniques applied successfully here to the spermidine-DNA torus in vitro viral DNA model system suggest themselves as valuable tools in investigating the internal organization of DNA in dsDNA bacteriophage or viral pathogens gently and partially lysed under DNA collapse conditions.

K.A.M. acknowledges CA 23108 NCI, DHEW; NIH GM 25886 and AI 17586, DHEW; Research Corp. 8859 and BRSG 05392 DHEW. G.C.R. acknowledges CA 23108 NCI, DHEW.

Ames, B.N., Dubin, D.T. and Rosenthal, S.M. (1958) Polyamines in certain Bacterial Viruses. Science. 127:814.
Chattoraj, D.K., Gosule, L.C. and Schellman, J.A. (1978) DNA Condensation with Polyamines II. Electron Microscopic Studies. J. Mol. Biol. 121:327.
Furlong, D., Swift, H. and Roizman, B. (1972) Arrangement of Herpesvirus DNA in the core. J. of Virology. 10:1071.
Gerhard, B. and Warren, R.A.J. (1982) Reactivity of the

α-Putrescinylthymine Amino Groups in φW-14 DNA. Biochemistry. 21:5458.

Haas, R., Murphy, R.F. and Cantor, C.R. (1982) Testing Models of the Arrangement of DNA Inside Bacteriophage λ by Crosslinking the packaged DNA. J. Mol. Biol. 159:71.

Klimenko, S.M., Tikchonenko, T.I. and Andreev, V.M. (1967) Packing of DNA in Phage T2. J. Mol. Biol. 23:523.

Marx, K.A. and Reynolds, T.C.(1982) Spermidine-condensed φX-174 DNA Cleavage by Nuclease: Torus Cleavage Model and Evidence for Unidirectional Circumferential DNA Wrapping. Proc. Nat'l. Acad. Sci. USA. 79:6484.

Marx, K.A. and Reynolds, T.C. (1983) Ion Competition and Micrococcal Nuclease Digestion Studies of Spermidine-Condensed Calf Thymus DNA: Evidence for Torus Organization by Circumferential DNA Wrapping. Biochim. Biophys. Acta. 741:279.

Marx, K.A. and Ruben, G.C. (1983) Evidence for Hydrated Spermidine-Calf Thymus DNA Toruses Organized by Circumferential DNA Wrapping. Nuc. Acids Res. 11:1839.

Marx, K.A. and Ruben, G.C. (1984) Studies of DNA Organization in Hydrated Spermidine-Condensed DNA Toruses and Spermidine-DNA Fibres. J. Biomolecular Structure and Dynamics. I, No. 5:1109.

McDougall, J.K., Galloway, D.A. and Fenoglio, C.M. (1981) Footprints of Herpes Simplex Virus in Transformed Cells and in Cervical Carcinoma. in Nahmias et. al. (eds.): "The Human Herpesviruses". New York:Elsevier, p. 245.

Miller, G. (1981) Oncogenesis by Epstein-Barr Virus. in Nahmias et. al. (eds.): "The Human Herpesviruses". New York: Elsevier, p. 229.

Post, C.B. and Zimm, B.H. (1982) Light-Scattering Study of DNA Condensation:Competition Between Collapse and Aggregation. Biopolymers. 21:2139.

Richards, K.E., Williams, P.C. and Calendar, R. (1973) DNA Packing in Bacteriophage Heads. J. Mol. Biol. 78:255.

Ruben, G.C. and Marx, K.A. (1984) Parallax Measurements on Stereomicrographs of Hydrated Single Molecules, Their Accuracy and Precision at High Magnification. J. Electron Microscopy Technique. 1, No. 4: in press.

Widom, J. and Baldwin, R.L. (1980) Cation-induced Toroidal Condensation of DNA. J. Mol. Biol. 144:431.

Widom, J. and Baldwin, R.L. (1983) Tests of Spool Models for DNA Packaging in Phage Lambda. J. Mol. Biol. 171:419.

II. STRUCTURE AND REACTIVITY OF CARCINOGENS AND DNA LESIONS

**Molecular Basis of Cancer, Part A: Macromolecular
Structure, Carcinogens, and Oncogenes, pages 143–152**

STRUCTURES OF DNA CONTAINING PSORALEN CROSSLINK AND   THYMINE
DIMER

Sung-Hou Kim, David A. Pearlman, Stephen R. Holbrook*
and David Pirkle

Department of Chemistry and
*Lawrence Berkeley Laboratory
University of California
Berkeley, California 94720

UV irradiation by itself or in conjunction with other
chemicals can cause covalent damages to DNA in living cells.
To overcome the detrimental effect of DNA damage, cells
developed a repair mechanism by which damaged DNA is
repaired. In the absence of such repair, cell malfunction
or cell death can occur.

Two most studied radiation-induced DNA damage are thymine dimer formation by UV irradiation and psoralen
crosslink by combination of psoralens and UV: In the former,
two adjacent thymine bases on a strand of DNA are fused by
forming cyclobutane ring, and in the latter, one pyrimidine
on one DNA strand is crosslinked to another pyrimidine on
the other strand via a psoralen. Our objective is to deduce
the structure of DNA segment which contains a psoralen
crosslink or a thymine dimer using the combination of
results of X-ray crystallographic studies, molecular model
building, and energy minimization. These structural
features may be important for understanding the biological
effects of such damages and for the recognition by the
repair enzymes.

METHOD

Our strategy was to start with x-ray crystallographic
results of the lesion and build DNA duplexes on both sides
of the lesion, then search for the structures that have low
energy by energy-minimization methods.

The form of the energy function used is:

$$E_{total} = \sum K_r(R-Ro)^2 + \sum K_\theta(\theta-\theta_0)^2 + \sum \frac{V_n}{2}[1-\cos(n\phi-\gamma)]$$

$$+ \sum_{i<j} [\frac{A_{ij}}{R_{ij}^{12}} - \frac{B_{ij}}{R_{ij}^6} + \frac{q_i q_j}{\epsilon R_{ij}}] + \sum [\frac{C_{ij}}{R_{ij}^{12}} - \frac{D_{ij}}{R_{ij}^{10}}]$$

where the summations are for all chemical bonds, bond angles, dihedral angles, non-bonded atom pairs and hydrogen bonds respectively. The standard parameters used in it are from Weiner et al. (1984), and those additional parameters necessary for the cyclobutane ring are from Rao et al. (1984). A dielectric constant of r was used, and non-bonded interactions between atoms separated by three bonds were scaled by a factor of 0.5 (Weiner et al., 1984). No partial charges were included for the psoralen molecule, and the psoralen was held to its crystallographic conformation (Peckler et al., 1982). by internal constraints of weight 2000.0 in all minimizations, All energy minimizations were carried out using the AMBER program (Weiner and Kollman, 1981) until either the root mean square gradient of energy with respect to atomic position was less than 0.1 kcal/mole-A, or both the rms change in position and the rms change in energy between two cycles of minimization were less than 10^{-8}. In no case was the rms gradient at the end of minimization greater than 0.25 kcal/mole-A.

For the initial stages of minimization, emphasis was placed on closing the long gaps between the two DNA strands on both sides of the lesion while maintaining reasonable distance and angle geometry throughout of the molecule. This was done using a series of minimizations in which the distance and valence angle terms in the potential energy function were heavily weighted. This, in essence, made torsion angles the only structural variable. While keeping the conformation of the lesion constrained to the respective crystal structures, each model was then energy-minimized in a series of steps in which the weight for angles and distances was lowered in the succession 100. --> 10 --> 5 --> 1. The structure was allowed to settle at each step before continuing. This gradual lowering of the angle and distance weights was done in order to allow strains of heavily weighted initial structure to be smoothly dissipated into the more relaxed structures. When refinement with unit weighting for the bond and angle terms was finished, the constraints on the geometries of the psoralen crosslink or thymine dimer were removed, and each structure was energy-minimized once more. For comparison purposes, a canonical B-DNA helix (Arnott and Hukins, 1972) of the same sequence without the lesion was also energy-minimized.

At this point, two more base pairs of regular B-form DNA were best fit to each end of all the models. The resulting 10-mer structures were then energy-minimized as described above.

RESULTS

As can be seen in Fig. 1, the resulting psoralen cross-linked structure and thymine dimer containing DNA structure are severely kinked compared to the energy minimized B-DNA. A comparison of torsion angles (Table 1) shows that major conformational changes in the psoralen structure relative to the energy-minimized B-form are primarily restricted to the psoralen-crosslinked thymine and subsequent two residues on the 3' end of the thymine nucleotide in each strand. This contrasts significantly to the bidirectional (both to 3' and 5' ends in both strands) distribution of conformational changes observed for the thymine dimer structure.

It is apparent, in the psoralen-DNA figure, that beside the crosslink itself, the major distortion occurs at the base pair between the crosslinked thymines and their complementary adenines: the base-pair plane of each of two central base pairs of the psoralen-DNA structure are bent by $10-19^{o}$ compared to near planar base-pairs of the energy-minimized B-form.

OVERALL HELIX DEFORMATIONS CAUSED BY PSORALEN CROSS-LINK

Our model shows that the psoralen cross-link causes very large changes, relative to the energy-minimized B form, in the calculated structural parameters (see Table 2). The kink angle for the psoralen structure is 46.5^{o}. The size of the kink is nearly the same as the angle between the two

RESIDUE		ζ	α	β	γ	δ	ε	X
1	PSORL	0.00	0.00	0.00	66.70	142.40	180.20	66.30
	B-DNA	0.00	0.00	0.00	67.30	144.10	182.90	72.00
2		258.10	291.90	178.90	58.20	132.70	178.60	55.40
		268.30	287.60	173.20	58.70	137.00	183.20	64.20
3		253.70	298.20	178.60	59.50	139.20	182.30	57.50
		231.80	298.70	173.70	61.60	143.20	183.50	56.30
4		242.80	298.00	163.90	71.90	151.30	209.40	46.20
		261.00	288.40	179.20	57.40	130.70	181.80	58.40
5		291.30	313.00	184.40	297.70	78.10	183.50	112.20
		257.90	292.70	176.70	58.60	139.80	190.00	62.60
6		266.70	183.50	176.20	185.50	152.80	174.50	74.10
		225.10	297.40	173.80	56.20	144.00	185.10	60.30
7		273.30	168.20	175.90	166.60	143.50	201.00	58.60
		266.60	288.90	176.40	56.40	141.60	197.30	68.10
8		206.80	302.90	162.60	54.10	147.30	185.70	51.30
		207.90	298.50	165.50	54.90	149.10	184.10	54.90
9		265.00	287.30	182.00	55.50	134.20	180.00	57.80
		268.70	286.10	183.70	58.20	146.40	186.50	68.40
10		0.00	296.20	178.10	57.30	148.30	0.00	61.80
		0.00	293.20	174.00	58.10	158.70	0.00	61.80
11		251.10	0.00	0.00	67.40	143.00	179.90	65.50
		235.20	0.00	0.00	67.30	144.10	182.90	71.90
12		256.70	292.70	179.50	58.90	134.90	182.90	55.20
		268.30	287.60	173.20	58.70	137.00	183.60	64.20
13		253.40	294.50	176.30	59.90	126.80	174.80	57.00
		231.60	298.70	173.70	61.60	143.20	183.50	56.30
14		260.40	295.10	157.20	83.30	151.00	211.00	42.60
		261.00	288.40	179.10	57.40	130.70	181.00	58.40
15		294.80	317.60	173.50	304.30	84.10	187.50	135.10
		257.90	292.70	176.70	58.60	139.80	190.00	62.60
16		293.00	177.20	188.20	178.00	84.90	172.30	48.70
		225.10	297.40	173.80	56.20	144.00	185.10	60.30
17		286.20	158.80	193.60	177.60	77.60	179.80	25.60
		266.60	288.90	176.40	56.40	141.60	197.30	68.10
18		285.70	303.80	175.50	61.80	143.60	184.10	55.30
		207.90	298.50	165.50	54.90	149.10	184.10	54.90
19		256.90	291.10	183.30	55.80	138.60	181.00	58.90
		268.70	286.10	183.70	58.20	146.40	186.50	68.40
20		258.10	296.20	177.40	57.40	148.10	0.00	61.10
		235.20	293.20	174.00	58.10	158.70	0.00	61.80

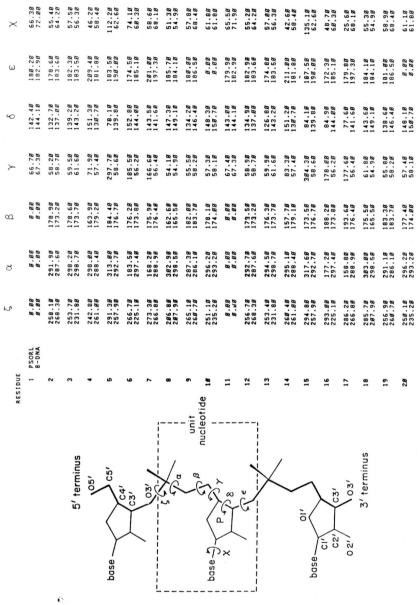

Table 1. Torsion angles in psoralen–DNA model. Residues 1 and 11 are 5' terminal residues. For each residue the top row is for psoralen-DNA model and the bottom row for energy-minimized B-DNA.

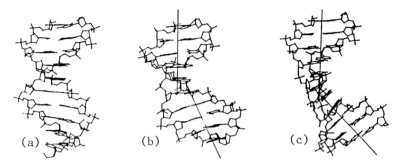

Figure 1. Structural models of (a) energy-minimized B-DNA, (b) thymine-dimer containing DNA, and (c) psoralen cross-linked DNA.

Table 2. Structural Parameters of Radiation-Damaged DNA.

	Psoralen-DNA	Thymine dimer-DNA
Unwinding angle	87.7°	19.7°
Kink angle	46.5°	27.0°
Displacement	3.5°	2.7 Å

crosslinked thymine bases (44.4°). The total unwinding angle covering the ten base-pairs in the model is 88.0° compared to the energy-minimized B form structure. A very large portion of this unwinding occurs at the cross-link site, where, due to the physical constraints of the thymine-psoralen-thymine crosslink, this structure is wound by 13.4° in a left handed sense, versus a 45.1° right handed step for the energy-minimized B form, i.e., unwinding of 58.5° at the lesion and rapid return to the values similar to those of the energy-minimized B-DNA (see Fig. 2a). The psoralen crosslink also causes two helices to be non-contiguous and displaced by 3.49 A.

OVERALL HELIX DEFORMATIONS CAUSED BY THYMINE DIMER

As can be seen in Figure 1, DNA containing a thymine dimer has a kink of about 30°. Table 1 lists the structural parameters describing the deformation caused by thymine dimer. The individual step turn angles (Fig. 2b) indicate that the unwinding caused by the dimer at the dimer site is

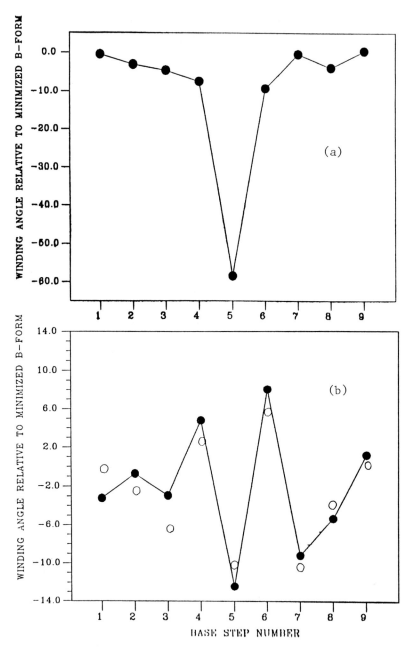

Figure 2. Step-by-step unwinding/winding angles in (a) psoralen crosslinked DNA and (b) thymine-dimer containing DNA with respect to the energy-minimized B-DNA (open circle for constrained model).

compensated for by overwinding at the adjacent base steps of about 1/2 the magnitude of the dimer step unwinding. The pattern of unwinding/winding here is quite different from that of the psoralen-DNA model.

Displacement distance for the helical axes is 2.66 A. It should be cautioned that the displacement parameters are extremely sensitive to the procedure used to obtain the helical axes: as the helices are not regular and the axes are only determined by the last two base pairs, one should be careful in interpreting these values.

DISCUSSION

It appears, from this work, that the introduction of a psoralen cross-link or thymine dimer in DNA brings about large conformational changes in the DNA helix (see Fig. 3) although precise magnitudes of such deformation may be subject to change depending on the limitations of the energy-minimization technique and uncertainties associated with parameters for the energy function used. Furthermore, it is well known that such techniques are not efficient at discovering energy minima far removed from the starting structure, and the likelihood of energy-minimization resulting in a conformation significantly removed from the starting model decreases as the complexity of the molecule being energy-minimized increases.

It is interesting that our thymine dimer-DNA structure is so grossly different overall from those of Rao et al (1984) who has recently attacked the problem of thymine dimer model building using the same energy force field. One probable reason for this lies in the method chosen for creating the starting model. We chose to fit separate 3 base pair helical segments onto both ends of a crystallographically determined thymine dimer and then minimize the resulting hexamer first, before extending it to a decamer. The length of hexamer was chosen as a DNA fragment probably long enough to accommodate all the significant local conformational changes due to the DNA damages while short enough that the energy-minimization method could indeed propagate them rather than get stuck in an unrealistic local minimum very close to the starting structure. Rao et al., on the other hand, started with a 12 base pair B-DNA helix and then attempted to use internal constraints to force the formation

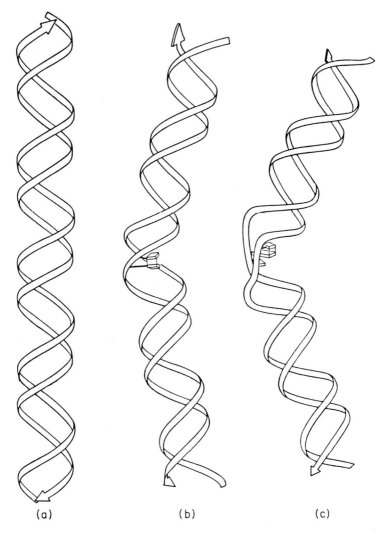

Figure 3. Schematic drawing of (a) B-DNA, (b) thymine dimer contraining DNA, and (c) psoralen crosslinked DNA.

of a dimer. As noted before, the minimization techniques available for such attempts suffer from an inability to force major tertiary structural changes. Thus, it was likely that since we started with a kinked and unwound structure, our final structure would contain some form of

kink and unwinding, and that Rao et al, whose initial structure was neither kinked nor unwound, would not realize a
kink or unwinding in their final structure. An experimental
result (see below) however is consistent with our model,
which predicts topological unwinding, but inconsistent with
the model of Rao et al. (1984), which predicts no topological unwinding.

At the present time, there is no experimental method to
directly determine type of structural distortion we derived
here. Experimental methods such as the band pattern shift
method of circular DNA was used to measure topological
unwinding angle due to psoralen adducts (-28°) (Weisehan and
Hearst, 1978) and thymine dimer (-14°) (Ciarrocchi and
Pedrini), but it is difficult to separate the effect of
duplex unwinding/winding from negative/positive supercoiling
due to successive kinking. Furthermore, in case of psoralen
adducts it is difficult to determine the proportion of
monoadducts and cross-links and respective structural
changes induced by them.

In summary these experiments and our results clearly
indicate the presence of distortion of DNA structure due to
these lesions. Such distortion may be important in understanding biological effects of these lesions and for repair
enzymes to recognize them.

The atomic coordinates of all three models are available on request to S.H.K.

ACKNOWLEDGEMENT

We are grateful to Prof. Peter Kollman at the University of California in San Francisco for the program AMBER,
their preprint on thymine dimer-DNA, and valuable consulta-
tion throughout this work. This work has been supported by
grants from NIH (GM31616, GM29287), NSF (PCM8019468), and
the Department of Energy.

REFERENCES

Arnott S, Hukins DWL (1972). Biochem Biophys Res Comm 47:1504.

Camerman N, Camermann A (1970). J Am Chem Soc 92:2523.

Ciarrocchi G, Pedrini A (1982). J Mol Biol 155:177.

Peckler S, Graves B, Kanne D, Rapoport H, Hearst JE, Kim SH (1982) J Mol Biol 162:157.

Rao S, Keepers J, Kollman PA (1984). Nuc Acid Res (in press).

Weiner PK, Kollman PA (1981). J Comp Chem 2:287.

Weiner S, Kollman PA, Case D, Singh U, Ghio C, Alagona G, Profeta S Jr., Weiner P (1984) J Am Chem Soc 106:765

Weisehan G, Hearst JE (1978). Proc Nat Acad Sci 75:2703.

Molecular Basis of Cancer, Part A: Macromolecular
Structure, Carcinogens, and Oncogenes, pages 153–171
© 1985 Alan R. Liss, Inc.

Conformations of DNA Adducts with Polycyclic Aromatic
Carcinogens

Suse Broyde* and Brian Hingerty+

*Department of Biology NYU, NY, NY 10003 and
+Health and Safety Research Division,
Oak Ridge Natl. Lab., Oak Ridge, TN 37830

INTRODUCTION

While it has been understood for some time
that the initiation of cancer is a multi-step
process, the widespread appreciation that a
somatic mutation is a critical event has gained
firm scientific support. Indeed, it has been
demonstrated that a point mutation in the DNA of
a proto-oncogene can turn that gene into an
actively transforming molecule (Land et al.
1983). The next question that arises then is,
"what causes the mutation?". It has long been
suspected that chemical carcinogens that link
covalently to the DNA can initiate cancer by
causing a mutation. The mutagenicity of a
number of such chemicals in various test systems
has in fact been demonstrated. More dramatic,
however, is the recent finding that nitroso-
methylurea induced mammary cancer in female rats
is actually associated with a G to A point
mutation in an oncogene (Sukumar et al. 1983).

Given the likelihood that a chemical
carcinogen initiates cancer via a mutation, we
would like to understand how such mutations are
produced. A number of steps take place
following the entry of a chemical into a cell,
which determine whether or not that substance is
mutagenic. These include various pathways of
metabolic activation or detoxification, the

reactions of the metabolites with DNA, and the interaction of each of the adducts that are formed with the replication apparatus and various repair systems (error-prone or error-free). The response of the replicative and repair enzymes to each damaging event in DNA is a critical factor in mutagenesis and cell trans-formation, one which is governed, we believe, by the local conformation of the modified DNA.

A particular carcinogen may form a number of adducts with DNA, only one of which may be the critical transforming moiety. We are interested in learning whether a unique conformation distinguishes mutagenic and carcinogenic lesions from benign ones. Accordingly, our attention has been centered on the influence of covalently linked polycyclic aromatic amines and hydrocarbons on DNA con-formation. Because of the difficulty associated with synthesizing and crystallizing carcinogen-DNA adducts, it has been, as yet, impossible to obtain experimental atomic resolution views of such structures above the nucleoside level. Surprisingly, to our knowledge there is only one carcinogen-nucleoside structure with intact base in the literature to date (Carrell et al. 1981). Therefore, the theoretical delineation of conformation is of particular importance, since it is the only one currently able to generate a molecular view.

We employ minimized semi-empirical potential energy calculations, with all torsion angles flexible, to obtain an energy ranked list of feasible conformers. The potentials employed are those devised by Olson and Srinivasan (1980, 1983), and their application to these studies has been described (Hingerty, Broyde 1982). A large number of trial starting conformations, ranging from 500 to 4,000 in our most recent work, are employed, yielding a satisfactory survey of conformation space for the modified deoxydinucleoside monophosphate we have been investigating. In particular, we have been studying the dCpdG sequence. This sequence is a mutational hotspot and a high reactivity locus for carcinogens of interest (Fuchs et al. 1981; Mizusawa et al. 1981; Yoon et al. 1982; Winkle et al. 1983; Fuchs, 1984). We have been investigating adducts with the aromatic amines acetylaminofluorene (AAF) and 4-aminobiphenyl (ABP), as well as the aromatic hydrocarbon benzo [a] pyrene-7,8-diol-9,10-epoxide (BP)(Figure 1).

AAF was an appropriate choice for an initial theoretical investigation because many solution studies of AAF modified DNA and DNA subunits have been carried out over the years. In vitro AAF is linked primarily to the C-8 of guanine (Kriek et al. 1967), while a minor adduct forms with guanine N^2 (Kriek 1972). In vivo, the majority of C-8 adducts are deacetylated (AF) (Kriek 1969; Irving, Veazey 1969). The solution studies indicate that AAF-modified DNA of random sequence adopts a conformation known as base-displacement (Grunberger et al.) or insertion-denaturation (Fuchs, Daune 1972), in which the carcinogen is stacked with the adjacent base and the guanine is syn. However, conformational details of the DNA backbone that define carcinogen-base stacking were not known. More recent solution studies also indicate that AAF induces a transition to the Z form in modified poly (dG-dC).poly(dG-dC) (Sage, Leng 1980; Santella et al. 1981), again without conformational details. These results apply to the guanine C-8 linked major adduct. Nothing is known about the conformation of the N^2 linked minor adduct, other than that it causes little denaturation (Yamasaki et al. 1977).

RESULTS AND DISCUSSION

Our calculations for dCpdG modified with AAF at guanine C-8 reveal base displacement as the energetically preferred state (Hingerty, Broyde 1982; Broyde, Hingerty 1983). Moreover, a large number of different DNA backbone conformations can produce carcinogen-base stacking. The two most important conformers are

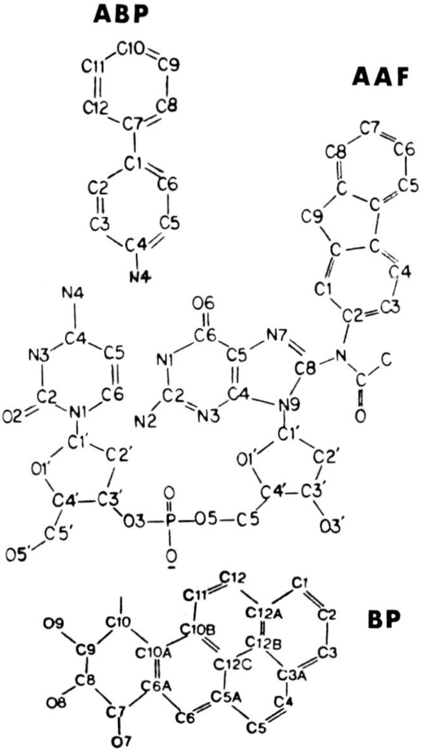

Figure 1. Structure of the AAF adduct with guanine C-8 of dCpdG. The AF adduct has hydrogen in place of acetyl. AAF also links to guanine N^2 via C-3. ABP links to guanine C-8 via its amino group. BP links to guanine N^2 via its C-10.

shown in Figure 2. One is a distorted B form and the other a distorted Z form. In all the carcinogen-base stacked conformations the guanine is syn, as previously suggested from model building (Grunberger et al. 1970), and the backbone torsions are altered from those found in standard helices. Incorporation of these states into the B form found in solutions of random sequence DNA leads to the kinking and denaturation that solution studies had suggested (Fuchs, Daune 1974).

Our calculations also located local minimum energy conformations that are similar in all details to the dCpdG residue of Z-DNAs (Wang et al. 1981) (Figure 3). These conformers can readily be incorporated into the Z helix, placing the carcinogen in a flexible position external to the helix without distortion. In addition, we have recently constructed a base displaced Z-DNA model, with the carcinogen inserted into the helix, using the distorted Z type conformer shown in Figure 2b incorporated into Z_{II}-DNA (Broyde, Hingerty 1984). Only the base pair at the modification site is ruptured in this model. Experimental results indicate little helix denaturation in AAF modified Z-DNA (Santella et al. 1981). Two types of AAF modified Z DNA have, in fact, recently been observed in immunogenic studies (Hanau et al. 1984). We suggest that these may be represented by the external and the inserted AAF conformations.

In the case of the C-8 AAF adduct, no minimum energy conformations were computed that are like the A or B helix in every respect. By contrast, our results for the deacetylated AF adduct present a different picture (Broyde, Hingerty 1983). In this adduct unperturbed A and B type conformers with guanine anti were computed among the lowest energy states (Figure 4a), together with low energy syn conformers like those found for the acetylated AAF adduct. Solution studies have also suggested an important guanine anti component for the AF

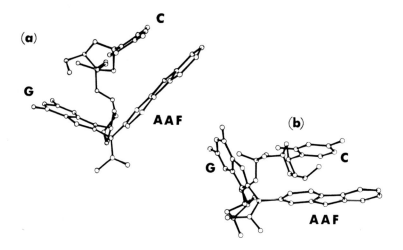

Figure 2. Base displaced conformations of C-8 AAF adduct. (a) is a distorted B form and (b) is a perturbed Z form. The guanines are syn.

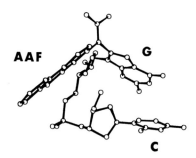

Figure 3. C-8 AAF adduct in Z-DNA conformation of dCpdG.

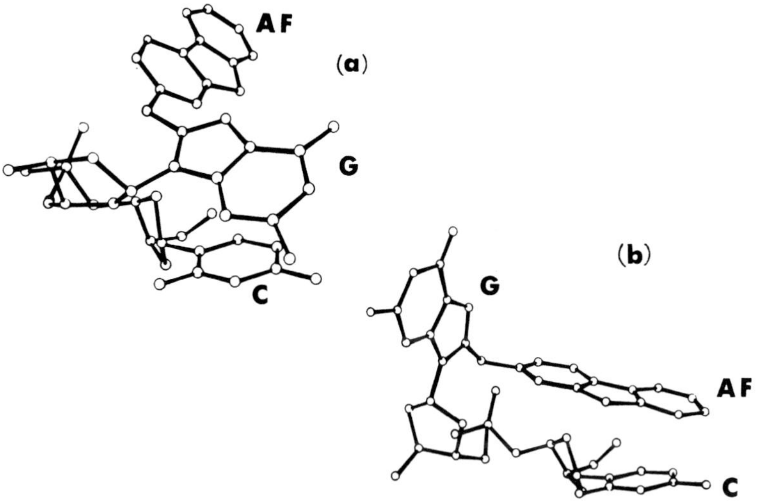

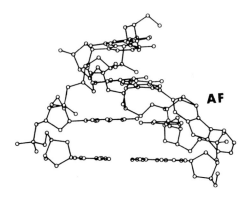

Figure 4. AF adduct to guanine C-8. (a) is a B-DNA like conformer. (b) is a perturbed B form. The guanines are anti.

Figure 5. AF modified B-DNA.

adduct (Evans et al. 1980; Leng et al. 1980; Santella et al. 1980), as have force field calculations for the nucleoside adduct (Lipkowitz et al. 1982). The computed guanine anti conformers simply place the carcinogen at the B helix exterior in the major groove when incorporated in the larger polymer (Figure 5). Furthermore, a second type of guanine anti low energy conformation was computed which had carcinogen-base stacking (Figure 4b). Interestingly, this newly discovered guanine anti base displaced state differs from the normal A or B helix only in the C5'-O5' torsion, which is rotated about 40 degrees from its usual trans orientation towards gauche minus. This simple movement has the effect of inserting the carcinogen so that it is stacked with the adjacent base in one direction, causing a kink in the helix axis, but no denaturation.

4-Aminobiphenyl also forms a predominant adduct with guanine C-8 (Beland et al. 1983). It chemically resembles the aminofluorene adduct except for the added degree of flexibility at the torsion linking the two phenyl rings. However, no information has been previously available about the conformational effect of this carcinogen. Our calculations for the dCpdG-ABP adduct reveal an overall similarity with the AF adduct: a pair of low energy A or B-like guanine anti conformers, one type with base-base stacking and a second with carcinogen-base stacking, in addition to the syn guanine carcinogen-base stacked forms (Figure 6). Carcinogen-base stacking is somewhat less than in the AF adduct because the phenyl rings are twisted relative to one another. The dCpdG-ABP adduct has recently been synthesized in the laboratories of Professors Shapiro and Underwood at New York University, as part of a collaborative experimental and theoretical undertaking. The nmr and CD data do indicate some carcinogen-base stacking, as evidenced by enhancement of the CD spectrum and upfield shifts in the cytidine proton resonances relative to unmodified dCpdG, similar to that

observed for the AF adduct, but less than for
AAF (Santella et al. 1980).

A second important site for covalent
modification of guanines by polycyclic aromatic
carcinogens is at the guanine amino group. A
minor AAF adduct is formed at this site (Kriek
1972). In addition, the (+) anti isomer of
benzo [a] pyrene-7,8-diol-9,10-epoxide (BP) binds
selectively to guanine N^2 (Conney 1982). It is
of interest to learn whether there are conformational features common to these two adducts,
as well as to the guanine C-8 adducts. The
calculations indicate a unique conformation for
the N^2-AAF adduct. (Hingerty, Broyde 1983).
Its most important state is Z-like (Figure 7).
However, the preferred Z-type conformer cannot
be fitted into a Z helix, because of steric
close contacts by the bulky acetyl group. It is
possible, however, to incorporate this conformer
at a B-Z junction with the carcinogen located in
the groove in the Z direction, and all base
pairs intact. A slight bend in the helix axis
is the only perturbation. This suggests that
AAF linked to the guanine amino group may induce
a B-Z junction at an appropriate sequence, or
that it will react preferentially at B-Z
junctions. A or B type helical conformations
with carcinogen-base or base-base stacking are
of considerably higher energy. Experimental
information on the conformation of this adduct,
other than that it causes little denaturation
(Yamasaki et al. 1977), is not available.
Models have been presented which show that the
carcinogen can reside in a B helix groove (Kriek
1974; Beland 1978; Kadlubar 1980). Other models
show that carcinogen-base stacking is possible
with modification at guanine N^2 (Drinkwater et
al. 1978; Frenkel et al. 1978; Hogan et al.
1981). These would be appropriate for random
sequence DNA, while the present model would
apply primarily to alternating dC-dG regions.

By contrast, the (+) anti BP adduct with
dCpdG does not favor this Z conformation
(Hingerty, Broyde 1983). The longer, puckered

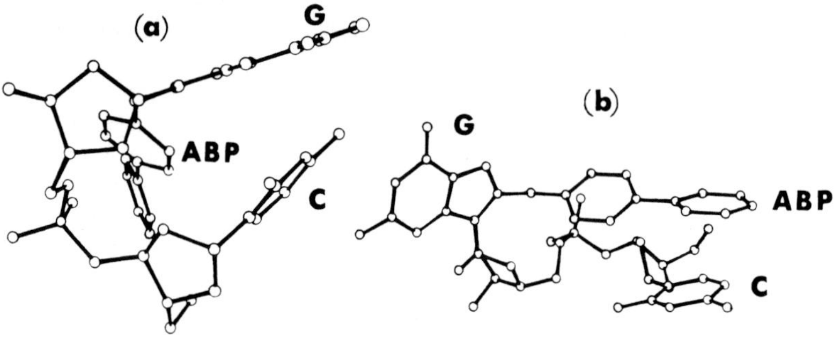

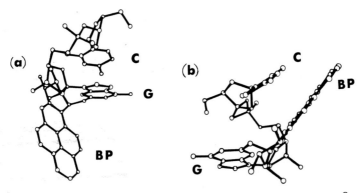

Figure 6. ABP adduct to guanine C-8. (a) is a B-DNA type conformer. (b) is a perturbed B form. The guanines are anti.

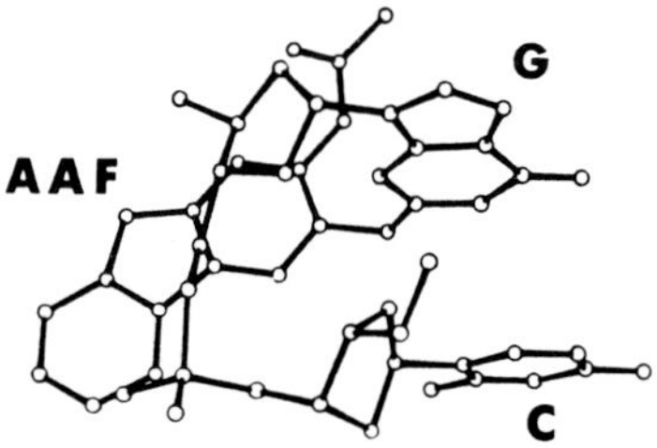

Figure 7. AAF adduct to guanine N^2. The DNA conformation is like the dCpdG residue of Z-DNA.

Figure 8. (+) anti BP adduct to guanine N^2. (a) is a B-DNA type conformer. (b) is a perturbed B form. The guanines are anti.

benzo[a]pyrene moiety does not fit readily into
the shallow Z groove. Instead, the most
important states are the A or B like carcinogen-
base stacked conformations (Figure 8b); this is
consistent with CD data on dinucleoside
monophosphates modified with (+) anti BP that
indicate carcinogen-base stacking (Frenkel et
al. 1978). Close in energy are forms of largely
similar backbone conformational characteristics
which place the carcinogen at the helix exterior
(Figure 8a). To interconvert the external form
to the carcinogen-base stacked conformation
requires only rotation of the guanine glycosidic
torsion from anti to high anti and rotation of
the C3' -O3' torsion from trans towards gauche
minus. Model building reveals that these two
states are readily interconvertible on the
polymer level as well. The inserted form is
kinked, but not seriously denatured, with
carcinogen-base stacking in one direction. The
two states may well be reversed in energy in
larger structures, in view of their closeness in
the deoxydinucleoside monophosphate (about 2
kcal./mole energy difference).

The biological properties of the adducts we
have studied have been investigated to some
extent. The AAF adducts are mutagenic, but the
mutagenicity of the C-8 adduct has not been
distinguished from that of the minor N^2 linked
constituent (Fuchs et al. 1983). However, it
has been established that the C-8 adduct is
primarily repaired (Kriek 1974) while the N^2
adduct is primarily persistent (Kriek et al.
1974; Howard et al. 1981). In vivo, the
majority of C-8 adducts are present as the
deacetylated AF. These AF adducts are largely
persistent in mammalian systems (Beland et al.
1982; Poirier et al. 1982), they are mutagenic
in the Salmonella assay and the number of
adducts correlates linearly with the number of
mutations (Beranek et al. 1982). The same is
true of the C-8 ABP adducts, although their
mutagenicity is less (Beland et al. 1983). The
(+) anti BP adduct to N^2 of guanine has actually
been identified as the tumorigenic lesion in

mammalian systems, it is the major BP adduct
(Conney 1982) and it is also persistant in some
mammalian systems (Kulkarni, Anderson 1984).

Thus, of the adducts that we have
investigated, three have been identified as
major adducts in vivo, as mutagens, and as
persistent in certain mammalian systems. They
are considered likely critical lesions. These
are the AF and ABP adducts to guanine C-8 and
the (+) anti BP adduct to guanine N^2. All three
share a low energy conformational feature not
found for the other adducts: a pair of preferred
A or B like conformers that are close in energy,
one with carcinogen-base stacking, and a second
with base-base stacking. The two states are
easily interconvertible. Simple, energetically
cheap movements about the C3'-O3' or C5'-O5'
bonds, from trans towards gauche minus, together
with rotation of the guanine glycosidic torsion
from anti to high anti in the case of the BP
adduct, will produce carcinogen-base stacking
from the normal base stacked A or B form. The
carcinogen-base stacked state is kinked but not
significantly denatured, with carcinogen-base
stacking occurring in one direction only. One
might envision that the carcinogen resides
primarily at the A or B type helix exterior, in
the groove, where it could escape timely repair
because it causes virtually no distortion.
However, the carcinogen could readily be re-
oriented so that it is stacked with an adjacent
base at a critical time during replication, and
thereby cause a mutation.

Our other computed conformers may also have
biological relevance. The B - Z junction model
for the N^2 - AAF adduct may explain the persistence of this adduct; the repair enzymes may
fail to recognize the buried location of the
carcinogen in the groove of an undenatured
helix. On the other hand, the gross distortion
to the B helix induced by base displacement in
the C-8 AAF adduct may account for the
recognition of this lesion by the repair
systems, as has been suggested previously (Kriek

1974). The Z helical conformations which are undeformed or only slightly altered, may be associated with the small fraction of persistent AAF C-8 adducts (Visser, Westra 1981). The AAF modified Z forms might occur in very short C-G domains that are mutational hotspots (Fuchs 1984), embedded in the B helix. Arnott and co-workers (1981) have shown that a single Z form dinucleotide can be merged smoothly into the B form. The syn guanine at such a site could be mutagenic.

CONCLUSION

Minimized semi-empirical potential energy calculations for a number of carcinogen adducts with dCpdG have yielded molecular views of the adduct conformations. The base displaced and Z type conformations of AAF adducts to guanine C-8 have been detailed. Model building shows that base displacement causes kinking and denaturation in the B helix, while the Z helix is largely unperturbed by modification with AAF, in agreement with experimental findings. The minor AAF adduct linked to guanine N^2 can reside at a B-Z junction, with the carcinogen buried in a groove in the Z direction, without causing denaturation. The syn guanine in these modified Z forms could be mutagenic, the lesion escaping repair because the helix is undeformed, while the distorted base-displaced conformers are repaired.

AF and ABP linked to guanine C-8 and (+) anti BP linked to guanine N^2 are currently believed to be critical lesions. They all have a pair of A or B type low energy states, one of which has base-base stacking with carcinogen at the helix exterior, and a second with carcinogen-base stacking. The two states are easily interconvertible. It is possible that the carcinogen may reside primarily at the unperturbed helix exterior where it escapes repair, but that carcinogen-base stacking may occur at a critical time during replication, leading to a mutation.

REFERENCES

1.   Arnott S, Chandrasekaran R, Hall I,
      Puigjaner L, Walker J, Wang M (1982). DNA
      secondary structures: helices, wrinkles and
      junctions. "Cold Spring Harbor Symposia on
      Quantitative Biology: Structures of DNA."
      XLVII p 53-65.
2.   Beland F (1978). Computer-generated
      graphic models of the N2-substituted
      deoxyguanosine adducts of 2-
      acetylaminofluorene and benzo[a]pyrene and
      the 06-substituted deoxyguanosine adduct of
      1-naphthylamine in the DNA double helix.
      Chem Biol Interactions 22:329.
3.   Beland F, Dooley K, Jackson C (1982).
      Persistence of DNA adducts in rat liver and
      kidney after multiple doses of the
      carcinogen N-hydroxy-2-acetyl-
      aminofluorene. Cancer Res 42:1348.
4.   Beland F, Beranek D, Dooley K, Heflich R,
      Kadlubar F (1983). Arylamine-DNA adducts
      in vitro and in vivo: Their role in
      bacterial mutagenesis and urinary bladder
      carcinogenesis. Environmental Health
      Perspectives 49:125.
5.   Beranek D, White G, Heflich R, Beland F
      (1982). Aminofluorene-DNA adduct formation
      in Salmonella typhimurium exposed to the
      carcinogen N-hydroxy-2-acetylaminofluorene.
      Proc Natl Acad Sci USA 79:5175.
6.   Broyde S and Hingerty B (1983).
      Conformation of 2-aminofluorene-modified
      DNA. Biopolymers 22:2423.
7.   Broyde S, Hingerty B (1983). An internal
      fluorene model for iodo-N-2-acetylamino-
      fluorene modified DNA. Chem Biol
      Interactions 47:69.
8.   Broyde S and Hingerty B (1984). Base
      displacement in the Z-DNA helix.
      Submitted.
9.   Carrell H, Glusker J, Moschel R, Hudgins W,
      Dipple A (1981). Crystal structure of a
      carcinogen-nucleoside adduct. Cancer Res
      41:2230.

10. Conney H (1982). Induction of Microsomal Enzymes by Foreign Chemicals and Carcinogenesis by Polycyclic Aromatic Hydrocarbons. Cancer Res 42:4875.

11. Drinkwater N, Miller J, Miller E, and Yang N (1978). Covalent intercalative binding to DNA in relation to the mutagenicity of hydrocarbon epoxides and N-acetoxy-2-acetylaminofluorene. Cancer Res 38:3247.

12. Evans F, Miller D, Beland F (1980). Sensitivity of the Conformation of deoxyguanosine binding at the C-8 position by N-acetylated and unacetylated 2-aminofluorene. Carcinogenesis 1:955.

13. Frenkel K, Grunberger D, Boublik M, Weinstein I (1978). Conformation of dinucleoside monophosphates modified with benzo [a] pyrene-7,8-dihydrodiol 9,10-oxide as measured by circular dichroism. Biochemistry 17:1278.

14. Fuchs RPP, Daune M (1972). Physical studies on deoxyribonucleic acid after covalent binding of a carcinogen. Biochemistry 11:2659.

15. Fuchs RPP, Daune M (1974). Dynamic structure of DNA modified with the carcinogen N-acetoxyN-2-acetylaminofluorene. Biochemistry 13:4435.

16. Fuchs R, Schwartz N, Daune M (1981). Hot spots of frameshift mutations induced by the ultimate carcinogen N-acetoxy-N-2-acetylaminofluorene. Nature 294:657.

17. Fuchs RPP, Koffel-schwartz N, Daune M (1983). N-acetoxy-N-2-acetylaminofluorene induced frameshift mutations- a comparison between the DNA modification spectrum and the mutation spectrum. In Friedberg, E., Bridges, B. (eds): "Cellular Response to DNA Damage": UCLA Symposia on Molecular and Cellular Biology- New Series, Vol 11, New York: Alan R. Liss, p 547.

18. Fuchs RPP (1984). DNA binding spectrum of the carcinogen N-acetoxy-N-2-acetylamino-fluorene significantly differs from the mutation spectrum. J Mol Biol In press.

19. Grunberger D, Nelson J, Cantor C, Weinstein I (1970). Coding and conformational properties of oligonucleotides modified with the carcinogen N-2- acetylamino-fluorene. Proc Natl Acad Sci USA 66:488.

20. Hanau L, Santella R, Grunberger D, Erlanger B (1984). An immunochemical examination of acetylaminofluorene-modified poly(dG-dC). poly(dG-dC) in the Z conformation. J Biol Chem 259:173.

21. Hingerty B, Broyde S (1982). Conformation of the deoxydinucleoside monophosphate dCpdG modified at carbon 8 of guanine with 2-(acetylamino)fluorene. Biochemistry 21:3243.

22. Hingerty B, Broyde S (1983). AAF linked to the guanine amino group: a B-Z junction. Nucleic Acids Res 11:3241.

23. Hingerty B, Broyde S (1983). A confor-mational analysis of the (+) anti BPDE adduct to the guanine amino group of dCpdG. Journal of Biomolecular Structure and Dynamics 1:905.

24. Hogan M, Dattagupta N, Whitlock J (1981). Carcinogen-induced alteration of DNA structure. J Biol Chem 256:4504.

25. Howard P, Casciano D, Beland F, Shaddock J (1981). The binding of N-hydroxy-2-acetyl-aminofluorene to DNA and repair of the adducts in primary rat hepatocyte cultures. Carcinogenesis 2:97.

26. Irving C, Veazey R (1969). Persisent binding of 2-acetylaminofluorene to rat liver DNA in vivo and consideration of the mechanism of binding of N-hydroxy-2-acetylaminofluorene to rat liver nucleic acids. Cancer Res 29:1799.

27. Kadlubar F (1980). A transversion mutation hypothesis for chemical carcinogenesis by N2-substitution of guanine in DNA. Chem Biol Interactions 31:255.

28. Kriek E, Miller J, Juhl U and Miller E
     (1967). 8-(N-2-fluorenylacetamido)
     guanosine, an arylamidation reaction
     product of guanosine and the carcinogen N-
     acetoxy-N-2-fluorenylacetamide in neutral
     solution. Biochemistry 6:177.

29. Kriek E (1969). On the mechanism of action
     of carcinogenic aromatic amines. I.
     Binding of 2-acetylaminofluorene and N-
     hydroxy-2-acetylaminofluorene to rat-liver
     nucleic acids in vivo. Chem Biol
     Interact 1:3.

30. Kriek E (1972). Persistent binding of a
     new reaction product of the carcinogen N-
     hydroxy-N-2-acetylaminofluorene with
     guanine in rat liver DNA in vivo. Cancer
     Res 32:2042.

31. Kriek E (1974). Carcinogenesis by aromatic
     amines. Biochem. et Biophys. Acta
     355:177.

32. Kulkarni M, Anderson M (1984). Persistence
     of benzo[a]pyrene metabolite: DNA adducts
     in lung and liver of mice. Cancer Res
     44:97.

33. Land H, Parada L, Weinberg R (1983).
     Cellular oncogenes and multistep carcino-
     genesis. Science 222:777.

34. Leng M, Ptak M, Rio P (1980). Conformation
     of acetylaminofluorene and aminofluorene
     modified guanosine and guanosine
     derivatives. Biochem Biophys Res Commun
     96:1095.

35. Lipkowitz K, Chevalier T, Widdifield M,
     Beland F (1982). Force field conforma-
     tional analysis of aminofluorene and
     acetylaminofluorene substituted
     deoxyguanosine. Chem Biol Interactions
     40:57.

36. Mizusawa H, Lee C, Kakefuda T, McKenney K,
     Shimatake H, Rosenberg M (1981). Base
     insertion and deletion mutations induced in
     an Escherichia coli plasmid by benzo[a]
     pyrene-7,8-dihydrodiol-9,10-epoxide. Proc
     Natl Acad Sci USA 78:6817.

37. Poirier M, True B, Laishes B (1982). Formation and removal of (guan-8-yl)-DNA-2-acetylaminofluorene adducts in liver and kidney of male rats given dietary 2-acetylaminofluorene. Cancer Res 42:1317.

38. Sage E and Leng M (1980). Conformation of poly(dG-dC).poly(dG-dC) modified by the carcinogen N-acetoxy-N-2-acetyl-N-aminofluorene and N-hydroxy-N-2-aminofluorene. Proc Natl Acad Sci USA 77:4597.

39. Santella R, Kriek E, Grunberger D (1980). Circular dichroism and proton magnetic resonance studies of dApdG modified with 2-aminofluorene and 2-acetyl-aminofluorene. Carcinogenesis 1:897.

40. Santella R, Grunberger D, Broyde S, Hingerty B (1981). Z-DNA conformation of N-2-acetylamino- fluorene modified poly(dG-dC).poly(dG-dC) determined by reactivity with anti cytidine antibodies and minimized potential energy calculations. Nucleic Acids Res 9:5459.

41. Santella R, Grunberger D, Weinstein I, Rich A (1981). Induction of the Z conformation in poly(dG-dC).poly(dG-dC) by binding of N-2-acetylaminofluorene to guanine residues. Proc Natl Acad Sci USA 78:1451.

42. Sukumar S, Notario V, Martin-Zanca D, Barbacid M (1983). Induction of mammary carcinomas in rats by nitroso-methylurea involves malignant activation of H-ras-1 locus by single point mutations. Nature 306:658.

43. Srinivasan A, Olson W (1980). Polynucleotide conformation in real solution- a preliminary theoretical estimate. Fed Proc Fed Am Soc Exp Biol 39:2199.

44. Srinivasan A, Olson W (1983). Polynucleotide conformation in real solutions: theoretical assessment of solvent effects. Conversation in Biomolecular Stereodynamics III:60.

45. Visser A, Westra J (1981). Partial persistence of 2-aminofluorene and N-acetyl-2-aminofluorene in rat liver DNA. Carcinogenesis 2:737.
46. Wang A, Quigley G, Kolpak F, van der Marel G, van Boom J, Rich A (1981). Left handed double helical DNA: variations in the backbone conformation. Science 211:171.
47. Winkle S, Combates N, Kiledjian M, Langieri G, Mallamaci M (1984). Biophys J 45:289a.
48. Yamasaki H, Pulkrabek P, Grunberger D, Weinstein I (1977). Differential excision from DNA of the C-8 and N2-guanosine adducts of N-acetyl-2-aminofluorene by single strand-specific endonucleases. Cancer Res 37:3756.
49. Yoon K, Shelegedin V, Kallenbach N (1982). Analysis of N-acetoxy-N-2-acetylaminofluorene induced frame-shifts in pBR322. Mutation Res 93:273.

ACKNOWLEDGEMENT

This work was supported jointly by PHS Grant #1 RO1 CA28038-04, awarded by the National Cancer Institute, DHHS (SB), DOE Contract #DE-ACO2-81 ER60015 (SB), and by the Office of Health and Environmental Research, U.S. Department of Energy, under Contract #DE-ACO5-84OR21400 with Martin Marietta Energy Systems, Inc. We thank Prof. R. Shapiro and Prof. D. Grunberger for many interesting discussions.

Molecular Basis of Cancer, Part A: Macromolecular
Structure, Carcinogens, and Oncogenes, pages 173–185
© 1985 Alan R. Liss, Inc.

A PERSPECTIVE ON MOLECULAR MECHANICAL AND MOLECULAR DYNAMICAL STUDIES INVOLVING DNA

P. Kollman, U. C. Singh, T. Lybrand, S. Rao
and
J. Caldwell

Department of Pharmaceutical Chemistry
School of Pharmacy,
University of California
San Francisco, CA 94143.

INTRODUCTION

The goals of our research efforts are to understand
the structural properties of DNA and its non-covalent
complexes and covalent adducts with other molecules at the
atomic level. To attempt to reach this goal, we have made
use of quantum mechanical and molecular mechanical
(molecular dynamical) methods, although the predominant
tool has been molecular mechanics. It is the goal of this
paper to give a general perspective on our work by
describing some technical aspects of the work, by giving
an overview of what the theory can and cannot do and by
describing the areas where there has been useful interplay
between theory and experiment in our studies.

It is our working hypothesis that for simulating
complex molecules, a molecular mechanical energy function
is very powerful and surprisingly accurate for studying
DNA or RNA itself and its non-covalent and covalent
complexes. Quantum mechanical methods are required to
characterize complete reaction pathways for covalent
attack, but molecular mechanical methods can still be used
in comparative studies of "strain" at selected points
along such pathways. We have spent considerable time in
improving the molecular mechanical models for studies of
nucleic acids (Weiner et al., 1984a,b), using information

on the charge distribution of molecules to derive
electrostatic potential based atomic charges (Singh et
al., 1984a). This is the major use we make of quantum
mechanical methods, since deriving reliable and accurate
atomic charges is important to finding accurate energies
at the molecular mechanical level. Ultimately, we
simulate and optimize the structures of systems with
hundreds or thousands of atoms and, to do so, we must
employ a simple, analytically differentiable function,
such as we describe in some detail in Weiner et al.,
(1984a). Most of our applications have involved
minimizing such a function to find the minimum energies
and structure and the vibrational frequencies at the
minimum, but we have recently incorporated molecular
dynamics in our molecular modeling program. This approach
uses the same energy function and derivatives employed in
minimization, and solves Newton's equations of motion
numerically using the energy gradients. Dynamics has the
advantage over minimization of going over energy barriers
and giving a more correct description of the system at any
temperature (minimization is equally "correct" only at
$0°K.$), but the disadvantage of much larger computer time
requirements and a data analysis problem.

It has been our approach to use molecular mechanics
(energy minimization) on a first pass to attack a
problem. Our future goals are to supplement this with
molecular dynamics to determine a more complete physical
picture. Below, we analyze what such molecular mechanical
calculations have been able to do to enable further
understanding of DNA structure and interactions.

Studies of DNA

In our earliest studies we carried out molecular
mechanics energy refinement on various sequences of A, B
and Z forms of DNA (Kollman et al., 1981, 1982; Tilton et
al., 1983). The general goals of these studies were
twofold; first, to understand the relative energies and
properties of the different families of DNA structure and,
secondly, to understand the sequence dependent energies
and structures within a given family. The first goal is
clearly much more difficult to reach, given that our
treatment of counterions and solvent was so primitive.
The dependence of DNA structure on solvent and counterion

environment suggests that high salt (lowered water activity) favors Z or A structures over B (depending on sequence) and, qualitatively, the calculations are consistent with this, in that inclusion of counterions in the calculation does lower the energy of the Z and A structures relative to B. However, the energy differences are very large, and don't allow a prediction of the quantitative dependents of DNA conformation on ionic strength and solvent.

The calculations have been more successful in understanding sequence dependent energies within a DNA family or "double differences", in which one compares two sequences within a family with the two sequences of another. Briefly, we have been quite successful in reproducing the relative energies of BDNA sequence isomers as reflected in relative melting temperatures of DNA polymers, in "predicting" the average backbone angles of "B" DNA, when they are compared with X-ray structural data. The calculated sequence dependent relative energies of A-DNA polymers reproducing the relative melting temperatures of A-RNA polymers, suggesting that the 2'OH does not significantly influence relative sequence dependent stabilities in nucleic acids.

Our calculations found, that the addition of a 5-methyl group to cytosine would favor the B $\rightarrow$ Z transition in d $(C^{5m}GC^{5m}GC^{5m}G)_2)$, compared to d$(CGCGCG)_2$, consistent with the observation that the B $\rightarrow$ Z transition occurs at 50 mM salt for the former polymer and at 4M salt in the latter. The calculations suggested that the reason a 5 Me substitution favors Z is that there is an unfavorable intramolecular base-backbone interaction upon addition of the methyl group in B compared to Z, thus leading to a net stabilization of Z. This is not inconsistent with the greater stability (as indicated by melting temperatures) of the B form 5 MeC polymer compared to the unmethylated B polymer because the interstrand interactions in the B form are more attractive in the 5 MeC polymer than the unmethylated.

An alternative explanation for the 5 Me-C effect is based on solvent accessibility of this group in B and Z DNA and the fact that it is more buried in the Z form polymer. The role of steric (base-backbone) and

hydrophobic effects in causing the 5 effect on the B → Z
transition is being further analyzed in a collaborative
theoretical and experimental study with T. Jovin on other
5-X substituents (Rao et al., 1984a) which are not so
hydrophobic and for which there is no correlation between
size and hydrophobicity. A puzzling feature of the B → Z
stabilities is that alternating AT polymers do not easily
undergo the B → Z transition, despite the presence of a 5
methyl group in thymine. Kopka et al. (1983) have
suggested that this is due to the lack of a 2-NH$_2$ group in
Adenine. Their argument is that there is a stabilizing
effect of solvent on a pure A-T polymer in the B form due
to the strong negative electrostatic potential of N3 on A
and O2 (T), which is disrupted by a 2-NH$_2$. That this is
not the only factor in determining the B → Z transition is
clear from the inability of d(T(2NH$_2$A)T(2NHA)T(2NH$_2$A))$_2$
(Gaffney et al., 1984) to undergo the B → Z transition at
high salt and the fact that poly d(2NH$_2$A-T) · poly (2NH$_2$A-
T) undergoes such a transition with difficulty, if at all
(Jovin et al., 1983) the evidence for its Z form being
based only on immunological studies. An alternative
explanation for the tendency of AT polymers not to undergo
the B → Z transition is the fact, discussed in detail
below, that the AT polymers are inherently more flexible
and are in equilibrium between two different right handed
B helices with mono and dinucleotide repeat, whereas the
GC polymers have only one lowest energy (mononucleotide
repeat) B-DNA structure (Rao et al., 1984b). Both AT and
GC polymers would form similar, relatively rigid Z
structures, so it is the greater stability of the AT B
form which prevents its B → Z transition under conditions
where the GC polymer undergoes such a transition.

We also showed, on the basis of molecular mechanical
calculations (Kollman et al., 1982) that the energy cost
of putting a non-alternating sequence into the Z structure,
which requires forcing a pyrimidine into a syn
conformation, is not great, suggesting that a sequence
with mainly alternating G-C pairs might allow a small
number of non-alternating internal base pairs to stay in a
Z structure, a prediction which has apparently been
confirmed by subsequent experiments (Jovin et al., 1983,
Wells, this symposium).

Our calculations (Kollman et al., 1981) and Levitt's

(1978) also suggested average dihedral angle values for B-DNA somewhat different than those of Arnott et al (1976), which were used as starting geometries in many of the calculations; the X-ray structure of Drew et al (1981) supports the reasonableness of our values. Calculations varying the helix repeat (Kollman et al., 1983) suggest an interesting coupling between helix repeat and sugar pucker. Other molecular mechanical calculations on torsional angle coupling and base pair opening have yielded insights into the experimental NMR relaxation measurements and imino proton exchange rates in DNA (Keepers et al., 1982).

One of our most interesting recent applications of molecular mechanics to DNA involved the question of mononucleotide vs. dinucleotide repeat of DNA and its sequence dependence (Rao et al., 1984). Single crystal X-ray studies suggested d(ATAT)$_2$ had a dinucleotide repeat, (Viswamitra et al., 1978) with sugar puckers A(C3'endo) and T(C2'endo). NMR studies in relatively low salt on poly d(A-T) · poly d(A-T) found two P^{31} signals (Patel, et al., 1981) consistent with such a structure. In contrast poly d(G-C) · poly d(G-C) showed a single P^{31} resonance under low salt conditions (Cohen et al., 1981) suggesting a mononucleotide repeat. Raman studies on poly d(A-T)· poly d(A-T) and poly dA ·poly dT suggested both polymers to have ~ $\frac{1}{2}$ C2'endo and $\frac{1}{2}$ C3'endo sugars, (Thomas and Peticolas, 1983) but give no information on which sugar went with which base. Calculations by ourselves and Arnott (Kollman et al., 1981, 1983; Tilton et al., 1983, Arnott, 1983) suggested different sugar puckers in dA$_n$· dT$_n$, with Kollman et al suggesting that the lowest energy structure was A(C2'endo), T(C3'endo) and Arnott et al suggesting A(C3'endo),T(C2'endo). Recently, we have carried out a more extensive (Rao et al., 1984b) set of molecule mechanics calculations on d(CGCGCG)$_2$, d(GCGCGC)$_2$, d(TATATA)$_2$, d(ATATAT)$_2$ and dA$_6$ ·dT$_6$, employing dihedral angle constraints to examine the structure and energy of the various sugar pucker combinations. In d(ATATAT)$_2$, the lowest energy structure was A(C3'endo)T(C2'endo) with the mononucleotide repeat structure A(C2'endo)T(C2'endo) 3 kcal/mole less stable. In d(TATATA)$_2$, these two were the lowest energy, but the order of stabilities were reversed and the uniform sugar model was 2 kcal/mole more stable than A(C3'endo)T(C2'endo). In d(GCGCGC)$_2$ and d(CGCGCG)$_2$, the uniform C2'endo model was lower in energy than other possibilities by 5-10 kcal/mole and in $dA_6 \cdot dT_6$, the order of stabilities was: A(C2'endo)T(C3'endo) 0, A(C2'endo)T(C2'endo) = + 2 kcal/mole and A(C3'endo)T(C2'endo) = + 10 kcal/mole.

What was particularly satisfying about these calculations was not only that they were consistent with experimental observations (poly d(A-T) • poly d(A-T) dinucleotide repeat; poly d(G-C) • poly d(G-C), mononucleotide repeat at relatively low salt and poly dA • poly dT, $1/2$ C2'endo and $1/2$ C3'endo), but the energy component analysis showed clearly why the relative energies came out the way they do. Briefly, there are three important energy terms which contribute: (1) intrinsic sugar pucker energy, which for deoxyribose is ~ 0.5 kcal/mole more stable C2'endo than C3'endo; (2) phosphate-phosphate repulsion, which is ~ 1-2 kcal/mole larger if the intervening sugar is C3'endo and (3) a favorable thymine-5'-phosphate interaction, which is ~ 1-2 kcal/mole more favorable if the sugar on the 5' end of the thymine is C3' endo. Terms (1) and (2) explain why poly d(G-C) prefers C2' endo sugar throughout. Term (3) explains at the same time why poly d(A-T)•poly d(A-T) prefers conformations which are A(C3'endo)T(C2'endo) and poly dA•poly dT prefers conformations which are A(C2'endo)T(C 3'endo), since these combinations allow the most favorable thymine backbone interactions. Term (2) rationalizes the fact that at extremely low salt, (Sarma, this symposium) poly d(A-T)•poly d(A-T) reverts to a mononucleotide repeat, since such conditions would favor pure C2'endo geometries.

DNA - Non Covalent Complexes

Our earliest foray into molecular mechanics was a study of ethidium-deoxy-dinucleoside phosphate interactions (Nuss et al., 1979) and, we and others (Pack and Loew, 1978; Broyde 1978; Ornstein and Rein, 1979, Miller et al., 1980) using different methods were able to reproduce the experimental preference of ethidium for C-3'-5'-G sites over G-3',5'-C and demonstrate that this preference was due to differences in stability of the nucleic acid sites rather than to differences in drug-DNA interactions. These earliest studies of ours were too limited in their geometry optimization, so we switched to complete optimization in cartesian coordinates. We then examined the sugar pucker preference of the intercalation sites in deoxyribodinucleoside complexes of proflavine (Dearing et al. 1981) and acridine orange and the sequence dependence of intercalation of 4-Nitroquinoline N-oxide (Lybrand et al., 1981) into deoxyribodinucleoside complexes. In the latter study, the importance of complete optimization of the system became clear when we found rather distorted non-classical intercalation geometries to be of the lowest energy and we are currently examining intercalation of this drug at the hexanucleotide level (Lybrand et al., 1984a).

Recently, we have gone back to the ethidium intercalation problem and have carried out studies of its intercalation with base-paired deoxyrinucleosides and base-paired deoxyhexanucleosides (Lybrand et al., 1984b). The most complete model we used (a recently developed all-atom force field) (Weiner et al, 1984b) was able to completely rationalize the experimental data of both Kastrup et al (1978) and the binding studies of Bresloff and Crothers (1981).

We are also studying the intercalation of actinomycin D into sequences $d(GCXYGC)_2$ where XY = GC,AT,CG,TA. Consistent with experiment, we find a strong preference for the XY = GC site and are able to rationalize this in terms of specific drug - DNA interactions. Our model is only a modest modification of that suggested by Sobell, but we do not find a strong preference for mixed (C3' endo - C2' endo) sugar puckering at the intercalation site. In collaboration with S. Brown and R. Shafer, who are studying $d(ATGCAT)_2$: Act D with 2D NMR, we are also studying this complex with molecular mechanics methods and hope to derive a complete picture of it which fits all the distance data from the NMR and is of suitable low energy (Lybrand et al., 1984c).

A comparison of non-intercalating and intercalating drug-DNA interactions has been part of the motivations for our studies of netropsin-DNA interactions, (Caldwell and Kollman, 1984a) and we have been successful in rationalizing the preference of this drug for AT over GC sequences and in finding a geometry of binding to

d(CGCGAATTCGCG)$_2$ consistent with Patel's (1982) NOE
measurements on this complex.

Mismatched and Covalently Modified DNA

We have carried out molecular mechanical studies on
analogs of d(CGCGAATTCGCG)$_2$ in which the GC base pair at
the third position is replaced by "mismatched" GA, AC, TC
and GT as well as an analog in which an extra A is
inserted into the helix of one strand (Keepers et al.,
1984). Our studies were directed at further understanding
the NMR studies of Patel and co-workers and were
successful in this. For the GT mismatch, a "wobble" base
pair with GNH$_1$....TO2 and GO6....TH1 H-bonds was formed
upon energy refinement starting from Arnott structure,
completely consistent with experiment. We found that one
could form low energy (2 H-bond) structures of the GA base
pair inside the helix with both bases anti, as well as one
with adenine syn, consistent with experimental
inferences. We found a new AC pair, different from the
one suggested by Rein et al., (1983) and which helps
rationalize the lack of an NOE between the adenine C2H and
the imino protons of the GC base pairs above and below.
The TC mismatch is calculated to be the least stable,
consistent with experiment, but the experimental data does
not allow one to test the reasonableness of our calculated
structures.

Stimulated by the experimental studies of Kuznich et
al., (1983) we have compared the structure and stabilities
of 60 Me guanine (OMG) modified polymers d(CG(OMG)CG)$_2$,
d(CGT(OMG)CG)$_2$, d(CGCGAATTC(OMG)CG)$_2$ with "normal" CG base
pairs and have been able to reproduce the relative
stabilities of these altered polymers (Caldwell and
Kollman, 1984b) as well as predicting the detailed
structure of a OMG-C and OMG-T base pair upon complete
energy refinement. Along similar lines, we have studied
mitomycin DNA interactions. Mitomycin is a clinically
effective anti-cancer drug, which apparently acts by
alkylating the 60 position of guanine. By carrying out
computer graphics model building and molecular mechanical
optimization on the non-covalent monolinked and cross-
linked complex of mitomycin with DNA, we are able to show
how this molecule can form low energy non-covalent
complexes with DNA (Singh et al., 1984b). This complex

places the mitomycin reactive aziridinum group in excellent position to attack a guanine 60, and, subsequent to this attack, places its reactive amidoester carbon in excellent position to attack the guanine 60 on the opposite strand of d(G-C) • d(G-C). The calculations thus allow one to build a detailed structural model of mitomycin - adducts, which ratinalizes the DNA sequence specificity of these molecules and their ability to crosslink DNA without much structural perturbation of the DNA.

Ultraviolet light is known to cause crosslinking of pyrimidine bases within DNA through the formation of a highly strained cyclobutane ring. We were interested in this crosslinked DNA because of suggestions that it would cause a large kink in the DNA structure. We thus studied d(CGCGAAT[   ]TCGCG) •d(CGCGAATTCGCG) ([   ] denotes cyclobutane dimer) and compared its properties to those of d(CGCGAATTCGCG)$_2$. We were able to demonstrate that one can form such a dimer with no <u>large</u> kink and no large distortion of the DNA structure (Rao et al., 1984c). One cannot definitely say that such is the lowest energy structure (since we examined only a limited number of possibilities). NMR experiments on psoralen cross-linked DNA presented at this symposium by Kim suggest that cyclobutane dimer formation via psoralen does <u>not</u> disrupt the AT base pairs at which cyclobutane dimer is formed supportive of our results, but experiments on a single TT dimerized structure are required to definitely establish this (Rao et al., 1984d). We are now extending our studies to 6-4 photodimers, which have been implicated (Hazeltine, 1983) as the ultimate mutagen after obligatory pyrimidine cyclobutane dimer repair and hope that such calculations will give insight into the nature of 6-4 dimer modified DNA.

A final set of calculations involve benzypyrene diol epoxide adducts to DNA (Rao et al., 1984e). We have shown that one can model build and energy refine stereochemically reasonable covalent adducts which sit in the minor groove of DNA; further analysis of the stereochemistry of this process and its dependence on aromatic hydrocarbon structure is continuing.

Molecular Dynamics Calculations

    We have recently acquired the ability to carry out molecular dynamics simulations and have applied this approach to the sequence d(CGCGA) • d(TCGCG), which we have simulated in the presence and absence of large "hydrated" cations (Singh et al., 1984c). The simulations were able to qualitatively reproduce the helix repeat, twists and tilts of the bases, torsional angles and sugar puckering observed in X-ray and NMR studies of BDNA and to suggest some interesting long range correlations between dihedral angle motions. Our long range goal is to compare the results of such simulations on normal BDNA, with mismatched base pair analogs, thymine dimer and mitomycin covalently modified adducts and ethidium, 4NQO and netropsin non-covalent complexes. We hope that such studies will further our understanding of the structural and energetic properties of DNA.

Acknowledgements:

    We are grateful to the NIH (CA-25644) for research support to PAK and for support of the UCSF Computer Graphics Lab (RR-1081), R. Langridge, director and T. Ferrin, facilities manager.

References
Arnott S, Campbell-Smith P and Chandrasekharan R (1976). CRC Handbook of Biochemistry, G. Fasman, ed., CRC Press, Cleveland, Ohio, vol. 2, p. 411-422.
Arnott S, Chandresekharan R, Banerjee AK, He R, Walker JK (1983). J. Mol. Struct. Dyn., 1: 437.
Bresloff JL and Crothers DM (1981) Biochem 20:3547.
Broyde S and Hingerty B (1979) Biopoly 18:2905.
Caldwell J and Kollman P (1984a). Molecular Mechanical Studies of 6OMe Guanine Modified DNA. Nucleic Acid Res (to be submitted).
Caldwell J and Kollman P (1984b). Molecular Mechanical Studies of Netropsin-DNA Interactions. Nucl Acid Res (to be submitted).
Cohen JS, Wooten JS and Chatterjee CL (1981). Biochem, 20:3049.
Dearing A, Weiner P and Kollman P (1981) Nucl Acid Res. 9:1483.
Drew HR, Wing RE, Takano T, Broka C, Tanaka S, Itakura K

and Dickerson RE (1981). Proc Nat Acad Sci 78:2179.

Gaffney B, Marky LA and Jones RA (1984). Tetrahedron, 40:3.

Jovin, TM Hazeltine W,(1983). Cell 33:13.

McIntosh LP, Arndt-Jovin DJ, Zarling DA, Robert-Nicourd M. van de Sande JH, Jorgenson KF and Eckstein F (1983). J Biomol Struct Dyn 1:21.

Kastrup RV, Young MA and Krugh TR (1978). Biochem 17:4855.

Keepers J, Kollman P, Weiner P and James T (1982). Proc Nat Acad Sci 79:5537.

Keepers J, Schmidt P, James TL and Kollman PA (1984). Molecular Mechanical Studies of the Mismatched Base Analogues of d(CGCGAATTCGCG)$_2$:d(CGTGAATTCGCG)$_2$, d(CGAGAATTCGCG)$_2$, d(CGCGAATTCACG)$_2$, d(CGCGAATTCTCG)$_2$ and d(CGCAGAATTCGCG): d(CGCGAATTCGCG). Biopolymers (in press).

Kollman P, Dearing A and Weiner P. (1981), Biopoly 20:2583.

Kollman P, Weiner P, Quigley G and Wang A (1982). Biopoly 21:1945.

Kollman P, Keepers JW and Weiner P (1982) Biopoly 21:2345.

Kopka ML, Fratini AV, Drew HR and Dickerson RE (1983) J Mol Biol 163:129.

Kuznich S, Marky LA and Jones RA (1983) Nuc Acid Res 11:3393.

Levitt M (1978) Proc Nat Acad Sci 75:640.

Lybrand TP Dearing A Weiner P and Kollman P (1981) Nucl Acids Res 9:6995.

Lybrand TL and Kollman PA (1984a) Molecular Mechanical Studies of 4 Nitroquinoline N-oxide Intercalation into Hexanucleotides of Varying Sequences. Nucl Acid Res (to be submitted).

Lybrand TL and Kollman PA (1984a) Molecular Mechanical Studies of Ethidium Intercalation into Di and Hexa Nucleotides Nucl Acid Res (to be submitted).

Lybrand TL and Kollman PA (1984b). Molecular Mechanical Studies of Actinomycin D Intercalation into Hexa-Nucleotides. J Mol Biol (to be submitted).

Miller KJ Brodzinsky R and Hall S (1980). Biopoly 19:2091.

Nuss ME Marsh FJ and Kollman PA (1979). J Amer Chem Soc 101:825.

Ornstein RL and Rein R (1979). Biopoly 18, 2821.

Pack GR and Loew GH (1978). Biochim Biophys Acta 519, 163.

Patel DJ, Kozlowski SA, Suggs JW, and Cox SD (1981) Proc Nat Acad Sci 78:4063.

Patel D (1982). Proc Nat Acad Sci 79:6424.

Patel DJ Kozlowski SA Marky LA Broka C Rice JA Itakura K and Breslauer KJ (1982). Biochem 21:428, 437, 445.

Patel DJ, Kozlowski SA, Ikuta S and Itakura S (1984) Deoxyadenosine-Deoxycytidine Pairing in the d(CGCGAATTCACG) Duplex: Conformation and Dynamics at and Adjoint to the dA.dC Mismatched Site (1984). Biochem (in press).

Rao SN and Kollman PA (1984a). Molecular Mechanical Studies of Unusual Bases in DNA and their effect on the B DNA Equilibrium. Unpublished Results.

Rao SN and Kollman PA (1984b) On the Role of Uniform and Mixed Sugar Puckers in DNA Double Helical Structures. J Amer Chem Soc (submitted).

Rao SN and Kollman PA (1984c). The Structure of d(CGCGAAT[ ]TCGCG) d (CGCGAATTCGCG). The Incorporation of Thymine Photodime into a B-DNA Helix. Nucl Acid Res (in press).

Rao SN and Kollman PA (1984d). Studies of 6-4 Photodimers Incorporated into B-DNA Helices. Unpublished results.

Rao SN, Herina D and Kollman PA (1984e). Studies of Benzpyrenediolepoxide covalent adducts to DNA. Unpublished results.

Rein R, Shibata M, Gardino-Juarez R and Kreber-Emmons T (1983). Structure and Dynamics: Nucleic Acids and Proteins. E. Clementi and R. Sarma, ed., Adenine Press, pp. 269-288.

Singh UC and Kollman PA (1984a). J Comp Chem 5:129.

Singh UC, Rao SN and Kollman PA (1984b). The Structure of Mitomycin C-DNA Complexes: Non-Covalent Binding, O6 Guanine Covalent Attack and Inter-strand Crosslinking. J Amer Chem Soc (submitted).

Singh UC, Weiner SJ, and Kollman PA (1984c). Molecular Dynamics Simulations of d(CGCGA): d(TCGCG) with and without "Hydrated" Counterions. Proc Nat Acad Sci (submitted).

Thomas GA and Peticolas WL (1983) J Amer Chem Soc 105:993.

Tilton R, Weiner T and Kollman P (1982). Biopolymers 22:969.

Viswamitra MA, Kennard O, Jones PG, Sheldrik GM, Salisbury SA, Falwello L and Shakked Z (1978). Nature, 273:687.

Weiner SJ, Kollman PA, Case D, Singh UC, Ghio C, Alagona G, Profeta S and Weiner P (1984a). J Amer Chem Soc

106:765.
Weiner SJ, Kollman PA, Case D, Nguyen D (1984b) An all
atom force field for Simulations of Proteins and Nucleic
Acids. J. Comp Chem (to be submitted).

Molecular Basis of Cancer, Part A: Macromolecular Structure, Carcinogens, and Oncogenes, pages 187–197
© **1985 Alan R. Liss, Inc.**

STEREOSELECTIVITY OF BENZO[A]PYRENE DIOL EPOXIDES BY DNA FOR ADDUCT FORMATION WITH N2 ON GUANINE

Kenneth J. Miller, Eric R. Taylor,
Josef Dommen, and Jonathan J. Burbaum

Department of Chemistry
Rensselaer Polytechnic Institute
Troy, N.Y. 12181

A summary of a theoretical study is presented for the binding of the four diastereoisomers of benzo[a]pyrene diol epoxides (BPDEs) to N2 on guanine. Molecular models for stereoselectivity involving intercalation and intercalative covalently bound forms are presented. Molecular mechanics calculations provide the energetics which suggest possibilities for the formation of each of the DNA–BPDE complexes. Stereographic projections are used to illustrate the molecular structures. The results of previous calculations on intercalation and adduct formation of BPDE I(+) in kinked DNA (Taylor, Miller 1983) are extended to include the four diastereoisomers I($\pm$) and II($\pm$). The theoretical model is consistent with the observed experimental data. Our results show that BPDE I(+) is preferred and BPDE II(+) is somewhat favored, whereas, I(−) and II(−) are not accommodated for adduct formation with N2 on guanine.

The carcinogenic and mutagenic activities of benzo[a]pyrene involves its conversion to the benzo[a]pyrene diol epoxides, BPDEs (Sims, et al. 1974; Huberman, et al. 1976; Meehan, et al. 1976; Weinstein, et al. 1976; Koreeda, et al. 1976; King, et al. 1976). These chemically reactive BPDEs are involved in covalent binding to DNA (Brooks, Lawley 1964; Ames, et al. 1972; McCann, et al. 1975). In particular binding to N2 on guanine (Weinstein, et al. 1976; Meehan, et al. 1977) is most extensive (Jeffrey, et al. 1976; Jennette, et al. 1977; Meehan, et al. 1979) and it is assumed to be the carcinogenic event. Studies involving the four diastereoisomers (+)7β,8α-dihydroxy-9α,10α-

epoxy-7,8,9,10-tetrahydrobenzo[a]pyrene, BPDE I(+), and (-)7β, 8α –dihydroxy– 9β, 10β–epoxy– 7, 8, 9, 10–tetrahydro–benzo[a]pyrene, BPDE II(-), as well as the optical enantiomers BPDE I(-) and BPDE II(+), demonstrate a correlation between binding to N2 on guanine and the stereoselectivity of the BPDE I(+) isomer (Weinstein, et al. 1976; Meehan, et al. 1977; Jeffrey, et al. 1976).

Recent experimental observations show that the BPDE I(+) intercalates prior to adduct formation to N2 on guanine (Geacintov, et al. 1981; Gagliano, et al. 1982; Meehan, et al. 1982; MacLeod, Selkirk 1982). In addition the adduct is observed to unwind the DNA by ca 30° while the intercalated form unwinds the DNA by only 13° (Gamper, et al. 1980; Meehan, et al. 1982). The observation that after adduct formation the pyrene moiety is not perpendicular to the helical axis of DNA has suggested outside binding (Geacintov, et al. 1978). Detailed studies of the local region suggests a kinked receptor site (Hogan, et al. 1981).

The stereoselectivity of the BPDEs for adduct formation with N2 on guanine may be viewed in terms of the ability of the individual diastereoisomers to fit into the receptor site and the ease in which the DNA can undergo a change to the site. A stepwise procedure is used in the analysis, and the energy required to accomplish each step is calculated. The process which is used to define the change begins with the alteration of DNA to an intercalation site (I) followed by a bending of the DNA to produce a kinked site (K)

$$\uparrow \left. \begin{matrix} BP_2 \\ BP_1 \end{matrix} \right\downarrow \xrightarrow{\Delta E^I_{DNA}} \uparrow \left. \begin{matrix} BP_2 \\ BP_1 \end{matrix} \right\downarrow \xrightarrow{\Delta E^K_{DNA} - \Delta E^I_{DNA}} \uparrow \left. \begin{matrix} BP_2 \\ BP_1 \end{matrix} \right\downarrow$$

where

$$\Delta E^R_{DNA} = E^R_{DNA} - E^{B-DNA}_{DNA}$$

is the energy required to form a receptor site R (I and K) relative to B–DNA. The details of the molecular mechanics calculations are described elsewhere (Miller, et al. 1980).

A mathematical technique has been used to obtain atomic coordinates for intercalation (Miller, Pycior 1979; Miller, 1981) and kinked sites (Taylor, Miller 1983). These states allow for the analysis of the process of intercalation of the BPDEs as a first step followed by an adjustment of the base pairs to non-planar orientations (kink) to accommodate the proper hybrid configurations about C10 on BPDE and N2 on guanine for covalent bond formation. Because attention is focused on binding to N2 on guanine, two orientations along the DNA must be considered: 3' and 5' binding. They are illustrated with the BPDEs involved in intercalation and co-valent intercalative binding between G•C (or C•G) and BP_2.

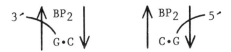

The arrow denotes the 5' → 3' direction along the backbone, i.e., 5'(sugar)3' or equivalently 3'(p)5'. The diagram corresponds to viewing the DNA into the minor groove as seen in all figures in this paper. Therefore the energy of opening the DNA to sites favoring 3' or 5' binding provides the contribution of the DNA to the process.

Once the site is created, the ability of each BPDE to fit into the receptor is examined. Two processes are considered: intercalation and covalent intercalative binding.

$$\uparrow \begin{array}{c} BP_2 \\ \\ BP_1 \end{array} \downarrow + BPDE \xrightarrow{\Delta E^R_{BPDE}} \uparrow \begin{array}{c} BP_2 \\ BPDE \\ BP_1 \end{array} \downarrow$$

By calculating the energy changes for the intercalation process, the preference for orientation of the epoxide in the major or minor groove can be determined. This step provides a rationale for the first step in covalent binding by examining whether the reacting atoms are in proximity to each other. The important step in diastereoselectivity is the ability of the BPDEs to fit into the site once a co-valent bond has formed. The conformations of the benzo ring are important in the fit of each of the diastereoisomers to the kink site. They modify the orientation of the double bond of the benzo ring and hence the entire pyrene moiety.

Therefore, this paper will report on the study of (1) Conformations and energies of the benzo ring after adduct formation, (2) Base sequence preference for the generation of receptor sites, (3) Intercalation of the BPDEs and (4) Stereoselectivity of the BPDEs by the DNA. The overall process favors the chair diequatorial conformation of BPDEs bound to a pyrimidine(p)purine sequence along the 5´ direction of DNA with BPDE I(+) selected by the DNA.

The parameters which define the orientation of the BPDE adduct to N2 on guanine are given in Fig. 1 in terms of the reaction coordinates R, α, β, γ, δ and ε. Minimum energy conformations of the benzo ring in the chair (C) and boat (B) forms each with the 07 and 08 diols in diaxial (da) and diequatorial (de) orientations were used in each step of the

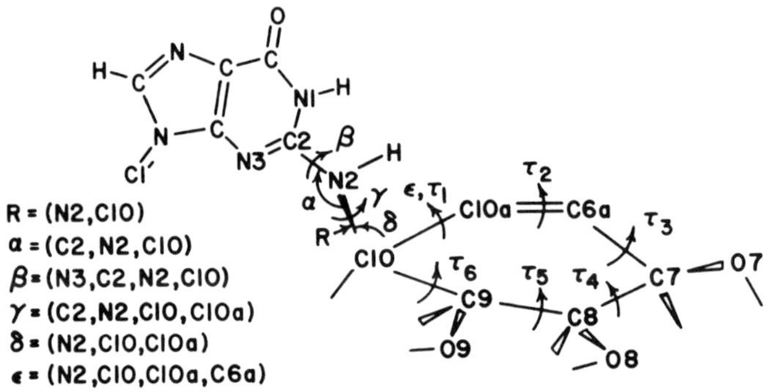

R = (N2,ClO)
α = (C2,N2,ClO)
β = (N3,C2,N2,ClO)
γ = (C2,N2,ClO,ClOa)
δ = (N2,ClO,ClOa)
ε = (N2,ClO,ClOa,C6a)

Fig. 1 Reaction coordinates for addition of BPDE to N2 on guanine. The torsional angles τ_1, τ_2, τ_3,... define the pucker of the benzo ring.

study. The role of the intercalation process in the orientation of the reactive epoxide in the region of N2 on guanine was explored. Each of the diastereoisomers in the Cda and Cde conformations were inserted into three intercalation sites with unwinding angles of 7°-12°, 14°-18° and 25°-32° (Miller 1981). The most favored site was IB (Miller, et al. 1979) which yields a small unwinding angle

(7-12°) in agreement with the observed value of 13° (Meehan, et al. 1982). Intercalation into both grooves occurs. For the case of minor groove binding the epoxide is oriented adjacent to N2 on guanine in a CpG sequence. In Fig. 2 the BPDE I(+) Cde isomer is shown inserted into a space filling model in which steric contours define the excluded region of

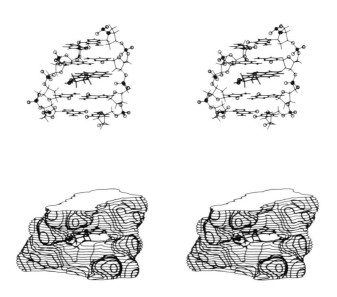

Fig. 2. BPDE I(+) intercalated in a CpG sequence of DNA. Relative values of electrostatic potential energy contours are denoted by ▬ (positive), ▬ (intermediate) and ▬ (negative).

the DNA and on which electrostatic contours are drawn. The epoxide lies in the most negative electrostatic region of the DNA. This observation suggests that among the cations which may be associated with this region of the DNA, hydrogen ions are available for the conversion of the BPDE to a reactive carbonium ion. To complete the formation of a chemical bond with proper hybrid configurations, the DNA must undergo a further change to a kinked site.

The formation of receptor sites must be studied for each of the base sequences. In Table 1, the energies required to open DNA to an intercalation site are reported for DNA duplex units containing at least one G·C base pair. The most stable base sequences (Ornstein, Rein 1979; Miller 1981) are the pyrimidine(p)purine ones: TpG and CpG. These lead to 5´ binding. The 3´ binding can result only from GpC, GpT and GpG sequences which are less stable by 10 kcal. This binding orientation is less likely to occur if the intercalation process preceeds covalent bond formation.

In the final step in which covalent bond formation occurs, the DNA undergoes a further change. Consistent with experimental data that the pyrene moiety is not perpendicular to the helical axis (Hogan, et al. 1981; Geacintov, et al. 1978) we have the base pairs form a kink (Taylor, Miller

Table 1. Energy, ΔE_{DNA}^{ν} in kcal/ duplex, required to alter B-DNA to receptor sites.[a]

Sequence	Intercalation	Kink Cons.	Kink Non-cons.	Binding Orient.
A·T ↑C·G↓	20.0	15.5	10.8	5´
G·C ↑C·G↓	20.5	17.4	12.1	5´
A·T ↑G·C↓	23.8	17.8	15.2	3´
G·C ↑G·C↓	24.7	20.2	17.0	3´,5´
T·A ↑C·G↓	26.2	23.8	19.6	5´
C·G ↑G·C↓	30.7	24.5	23.6	3´
T·A ↑G·C↓	29.6	25.6	23.5	3´

[a]Energies reported are for intercalation site IB (Miller 1981) and kinked sites for C(2´)-endo sugar puckers (conservative) and alternating C(2´)-endo to C(3´)-endo (non-conservative) sugar puckers (Taylor, Miller 1983).

1983). Once again, the trends in the stability favor TpG and CpG and hence 5′ binding as seen from the results in Table 1. Two sequences of sugar puckers are possible: (1) B-DNA can bend 39° to yield a kink in which the sugar puckers and glycosidic bonds remain unchanged (conservative conformational change). (2) B-DNA can bend with an accompanying change in sugar puckers to the alternating C(2′)-endo to C(3′)-endo forms and with a change in glycosidic angles analogous to an intercalation site (non-conservative conformational change). Of the two conformational changes, the non-conservative one provides a pathway which is favored and allows an explanation of the experimental data of intercalation followed by covalent binding (Geacintov, et al. 1981; Meehan, et al. 1982; MacLeod, Selkirk 1982).

Table 2. Binding of diastereoisomers of BPDE to N2 on guanine in the 3′- and 5′-orientations in a kinked site (K).[a]

BPDE Adduct	Benzo Ring	3′-orientation			Benzo Ring	5′-orientation		
		β	γ	δE^K_{BPDE}		β	γ	δE^K_{BPDE}
I(+)	Cde:	−68	−21	16.4	Cde:	70	102	0.0
II(+)	Cda:	−60	−5	13.6	Cda:	70	99	4.8
I(−)	Cde:	−77	−73	64.5	Cde:	56	97	10^4
II(−)	Cda:	−77	−74	68.5	Cda:	54	95	10^5

[a]The intermolecular energy, δE^K_{BPDE} (kcal), between each BPDE and kinked DNA as well as β, γ (deg) and the benzo ring conformation are reported relative to the global minimum.

An analysis of the energy changes for the creation of receptor sites favors 5′ binding for both the intercalation and kink sites. The intercalation process orients the

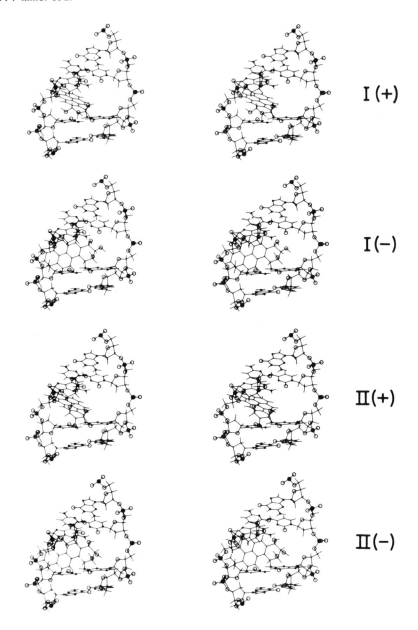

Fig. 3 Covalently bound diastereoisomers of the BPDEs with kinked DNA. Optimum conformations for 5´ binding are illustrated.

epoxide in position for subsequent adduct formation.
Stereoselectivity has not emerged. It appears when the BPDE
are placed in position for covalent bond formation. The
energies were calculated for adduct formation with each of
the four conformations of the benzo ring in each of the diastereoisomers. The minima for 3´ and 5´ (preferred, Fig. 3)
binding are listed in Table 2. Not only does the B-DNA ad-
just to receptor sites favoring 5´ binding, but also, adduct
formation favors 5´ binding. BPDE I(+) is the most favored
isomer in the formation of a covalent bond. Interestingly,
the BPDE II(+) also exhibits favorable non-bonded contacts
between the DNA and pyrene moiety. Experimental results
(Undeman, et al. 1983) with racemic BPDE I(±) and BPDE II(±)
show two types of binding. The first is favored by the I(±)
isomers and the second by the II(±) isomers. We suggest
that BPDE II(+) also forms an adduct with N2 on guanine.

The present model demonstrates that the process of
stereoselectivity entails the relative stability of CpG and
TpG receptor sites in DNA, the favorable positioning of the
epoxide during intercalation for subsequent covalent binding
to N2 on guanine and finally the accessibility of the BPDEs
to the environment of the DNA at the site of N2 adduct formation. In our model all of these processes favor 5´
binding of the BPDE I(+) and BPDE II(+) enantiomers and exclude the BPDE I(−) and BPDE II(−) enantiomers from covalent
bond formation with N2 on guanine. A paper containing a more
detailed analysis of this work is in preparation.

The authors acknowledge the grant of computer time from
Rensselaer Polytechnic Institute and support by the National
Institutes of Health under Grant CA-28924.

Ames BN, Sims, P, Grover PL (1972). Epoxides of carcinogenic polycyclic hydrocarbons are frameshift mutagens.
Science 176:47.
Brooks P, Lawley PD (1964). Evidence for the binding of
polynuclear aromatic hydrocarbons to the nucleic acids of
mouse skin: Relation between carcinogenic power of
hydrocarbons and their binding to deoxyribonucleic acid.
Nature 202:781.
Gagliano AG, Geacintov NE, Ibanez V, Harvey RG, Lee HM
(1982). Application of fluorescence and linear dichroism
techniques to the characterization of the covalent adducts
derived from interaction of (±)-trans-9,10-dihydroxy-

anti-11,12-epoxy-9,10,11,12-tetrahydrobenzo[e]pyrene with DNA. Carcinogenesis 3:969.

Gamper HB, Straub K, Calvin M, Bartholomew JC (1980). DNA alkylation and unwinding induced by benzo[a]pyrene diol epoxide: Modulation by ionic strength and superhelicity. Proc Natl Acad Sci (USA) 77:2000.

Geacintov NE, Gagliano A, Ivanovic V, Weinstein IB (1978). Electric linear dichroism study of the orientation of benzo[a]pyrene-7,8-dihydrodiol 9,10-oxide covalently bond to DNA. Biochemistry 17:5256.

Geacintov NE, Yoshida H, Ibanez V, Harvey RG (1981). Non-covalent intercalative binding of the 7,8-dihydroxy-9,10-epoxybenzo(a)pyrene to DNA. Biochem Biophys Res Commun 100:1569.

Hogan ME, Dattagupta N, Whitlock Jr. JP (1981). Carcinogen-induced alteration of DNA structure. J Biol Chem 256:4504.

Huberman E, Sachs L, Yang SK, Gelboin HV (1976). Identification of mutagenic metabolites of benzo[a]pyrene in mammalian cells. Proc Natl Acad Sci (USA) 73:607.

Jeffrey AM, Jennette KW, Blobstein SH, Weinstein IB, Beland FA, Harvey RG, Kasai H, Miura I, Nakanishi K (1976). Benzo[a]pyrene nucleic acid-derivative found in vivo: structure of a benzo[a]pyrene tetrahydrodiol epoxide-guanosine adduct. J Amer Chem Soc 98:5714.

Jennette KW, Jeffrey AM, Blobstein SH, Beland FA, Harvey RG, Weinstein IB (1977). Nucleoside adducts from the in vitro reaction of benzo[a]pyrene-7,8-dihydrodiol 9,10-oxide or benzo[a]pyrene 4,5-oxide with nucleic acids. Biochemistry 16:932.

King HW, Osborne MR, Beland FA, Harvey RG, Brookes P (1976). (±)-7α, 8β-Dihydroxy- 9β, 10β-epoxy-7, 8, 9,10-tetrahydro-benzo[a]pyrene is an intermediate in the metabolism and binding to DNA of benzo[a]pyrene. Proc Natl Acad Sci (USA) 73:2679.

Koreeda M, Moore PD, Yagi H, Yeh, HJ, Jerina DM (1976). Alkylation of polyguanylic acid to the 2-amino group and phosphate by the potent mutagen (±)-7β,8α-dihydroxy 9β,10β-epoxy 7,8,9,10-tetrahydro benzo[a]pyrene. J Amer Chem Soc 98:6720.

McCann J, Choi E, Yamasaki E, Ames BN (1975). Detection of carcinogens as mutagens in the Salmonella/microsome test: Assay of 300 chemicals. Proc Natl Acad Sci (USA) 72:5135.

MacLeod MC, Selkirk JK (1982). Physical interactions of isomeric benzo[a]pyrene diol-epoxides with DNA. Carcinogenesis 3:287.

Meehan T, Straub K, Calvin M (1976). Elucidation of hydrocarbon structure in an enzyme-catalyzed benzo[a]pyrene-
poly(G) covalent complex. Proc Natl Acad Sci (USA)
73:1437.

Meehan T, Straub K, Calvin M (1977). Benzo(a)pyrene diol
epoxide covalently binds to deoxyguanosine and deoxyadenosine in DNA. Nature 269:725.

Meehan T, Straub K (1979). Double-stranded DNA stereoselectivity binds benzo(a)pyrene diol epoxides.
Nature 277:410.

Meehan T, Gamper H, Becker J (1982). Characterization of
reversible, physical binding of benzo[a]pyrene derivatives
to DNA. J Biol Chem 257:10479.

Miller KJ, Pycior JF (1979). Interactions of molecules
with nucleic acids. II. Two pairs of families of intercalation sites, unwinding angles, and the neighbor-
exclusion principle. Biopolymers 18:2683.

Miller KJ, Brodzinsky R, Hall S (1980). Interactions of
molecules with nucleic acids. IV. Binding energies and
conformations of acridine and phenanthridine compounds in
the two principal and in several unconstrained dimer-
duplex intercalation sites. Biopolymers 19:2091.

Miller KJ (1981). Three families of intercalation sites
for parallel base pairs: a theoretical model. In Sarma
RH (Ed): "Proceedings of the Second SUNYA Conversation in
the Discipline Biomolecular Stereodynamics", Vol II. New
York: Adenine Press, p 469.

Ornstein R, Rein R (1979). Energetics of intercalation
specificity. I. Backbone unwinding. Biopolymers 18:1277.

Sims P, Grover PL, Swaisland A, Pal K, Hewer A (1974).
Metabolic activation of benzo(a)pyrene proceeds by a diol-
epoxide. Nature (London) 252:326.

Taylor ER, Miller KJ (1983). Interactions of molecules with
nucleic acids. X. Covalent intercalative binding of the
carcinogenic BPDE I(+) to kinked DNA. J Biomolec Struct
and Dynamics 1:883.

Undeman O, Lycksell P-O, Graslund A, Astlind T, Ehrenberg A,
Jernstrom B, Tjerneld F, Norden B (1983). Covalent complexes of DNA and two stereoisomers of benzo(a)pyrene 7,8-
dihydrodiol 9,10-epoxide studied by fluorescence and
linear dichroism. Cancer Res. 43: 1851.

Weinstein IB, Jeffrey AM, Jennette KW, Blobstein SH, Harvey
RG, Harris C, Autrup H, Kasai H, Nakanishi K (1976).
Benzo[a]pyrene diol epoxides as intermediates in nucleic
acid binding in vitro and in vivo. Science 193:592.

Molecular Basis of Cancer, Part A: Macromolecular
Structure, Carcinogens, and Oncogenes, pages 199–206
© 1985 Alan R. Liss, Inc.

NMR STUDIES OF CARCINOGEN-MODIFIED DNA MODEL COMPOUNDS

Harold C. Box, Ph.D., Minoti Sharma, Ph.D.
and James L. Alderfer, Ph.D.

Biophysics Department
Roswell Park Memorial Institute
Buffalo, New York 14263

INTRODUCTION

Chemical carcinogens produce a variety of lesions in DNA. A particular chemical carcinogen will generally cause several different lesions. Ionizing and non-ionizing radiations also produce a variety of DNA lesions. Biological tests for carcinogenesis are unable to associate a biological endpoint with any specific type of DNA damage. It is useful therefore to examine carcinogenic effects at the level of molecular structure and function. In a molecular approach one has the advantage of being able to evaluate one lesion at a time for its effect on the conformation and function of DNA (Grunberger and Santella, 1983). A central consideration in such investigations is how the carcinogen-induced lesion may compromise the DNA's capacity to properly base pair. Inability to properly base pair may introduce an heritable change into the genome and thus provide the molecular basis of initiation.

NMR spectroscopy affords a means for examining many aspects of nucleic acid conformation and function. It is interesting to compare the information that is obtained from NMR spectroscopy and X-ray diffraction studies of molecular structure presuming the measurements are made on solutions and single crystals respectively. The crystallographer generally observes the molecule in a single conformation and is able to provide a complete description of conformation in terms of atomic coordinates. The observations of the NMR spectroscopist, on the other hand, indicate the conformational preferences of the molecule and the

information is obtained piecemeal. Figure 1 indicates some
of the functional and conformational features that can be
inferred from H-1, C-13 and P-31 NMR studies on model systems of nucleic acids. H-1 NMR measurements on exchange-
able hydrogen can provide information on base pairing
configurations. Chemical shift data, H-1 and C-13, are
useful indicators of stacking arrangements between conju-
gated moieties. Carbohydrate proton spin-spin couplings
provide information on the conformation of the carbohydrate moieties. Selected carbohydrate C-13 chemical
shifts are indicative of the conformation of a nucleoside
about its glycosidic bond. P-31 NMR provides information
concerning the conformation of the backbone. In recent
years, as NMR technology continues to develop, Nuclear
Overhauser Enhancement (NOE) and two-dimensional NMR
techniques are being used to deduce spatial and bonding
relationships between protons. Thus, the NMR approach to
the study of carcinogen-modified DNA is highly variegated.
This report will focus on the usefulness of C-13 and P-31
NMR spectroscopies in studies of carcinogen-modified model
DNA compounds.

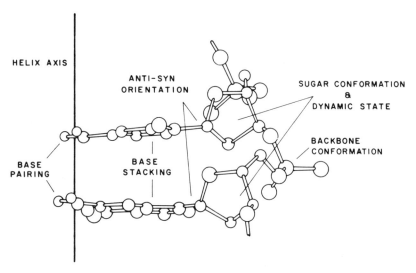

Fig. 1. Conformational features of DNA molecules.

C-13 AND P-31 NMR STUDIES

Since the natural abundance of C-13 is only 1% and the magnetic moment of the C-13 nucleus is one-fourth that of the proton, the sensitivity of C-13 NMR is about three orders of magnitude less than that of H-1 NMR spectroscopy. This is an important practical consideration in the application of C-13 NMR to the study of carcinogens. In preliminary studies on carcinogen-modified dinucleoside monophosphates it was found that 10-20 mg samples were required to make such studies feasible (Alderfer et al., 1984). Measurements were made at 50 MHz and the average duration of a run required to obtain quality C-13 NMR spectra was 16 hrs. Limitations imposed by poor sensitivity must be compensated for as far as possible by using samples of optimum size and concentration. Fortunately, the continued development of the triester method of oligodeoxynucleotide synthesis indicates that sufficient quantities of representative lengths of DNA bearing specific lesions can be obtained to make such studies worthwhile.

Grunberger and colleagues (Grunberger et al., 1970; Nelson et al., 1971) initiated the study of carcinogen-induced conformational effects by means of NMR in their well known investigation of AAF (acetylaminofluorene)-modified ribose dinucleoside monophosphates. They demonstrated that the fluorene moiety displaced guanine in stacking with adenine. The base displacement model of AAF's mode of action was enunciated. These early studies were limited, of course, to H-1 NMR measurements. We decided to investigate what further information might be gleaned from C-13 and P-31 NMR measurements on DNA model systems.

The dinucleotides dpApG and dpGpA were reacted with acetoxyacetylaminofluorene and the AAF adduct formed at the 8 position of guanine was isolated (Box et al., 1984). There are five carbon atom resonances in purine bases that can be monitored for chemical shift changes. All five adenine carbon atom resonances in AAF-modified dpApG and in AAF-modified dpGpA exhibited upfield shifts when compared with unmodified dpApG and dpGpA. The average chemical shift change was -.80 PPM for the former and -.30 PPM for the latter. Similarly, most carbon atom resonances of the fluorene moiety exhibited an upfield shift when compared with the corresponding AAF-modified monomer. The average

chemical shift change for the fluorene carbon atoms (ex-
cluding those resonances which are motionally broadened)
was -.84 for AAF-modified dpApG and -.02 for AAF-modified
dpGpA. These chemical shift changes are clearly indicative
of stacking between the adenine base and fluorene moieties.

Among the carbohydrate carbon atom resonances the C2'
resonance exhibited the most pronounced change in chemical
shift. The C2' resonance shifted -2.52 PPM upfield in AAF-
modified dpApG compared with the unmodified dinucleotide.
In AAF-modified dpGpA the corresponding chemical shift
change was -2.36. Uesugi and Ikehara (1977) observed analogous upfield shift changes of the C-13 resonance in a
variety of purine nucleosides substituted at the 8 position. The C-13 chemical shift changes seemed not to be
related to the nature of the substituent. These authors
ascribe the chemical shift change to a change in conformation, namely a rotation about the glycosidic bond. Instead
of the anti conformation typical of unsubstituted purines,
the modified molecules tend toward a syn conformation.
Presumably a similar conformational change occurs in AAF-
modified dinucleotides.

The P-31 resonances of the phosphodiester linkages in
AAF-modified dpApG and AAF-modified dpGpA are shifted downfield with respect to the unmodified dimers. In the former
the change in chemcal shift is 0.96 and in the latter it is
0.23. Phosphodiester downfield shifts are associated with
a change in the conformation from the usual gauche, gauche
conformation of a nucleic acid toward a gauche, trans conformation (Gorenstein, 1978; Alderfer and Hazel, 1981).
This type of conformational change results in extension of
the backbone structure of the nucleic acid.

The picture that emerges from C-13 and P-31 studies of
AAF-modified dinucleotides is in conformity with the base
displacement model originally proposed (Grunberger et al.,
1970; Nelson et al., 1971) but provides considerably more
detail. Summarizing, base carbon atom C-13 chemical shift
data clearly indicate stacking of the adenine and fluorene
moieties, carbohydrate C2' chemical shifts are indicative
of a preference for the syn conformation about the glycosidic bond and P-31 chemical shifts are indicative of tendency toward a guache, trans conformation of the backbone.
It is interesting to note that all of the indices used to
monitor these changes are larger for AAF-modified dpApG

than for AAF-modified dpGpA.

PROSPECTUS

Preliminary attempts to use C-13 and P-31 NMR spectroscopies to obtain information on the conformation of
carcinogen-modified DNA have been encouraging. There may
be other aspects of conformation, in addition to those
already discussed, that can be deduced from C-13 spectra.
Figure 2 illustrates the carbohydrate portion of a dinucleotide (dpGpA). As one might expect, the carbon atoms within three bond lengths of a backbone phosphorus atom exhibit
carbon-phosphorus spin-spin coupling. Thus the C2', C3'
and C5' resonances of deoxyguanosine and the C4' and C5'
resonances of deoxyadenosine exhibit doublet splittings.
The C4' nucleus of guanosine experiences both phosphorus
nuclei and exhibits a further splitting. Although not
readily apparent in Figure 2a (lower trace), these spin-
spin splittings are generally measureable in the unmodified
dimer. Alderfer and Ts'o (1977) have discussed the relationship of carbon-phosphorus splittings to conformation.
Our interest would be, of course, to relate changes in
carbon-phosphorus splittings to changes in conformation
induced by the carcinogen. However, a difficulty arises.
Selective broadening of C-13 carbohydrate resonances occurs
in AAF-modified dimers which is of the same order of magnitude as the spin-spin splittings. Figure 2b (upper trace)
shows the effect of the AAF modification on dpGpA. It is
interesting to note that adenosine as well as guanosine
carbohydrate resonances may be broadened. In Figure 2, the
A3' resonance is a striking example. The broadening effects are due to conformational changes occurring on a time
scale appropriate to the NMR experiment and are reduced, of
course, at higher temperatures. The motional implications
of the observed broadenings are not yet clear. We have
observed, however, that these broadening effects are less
of an impediment to C-13 NMR measurements than to H-1 NMR
measurements, which may be another important reason for
pursuing ^{13}C NMR studies.

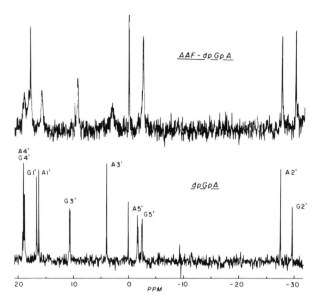

Fig. 2. Carbohydrate portion of the C-13 NMR spectrum of
AAF-modified dpGpA (upper trace) and of dpGpA
(lower trace).

It must be kept in mind that a serious practical limitation in the application of the C-13 NMR is the need for a
substantial quantity of the modified DNA model compound.
The extension of these studies to longer oligomers more
representative of DNA polymer would be highly desirable.
Figure 3 shows the C-13 NMR spectrum of the hexamer
dTACGTA. Evidently resolution of the individual carbon
atoms in each of the bases is still retained at this level.
Most carbohydrate carbon atoms, although generally split by
carbon-phosphorus spin-spin splittings, are also distinguishable. Initial efforts to obtain the AAF-modified hexamer indicate that sufficient amounts of material can be
obtained to carry out C-13 NMR studies and this work is in
progress.

ACKNOWLEDGEMENT

This work was supported by grant CA 29425 from the
National Cancer Institute.

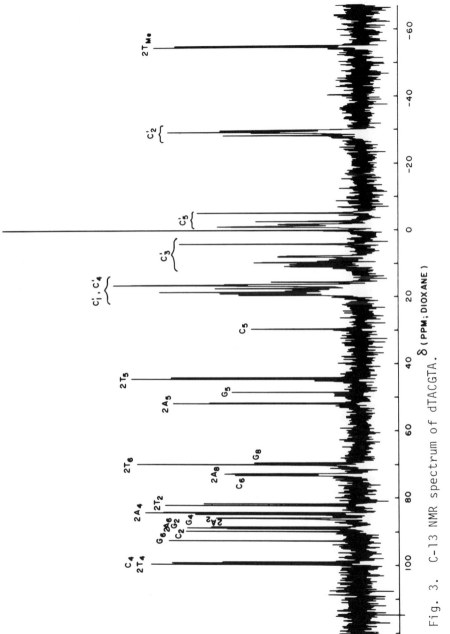

Fig. 3.   C-13 NMR spectrum of dTACGTA.

Alderfer JL, Lilga KT, French JB, Box HC (1984). Chem.-Biol. Interactions 48:69.

Alderfer JL, Hazel GL (1981). J. Amer. Chem. Soc. 103:5925.

Alderfer JL and Ts'o POP (1977). Biochemistry 16:2410.

Box HC, Lilga KT, French JB, Alderfer JL (1984) Chem.-Biol. Interactions, in press.

Gorenstein DG (1978). In Pullman B (ed) "Nuclear Magnetic Resonance Spectroscopy in Molecular Biology".

Grunberger D, Nelson JH, Cantor CR, Weinstein IB (1970). Proc. Natl. Acad. Sci. USA 66:488.

Grunberger D, Santella RM (1983), in "Genes and Proteins" in Oncogenesis".

Nelson JH, Grunberger D, Cantor CR, Weinstein IB (1971). J. Mol. Biol. 62:331.

Uesugi S, Ikehara M (1977). J. Amer. Chem. Soc. 99:3250.

**Molecular Basis of Cancer, Part A: Macromolecular
Structure, Carcinogens, and Oncogenes, pages 207–216
© 1985 Alan R. Liss, Inc.**

SEQUENCE SPECIFIC AND STEREOSELECTIVE COVALENT BINDING OF
TRANS-7,8-DIHYDROXY-ANTI-9,10-EPOXY-7,8,9,10-TETRAHYDRO-
BENZO[A]PYRENE TO DNA

Fu-Ming Chen

Department of Chemistry
Tennessee State University
Nashville, Tennessee 37203

The most widely studied polycyclic aromatic hydrocarbon
(PAH) is benzo[a]pyrene (BP) and there is strong evidence to
suggest that the ultimate carcinogenic metabolite is trans-
7,8-dihydroxy-anti-9,10-epoxy-7,8,9,10-tetrahydro-benzo[a]-
pyrene (anti-BPDE). Of the two enantiomers of anti-BPDE,
the (+) isomer is much more carcinogenic than the (-)
variety (Buening, et al 1978; Slaga, et al 1979) which
correlates well with the DNA binding ability of these two
enantiomers in vitro (Meehan, Straub 1979).

Anti-BPDE has been shown to preferentially form
covalent bonds to the exocyclic amino group of guanine
(Weinstein, et al 1976; Jeffrey, et al 1977). Experiments
with natural DNA has shown that such covalent binding is
quite stereo- selective, i.e. the preference of
(+)anti-BPDE, for the duplex DNA but is devoid of such
effect for the single-stranded form (Meehan, Straub 1979).
Such specificity is lost for anti-BPDE modification at the
adenine sites and the (+) and (-) enantiomers react equally
in either single- or double-stranded DNA. It has been
suggested that such stereoselectivity on the covalent
binding to the guanine base is the consequence of
stereospecific physical binding such as intercalation
(Meehan, Straub 1979).

There is, indeed, evidence to indicate that the
predominant mode of physical binding between anti-BPDE and
the duplex DNA is that of intercalation (Geacintov, et al
1981) which led to the suggestion that the covalent linkage
is preceded by intercalative physical binding (Meehan, et al

1982). There is also strong spectroscopic evidence to
suggest that the covalently linked anti-BPDE resides
external to DNA and presumably in the minor groove
(Geacintov, et al 1980; Lefkowitz, et al 1982). It is thus
puzzling that if intercalative physical binding precedes
chemical lesion why should the covalent adducts exhibit
external binding characteristics?

To help answer some of these questions, we have earlier
carried out physical binding studies with synthetic
polynucleotides using pyrene (Chen 1983) and
anti-BPDE-tetraol (anti-BPT) (Chen 1984) as model compounds
for anti-BPDE. Specifically, we were interested in finding
out the possible base sequence preference on such binding
since if intercalation is the dominant binding mode it
should depend on π-electron interactions between the pyrene
chromophore and the sandwiching bases. These studies reveal
that in neutral pH the intercalative binding modes of pyrene
and anti-BPT are important in poly(dA-dT):poly(dA-dT), much
less so in poly(dG-dC):poly(dG-dC) and
poly(dA-dC):poly(dG-dT), and negligible in poly(dG):poly(dC)
and poly(dA):poly(dT) solutions. Based on these
observations as well as the fact that intercalative binding
of anti-BPDE to the duplex DNA accelerates its hydrolysis to
tetraols (Geacintov, et al 1980), we have earlier speculated
that in neutral solutions intercalation may have little, if
any, to do with the chemical lesion of anti-BPDE to the
guanine base of DNA. It may, on the contrary, provide an
efficient pathway for detoxification at the intercalating
(dA-dT and/or dT-dA) sites through accelerated hydrolysis.
Chemical lesions presumably occur mainly at the external
sites and consequently the covalent adducts exhibit external
spectral characteristics.

To further clarify the interplay between the physical
binding and chemical lesion, covalent binding studies of
anti-BPDE to synthetic polynucleotides are hereby carried
out.

EXTENT OF COVALENT MODIFICATION ON POLYNUCLEOTIDES BY
ANTI-BPDE

Absorption spectra of anti-BPDE chemically bound to
various polynucleotides are shown in Figs. 1A and 1B.
Interesting features to be noted are: (1) poly(dG-dC):
poly(dG-dC) and poly(dG):poly(dC) exhibit the highest

binding abilities with the homopolymer slightly more
effective and their absorbance maxima are about 2-3 nm red
shifted from the corresponding tetraols; (2) Significant
binding occurs with poly(dA):poly(dT) and is more effective
than its sequence isomer poly(dA-dT):poly(dA-dT) and no
shift in absorption maxima are observed; (3) the spectrum of
anti-BPDE bound to poly(dA-dC):poly(dG-dT) is broadened and
the amplitudes are slightly lower than poly(dA):poly(dT);
(4) the spectrum of anti-BPDE adduct of natural DNA is
similar to those of dG-dC polymers with a 2-3 nm red shift;
(5) anti-BPDE attached to poly(G) exhibits almost
featureless spectrum with major contribution from the 350 nm
band being quite evident; (6) anti-BPDE can chemically bind
to Z-form poly(dG-dC):poly(dG-dC) (induced by 50 uM
hexaminecobalt) and the extent of binding as well as
spectral features are almost identical to those of
poly(dA):poly(dT) but not to the B-form poly(dG-dC):
poly(dG-dC).

Higher binding abilities of the two G:C polymers are to
be expected as anti-BPDE is known to be quite guanine
specific. The 2-3nm red shifts of pyrenyl absorption maxima
in these polynucleotides are consistent with earlier DNA
observations (Geacintov, et al 1982; Undeman, et al 1983).
Significant anti-BPDE modification on poly(dA):poly(dT) as
well as the large difference with its sequence isomer
poly(dA-dT): poly(dA-dT) are rather interesting and
unexpected as previous studies indicate adenine adducts to
be only minor products formed between anti-BPDE and native
DNA (Meehan, Straub 1979). The reduced binding to
poly(dA-dC):poly(dG-dT) as compared to the G:C polymers are
understandable in terms of the decreased guanine content and
the lower binding ability of the alternating dA polymer.
The spectral similarity of chemically reacted anti-BPDE in
natural DNA and G:C polymers are consistent with its guanine
specificity.

The distinct broad specturm exibited by anti-BPDE in
poly(G) is the consequence of important contribution from
the 8-nm red shifted spectrum. This is significant as it
suggests that stacking interactions between the pyrene
moiety and guanine base occurs in anti-BPDE modified
poly(G). The absence of such 8-nm red shifts in anti-BPDE
modified natural and synthetic duplex DNAs suggests that the
pyrene moiety does not intercalate into DNA in the classical
sense.

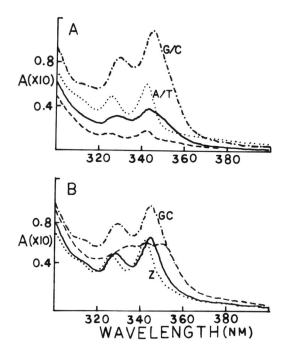

Fig. 1. Absorption spectra of covalently attached anti-BPDE
in (A): 0.1 mM poly(dG):poly(dC) (-.-.-); 0.1 mM poly(dA):
poly(dT) (. . . .); 0.1 mM poly(dA-dC):poly(dG-dT) (———);
0.1 mM poly(dA-dT):poly(dA-dT) (- - -). (B): 0.1 mM
poly(dG-dC):poly(dG-dC) (-.-.-); 0.1 mM Z-DNA (˙ ˙ ˙)
containing 50 uM hexaminecobalt (III); 0.2 mM natural DNA
(———); 0.05 mM poly(G) (- - -). All solutions are
prepared by adding 13.7 uL of 4.6 mM anti-BPDE stock
solution in tetrahydrofuran (THF) to 2.5 mL of a
polynucleotide solution with the concentration indicated
above. The mixture is then let stand for at least two hours
to ensure maximum modification and subsequently extracted
with ether (saturated with 10 mM sodium phosphate/10 mM
NaCl/1 mM EDTA/pH 7.0 buffer) for about 25 times to remove
the non-covalently bound tetraols. Absorbance measurements
were made with a Cary 210 spectrophtometric system using
cuvettes of 1 cm pathlength. Respective unmodified DNA
spectrum has been substracted out.

The smaller but significant modification on Z-form poly(dG-dC):poly(dG-dC) as compared to the B-form is also interesting and may be the consequence of the fact that now the reactive 2-amino group of guanine is residing in the deep groove thus making it less accessible for the ligand attack. Covalent attachments to other groups cannot be ruled out, however. The absence of a 2-3 nm red shift in contrast to its corresponding B form suggests that the pyrene moiety is in a microenvironment which is less perturbed by the bases as compared to adducts of B form poly(dG-dC):poly(dG-dC).

SEQUENCE DEPENDENT STEREOSELECTIVE COVALENT BINDING OF ANTI-BPDE

Although the extent and the absorption spectral characteristics of anti-BPDE modification on the two G:C polymers are quite similar, their corresponding CD spectra are strikingly different as can be seen in Fig. 2A. CD spectrum of anti-BPDE bound to poly(dG-dC):poly(dG-dC) exhibits strong negative maxima at 343 and 327 nm whereas that of poly(dG):poly(dC) shows positive long wavelength maximum with definite red shift. This red shift undoubtedly arises from partial spectral cancellation from the negative contributions of slightly shorter wavelengths as evidenced by the appearance of a weak 327 nm negative maximum. CD spectrum for anti-BPDE bound to DNA is similar to that of poly(dG-dC):poly(dG-dC) but with much reduced intensity and can partially be attributed to the spectral cancellation of these two sequences.

The CD spectra of anti-BPDE bound to other polynucleotides are at least an order of magnitude smaller than those of G-C polymers and the ones with detectable Cotton effects are shown in Fig. 2B (note the reduced scale). Consistent with the absorbance observation, broad negative CD bands are observed for poly(dA-dC):poly(dG-dT). Weak negative CD maximum at 352 nm is apparent in poly(G) solution as a consequence of stereoselective stacking interaction between the pyrene moiety and the guanine base. It is also interesting to note that negative CD maxima are detected for anti-BPDE bound to Z-DNA at 343 and 327 nm, same locations as those of absorbance. Although the order of magnitude smaller Cotton effects detected are, to be sure, partially due to the less extensive covalent binding of anti-BPDE to these polynucleotides (2-3 times less), it

cannot account for the bulk of optical inactivity. For
example, although poly(dA):poly(dT) is about half as
effective as poly(dG):poly(dC) in its chemical lesion to
anti-BPDE, no detectable Cotton effects are observed. One
is, thus, led to the conclusion that the covalent binding of
anti-BPDE to these polynucleotides are less stereoselective
than the G:C polymers.

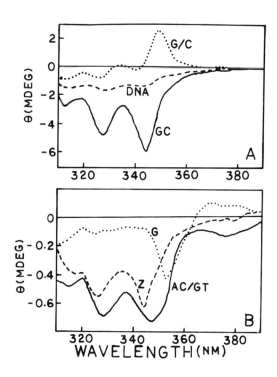

Fig. 2. CD spectra in the pyrene spectral region of some
anti-BPDE modified polynucleotide solutions. (A): 0.1 mM
poly(dG):poly(dC) (. . . .); 0.1 mM poly(dG-dC):poly(dG-dC)
(————); 0.2 mM DNA (- - -). (B): 0.1 mM poly(dA-dC):
poly(dG-dT) (————); 0.1 mM Z-DNA (- - -); 0.05 mM
poly(G) (. . . .). Note the ten times smaller ellipticity
scale in B. Solution preparations are as described in Fig.
1. CD measurements are made at room temperatures with JASCO
J-500A spectropolarimeter using a 2 cm cell.

To further investigate the stereoselective binding of
anti-BPDE to the two G:C polymers, difference CD spectra are
obtained by substracting the unmodified polynucleotide
spectra from the corresponding anti-BPDE modified ones and
the results are presented in Fig. 3 for the shorter
wavelength region. Consistent with the dramatic difference

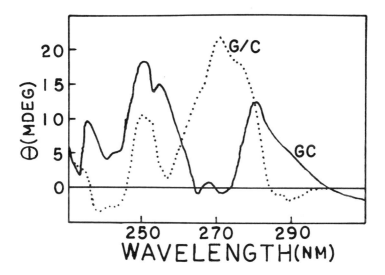

Fig. 3. Difference CD spectra between the anti-BPDE modified
and unmodified DNA solutions. 0.1 mM poly(dG-dC):
poly(dG-dC) (————) and 0.1 mM poly(dG):poly(dC) (. . .)
solutions.

in the pyrene spectral region, the difference CD spectra
below 300 nm are quite distinct for anti-BPDE bound to
poly(dG-dC):poly(dG-dC) and to poly(dG):poly(dC). The
positive CD maxima at 280 and 250 nm (Fig. 3) and negative
maxima at 343 and 327 nm (Fig. 2A) in the poly(dG-dC):
poly(dG-dC) adduct are consistent with the predominant
(+)anti-BPDE trans addition as observed in native as well as
poly(G) adducts (Jeffrey, et al 1977; Moore, et al 1977).
The difference spectrum below 300 nm for the
poly(dG):poly(dC) adduct does not appear to conform with any
reported CD on diastereomeric adducts of guanosine,
suggesting combined contribution from more than one
stereomeric addition. Indeed, the positive 346 nm band
(Fig. 2A) suggests a (-)anti-BPDE trans and/or (+)anti-BPDE

cis addition at C-10 position. The appearance of a negative
maximum at 327 nm and a positive maximum around 250 nm
indicate significant contribution from the trans addition of
(+)anti-BPDE. Quantitative characterization of these
adducts must await detailed HPLC analysis.

The preference for the (+) isomer at the guanine sites
of the native DNA (Pulkrabek, et al 1979; Meehan, Straub
1979) may thus be due to the fact that only the dG-dG
sequence exhibits significant binding to the (-) isomer.
The absence of detectable pyrenyl CD spectra for the
anti-BPDE modified poly(dA-dT):poly(dA-dT) and
poly(dA):poly(dT) is also consistent with the lack of
stereoselectivity at the dA sites of the natural DNA towards
anti-BPDE binding (Pulkrabek, et al 1979; Meehan, Straub
1979). The much weaker CD signal detected in the pyrene
spectral region for the anti-BPDE modified poly(G) suggests
reduced stereoselectivity and is consistent with the
observation that diastereomers are formed in approximately
equal amounts in the poly(G) system (Meehan, et al 1977).

The kinetics of anti-BPDE hydrolysis in various
polynucleotide solutions are also investigated by monitoring
the absorbance change at 342 nm. The hydrolysis in the
buffer solution is seen to exhibit a single exponential
increase in absorbance with a first order rate constant of
$3 \times 10^{-3} s^{-1}$. It is known that the rate of anti-BPDE
hydrolysis is markedly accelerated by the presence of DNA in
the solution (Geacintov, et al 1980). This is confirmed by
the appearance of all semilog kinetic plots for
polynucleotide solutions to curve below the buffer line. It
is apparant that multiple processes are involved as
evidenced by the curvatures in these plots (results not
shown). These curves, however, are unusual in that slight
convexities appear in most plots suggesting that not all the
processes are accompanied by absorbance increase. It is
noteworthy that poly(dA-dT):poly(dA-dT) enhances hydrolysis
more than poly(dA):poly(dT) and the similarity between the
hexaminecobalt induced Z-form poly(dG-dC):poly(dG-dC) and
the latter extends even to the kinetic behavior.

It is interesting to note that the lower anti-BPDE
modification of poly(dA-dT):poly(dA-dT) as compared to
poly(dA):poly(dT) is consistent with the dominant
intercalative binding of the former and the accelerated rate
of hydrolysis at these sites, thus giving credence to our

earlier speculation on the effect of intercalation on the
anti-BPDE detoxification. The slightly reduced extent of
modification for poly(dG-dC):poly(dG-dC) as compared to
poly(dG):poly(dC) may also be of similar origin.

The significant covalent binding of anti-BPDE to the
Z-form poly(dG-dC):poly(dG-dC) and its near identical
spectral characteristics to that of poly(dA):poly(dT) are
quite interesting. The identification of dominant adducts
of this complex should render important information on the
structure of Z-DNA as well as anti-BPDE reactive pathways.

Buening MK, Wislocki PG, Levin W, Yagi H, Thakker DR, Akagi
    H, Koreeda M, Jerina DM, Conney AH (1978). Tumorigenicity
    of the optical enantiomers of the diastereomeric
    benzo[a]pyrene 7,8-diol-9,10-epoxidex in newborn mice.
    Proc Natl Acad Sci USA 75:5358.
Chen FM (1983). Binding of pyrene to DNA, base sequence
    specificity and its implication. Nucleic Acid Res
    11:7231.
Chen FM (1984). Sequence specific binding of tetraols of
    benzo[a]pyrene-diol-epoxide to DNA in neutral and acidic
    solutions. Carcinogenesis (in press).
Geacintov NE, Ibanez V, Gagliano AG, Yoshida H, Harvey RG
    (1980). Kinetics of hydrolysis to tetraols and binding of
    benzo[a]pyrene-7,8-dihydrodiol-9,10-epoxide and its
    tetraol derivatives to DNA. Conformation of adducts.
    Biochem Biophys Res Commun 92:1335.
Geacintov NE, Yoshida H, Ibanez V, Harvey RG (1981).
    Non-covalent intercalative binding of
    7,8-dihydroxy-9,10-epoxy benzo[a]pyrene to DNA. Biochem
    Biophys Res Commun 100:1569.
Geacintov NE, Gagliano AG, Ibanez V, Harvey RG (1982).
    Spectroscopic characterizations and comparisons of the
    structures of the covalent adducts derived from the
    reactions of
    7,8-dihydroxy-7,8,9,10-tetrahydrobenzo[a]pyrene-9,10-oxide,
    and the 9,10-epoxides of 7,8,9,10-tetrahydrobenzo[a]pyrene
    and 9,10,11,12-tetrahydrobenzo[e]pyrene with DNA.
    Carcinogenesis 3:247.
Jeffrey AM, Weinstein IB, Jennette KW, Grezeskowiak K,
    Nakanishi K, Harvey RG, Autrup H, Harris C (1977).
    Structure of benzo[a]pyrene-nucleic acid adducts formed in
    human and bovine bronchial explants. Nature 269:348.
Lefkowitz SM, Brenner HC (1982). Distinct local
    environments of the pyrene chromophores in the covalent

deoxyribonucleic acid adducts of
   9,10-eppoxy-9,10,11,12-tetrahydrobenzo[e]pyrene and
   7,8-dihydroxy-9,10-epoxy-7,8,9,10-tetrahydrobenzo[a]pyrene
   elucidated by optically detected magnetic resonance.
   Biochemistry 21:3735.
Slaga TJ, Bracken WJ, Gleason G, Levin W, Yagi H, Jerina DM,
   Conney AH (1979). Marked differences in the skin tumor
   initiating activities of the optical enantiomers of the
   diastereomeric benzo[a]pyrene-7,8-diol-9,10-epoxides.
   Cancer Res 39:67.
Meehan T, Straub K (1979). Double-stranded DNA
   stereoselectively binds benzo[a]pyrene diol epoxides.
   Nature 277:410.
Meehan T, Gamper H, Becker JF (1982). Characterization of
   reversible, phsical binding of benzo[a]pyrene derivatives
   to DNA. J Biol Chem 257:10479.
Moore PD, Koreeda M, Wislocki PG, Levin W, Conney AH, Yagi
   H, Jerina DM (1977). In vitro reactions of the
   diastereomeric 9,10-epoxides of (+) and
   (-)-trans-7,8-dihydroxy-7,8-dihydrobenzo[a]pyrene with
   polyguanylic acid and evidence for formation of an
   enantiomer of each diastereomeric 9,10-epoxide from
   benzo[a]pyrene in mouse skin. ACS Symposium Series
   44:127.
Pulkrabek P, Leffler S, Weinstein IB, Grunberger D (1977).
   Conformation of DNA modified with dihydrodiol epoxide
   derivative of benzo[a]pyrene. Biochemistry 16:3127.
Pulkrabek P, Leffler S, Grungerger D, Weinstein IB (1979).
   Modification of deoxyribonucleic acid by a diol epoxide of
   benzo[a]pyrene. Biochemistry 18:5128.
Undeman O, Lycksell P-O, Graslund A, Astlind T, Ehrenberg A,
   Jernstrom B, Tjerneld F, Norden B (1983). Covalent
   complexes of DNA and two stereoisomers of benzo[a]pyrene
   7,8-dihydrodiol-9,10-epoxide studied by fluorescence and
   linear dichroism. Cancer Res 43:1851.
Weinstein IB, Jeffrey AM, Jennette KW, Blobstein SH, Harvey
   RG, Harris C, Autrup H, Kasai H, Nakanishi K (1976).
   Benzo[a]pyrene diol epoxides as intermediates in nucleic
   acid binding in vitro and in vivo. Science 193:592.

ACKNOWLEDGMENTS

     This work is supported by PHS Grant CA29817 and in
part by MBRS Grant S06RR08092.

**Molecular Basis of Cancer, Part A: Macromolecular
Structure, Carcinogens, and Oncogenes, pages 217–225**
© **1985 Alan R. Liss, Inc.**

A COMPARISON OF THE DNA INTERCALATIVE BINDING OF BAY
VERSUS K REGION METABOLITES OF BENZO(a)PYRENE

M. Abramovich*, I.S. Zegar*, A.S. Prakash*,
R.G. Harvey[+] and P.R. LeBreton*

*Department of Chemistry
 University of Illinois at Chicago
 Chicago, Illinois 60680
 and
[+]Ben May Laboratory for Cancer Research
 University of Chicago
 Chicago, Illinois 60637

SUMMARY

The DNA intercalating properties of trans-7,8-dihy-
droxy-7,8-dihydrobenzo[a]pyrene (1) and of trans-4,5-di-
hydroxy-4,5-dihydrobenzo[a]pyrene (2) have been compared
in UV absorption and in fluorescence emission and fluorescence lifetime studies. Molecules 1 and 2 represent
steric models of the two epoxide containing metabolites
of benzo[a]pyrene, trans-7,8-dihydroxy-anti-9,10-epoxy-
7,8,9,10-tetrahydrobenzo[a]pyrene (BPDE) and benzo[a]py-
rene-4,5-oxide. The former of these metabolites is a
highly carcinogenic bay region metabolite, the latter is
a much less carcinogenic K region metabolite. The association constant for intercalation for model 1 is 5,226
M^{-1}. This is more than 2.7 times greater than that for
molecule 2.

These results taken together with results form previous studies of bay and K region metabolite models of
benz[a]anthracene suggest that intercalation is important
to the overall carcinogenic activity of polycyclic aromatic hydrocarbons.

INTRODUCTION

The DNA intercalation of reactive epoxide containing polycyclic aromatic hydrocarbon metabolites is thought to be important to the carcinogenic activity of these molecules. (Zegar 1984, Shahbaz 1983, Yang 1983, Meehan 1982, Meehan 1981, Lin 1980, Meehan 1979) Physical intercalation prior to reaction may influence the sites of reaction (Lin 1980; Meehan 1979; Meehan 1981; Meehan 1982; Yang 1983) and the reactivity of the epoxide group (Geacintov 1982; MacLeod 1982).

Recent studies of nonreactive metabolite models of 7,12-dimethylbenz[a]anthracene indicate that the highly carcinogenic bay region metabolite models have intercalation binding constants which lie in the range 2.3–1.6 x 10^3 M^{-1} and are more than 4 times greater than those of less carcinogenic K region models (Shahbaz 1983). In these studies physical binding was separated from reactive binding by using metabolite models in which the reactive epoxide group was not present. Physical binding studies of the bay region diol epoxide of benzo[a]pyrene indicate that, in aqueous medium at pH values of 7.0-7.4, DNA intercalation readily occurs with an association constant in the range 6,500-12,000 M^{-1} (Geacintov 1982; MacLeod 1982).

In the study reported here we have compared the intercalative binding of bay and K region metabolites of benzo[a]pyrene by examining hydroxylated models of the reactive bay and K region epoxides trans-7,8-hydroxy-anti-9,10-epoxy-7,8,9,10-tetrahydrobenzo[a]pyrene and benzo[a]pyrene-4,5-oxide. The models studied are trans-7,8-dihydroxy-7,8-dihydrobenzo[a]pyrene (1) and trans-4,5-dihydroxy-4,5-dihydrobenzo[a]pyrene (2). Molecule 1 is especially interesting because it is a metabolic precursor of the bay region diol epoxide of benzo[a]pyrene. The structures of the reactive metabolites and of the nonreactive models used are given in Fig. 1. Previous binding studies with model 1 (Hsu 1981) indicate that in different solvent systems this molecule readily binds and inactivates single-stranded φX174 DNA.

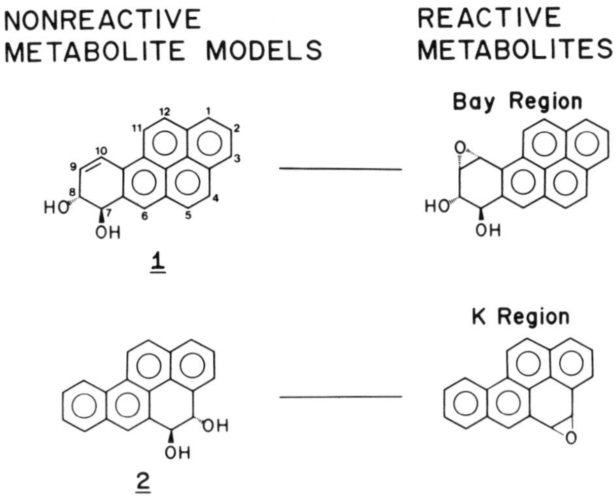

NONREACTIVE
METABOLITE MODELS

REACTIVE
METABOLITES

Bay Region

HO

OH

1

HO

OH

K Region

2

O

Fig. 1. Reactive metabolites formed from benzo[a]pyrene
and nonreactive metabolite models.

EXPERIMENTAL

Fluorescence quenching experiments were performed
with a Perkin Elmer 650-10 Fluorescence Spectrometer.
Fluorescence lifetime measurements were carried out with
a Photochemical Research Associates Model 2000 Nanosecond
Fluorescence Spectrometer. Absorption spectra were measured on a Cary 17 Spectrometer. Samples of molecules 1
and 2 were prepared using published methods (Harvey 1981;
Fu 1980; Harvey 1978). Calf thymus DNA was purchased
from Sigma Chemical Company.

All binding studies were carried out in a solvent
system consisting of double distilled water and methanol
(15% by volume). The solutions were maintained at a pH
of 7.1. The hydrocarbon concentrations were in the
range $10^{-6} - 10^{-7}$ M. DNA concentrations are reported in
terms of PO_4^- molarity calculated from an average base-

pair molecular weight of 617.8. This is based on a calf
thymus DNA composition which is 60% A-T base pairs (Adams
1981). DNA concentrations have been corrected for the
amounts of H_2O and Na^+ reported by the supplier for each
DNA batch. Denatured DNA was prepared by heating native
DNA to 95°C for 5 minutes. The denatured DNA exhibited a
hyperchromicity of 35% at 260 nm.

For molecules 1 and 2, Stern-Volmer plots were measured at excitation wavelengths of 350 and 328 nm respectively. The corresponding emission wavelengths were 402
and 388 nm. Lifetime studies were carried out at the
emission and excitation wavelengths given in Fig. 4.
Analysis of the lifetime data was carried out using a
least squares deconvolution method (Hui 1976).

RESULTS AND DISCUSSION

Figure 2 shows UV absorption spectra of molecules 1
and 2 with varying amounts of native DNA. Without DNA
the metabolite models have absorption maxima at λ_{free}.
For molecules 1 and 2 these occur at 365 and 323 nm respectively. As DNA is added a new 10-12 nm red shifted
band caused by complex formation is observed at $\lambda_{complex}$.
Complex formation is inhibited by DNA stabilizers. For
model 1 Fig. 2 shows that at $[PO_4^-] = 3.2 \times 10^{-4}$ M, the
intensity of the red shifted band is greatly reduced when
spermine is added. This is a spectral property which is
characteristic of intercalated complexes. (Meehan 1982;
Meehan 1981; Meehan 1979).

Association constants for intercalation are given in
Fig. 2. These have been obtained from double reciprocal
plots (MacLeod 1982) of $1/(\Delta A-\Delta A_0)$ versus $1/[PO_4^-]$. Here ΔA_0
is the difference in absorbances at λ_{free}
and $\lambda_{complex}$ measured without DNA, and ΔA is the difference measured with DNA. The estimated error in the intercalation binding constants obtained in this manner
is ±10%. The results indicate that for the bay region
model, molecule 1, the association constant is 2.7 times
greater than that for the K region model, molecule 2.

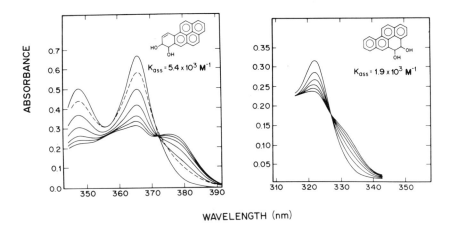

Fig. 2. Absorption spectra of trans-7,8-dihydroxy-7,8-di-
hydrobenzo[a]pyrene (1) and of trans-4,5-dihy-
droxy-4,5-dihydrobenzo[a]pyrene (2) in native DNA
at concentrations of 0.0, 8.0 x 10^{-5}, 1.6 x 10^{-4},
2.4 x 10^{-4}, 3.2 x 10^{-4} and 4.0 x 10^{-4} M. The
broken line shows a spectrum of molecule 1 with
DNA (3.2 x 10^{-4} M) and spermine (3.2 x 10^{-4} M).

Figure 3 contains Stern-Volmer plots and quenching
constants, K_{SV}, for the fluorescence quenching of molecules 1 and 2 by DNA. The results of Fig. 3 show that
fluorescence quenching which accompanies DNA binding is
strongly dependent upon DNA secondary structure. In denatured DNA the quenching is greatly reduced. These results indicate that like the UV red shift, fluorescence
quenching arises from intercalation (Shahbaz 1983; LePecq
1967). These results, which show that intercalation is
greatly reduced when DNA is denatured, are interesting in
view of previous results, which indicate that model 1
binds much better to single-stranded DNA than to double-
stranded DNA (Hsu 1981). The apparent contradiction be-

tween the two studies may be due to the fact that the earlier work examined total binding while this investigation focuses on intercalative binding.

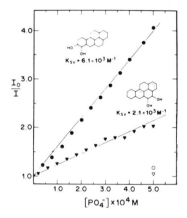

Fig. 3. Stern-Volmer plots and quenching constants derived from the fluorescence quenching of metabolite models 1 and 2 by native DNA (closed symbols) and denatured DNA (open symbols).

The Stern-Volmer quenching constants given in Fig. 3 are very similar to the binding constants obtained from UV absorption studies. This indicates that the quantum yields of the bound complexes are negligible compared to those of the free molecules. For models 1 and 2 the Stern-Volmer quenching constants are approximately equal to the intercalation association constants.

Fluorescence lifetime studies also support this conclusion. Figure 4 shows fluorescence decay profiles of molecules 1 and 2 measured with and without DNA. The results indicate that for both molecules the decay profiles with DNA are similar to those without DNA. This points out that the quantum yields of the intercalated complexes are small.

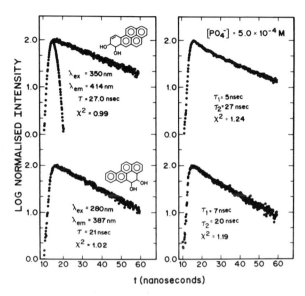

Fig. 4. Fluorescence decay profiles of metabolite models 1 and 2 measured with and without native DNA along with emission and excitation wavelengths, lifetimes and values of x^2 obtained from deconvolution of the data. The upper left-hand corner shows an instrument response profile.

An analysis of the lifetime data shows that without DNA, molecules 1 and 2 have single exponential decay laws with lifetimes of 27 and 21 nsec respectively. The similarity of the lifetimes measured with and without DNA indicate that dynamic quenching involving DNA does not play an important role in these experiments (Shahbaz, 1983).

For both molecules 1 and 2 the analysis of lifetime data obtained with DNA points out that there is a small contribution to the decay profile from a short lived component ($\tau = 5 - 7$ nsec). However in both molecules this component, which arises from complexes, contributes less than 12% to the total emission observed at $[PO_4^-] = 5 \times 10^{-4}$ M.

The carcinogenic activity of hydrocarbon metabolites depends upon several factors. These include the susceptibility of reactive metabolites to enzymatic detoxifica-

tion; the transport properties of metabolites from activation sites to reaction sites, and the reaction properties of metabolites at target sites.

Physical binding properties are also important.
Both the absorption and fluorescence studies indicate
that the intercalation binding constant of the bay region
model is significantly greater than that of the K region
model. The present studies along with previous studies
of metabolite models of 7,12-dimethylbenz[a]anthracene
suggest that intercalation is important to the mechanism
of polycyclic hydrocarbon carcinogenesis. Further studies will show whether π interactions associated with intercalation play a significant role in hydrogen carcinogenesis only because they influence epoxide reactivity
and reaction sites or whether these interactions also influence DNA function in biologically important ways.

Acknowledgment

The authors wish to thank the American Cancer Society and the National Institutes of Health for support of
this work.

REFERENCES

Adams, R. L. P., Burdon, R. H., Campbell, A. M., Leader,
    D. P., and Smellie, R. M. S. (1981) The Biochemistry of
    the Nucleic Acids, 9th Ed., Chapin and Hall, London.
Fu, P. P., Lee, H. M. and Harvey, R. G. (1980) J. Org.
    Chem. 45, 2797.
Geacintov, N. E., Yoshida, H. and Harvey, R. G. (1982)
    Biochemistry, 21, 1864.
Harvey, R. G. (1981) Acc. Chem. Res. 14, 218.
Harvey, R. G., Fu, P. P. (1978) Polycyclic Hydrocarbons
    and Cancer (Gelboin, H. V., Ts'o, P. O. P., Eds.) 1,
    pp. 133-165, Academic Press, New York.
Hsu, W.-T., Harvey, R. G., and Weiss, S. B. (1981) Bio-
    chem. Biophys. Res. Comm. 101 317.
Hui, H. M. and Ware, W. R. (1976) J. Am. Chem. Soc. 98,
    4718.
LePecq, J. B. and Paoletti, C. (1967) J. Mol. Biol. 27,
    87.
Lin, J. H., LeBreton, P. R., and Shipman, L. L. (1980) J.

Phys. Chem. 84, 642.

MacLeod, M. C., and Selkirk, J. K. (1982) Carcinogenesis, 3, 287.

Meehan, T., Gamper, H., and Becker, J. F. (1982) J. Biol. Chem. 257, 10479.

Meehan, T., Becker, J. F., and Gamper, H. (1981) Proc. Amer. Assoc. Cancer Res. 22, 92.

Meehan, T., and Straub, K. (1979) Nature 277, 410.

Shahbaz, M., Harvey, R. G., Prakash, A. S., Boal, T. R., Zegar, I. S., and LeBreton, P. R. (1983) Biochem. Biophys. Res. Commun. 112, 1.

Yang, N. C., Hrinyo, T. P. Petrich, J. W., and Yang, D. H. (1983) Biochem. Biophys. Res. Commun. 114, 8.

Zegar, I. S., Prakash, A. S., and LeBreton, P. R. (1984) J. Biomolecular Structure & Dynamics, submitted.

Molecular Basis of Cancer, Part A: Macromolecular Structure, Carcinogens, and Oncogenes, pages 227–237
© 1985 Alan R. Liss, Inc.

HALOGENATED OLEFINS AND THEIR EPOXIDES: FACTORS UNDERLYING CARCINOGENIC ACTIVITY

Peter Politzer, Patricia R. Laurence and
Keerthi Jayasuriya
Department of Chemistry
University of New Orleans
New Orleans, Louisiana, 70148, U.S.A.

BACKGROUND

In seeking to understand and predict the carcinogenic behavior of halogenated olefins, one is soon led to the study of the corresponding epoxides. This comes about because the initial metabolic step undergone by many halogenated olefins is microsomal epoxidation, and it is the resulting epoxides that are believed to be responsible for the carcinogenicities of many of the parent compounds (Rannug, Gothe, Wachtmeister 1976; Osterman-Golkar et al 1977; Banerjee, Van Duuren 1978; Bartsch et al 1979; Woo et al 1984).

One of the most extensively-studied of these epoxides is chlorooxirane (I), which is a metabolite of the well-established carcinogen vinyl chloride (II) (Van Duuren 1975; Rannug, Gothe, Wachtmeister 1976; Bartsch et al 1979; Infante 1981). Chlorooxirane is both a mono- and a bifunctional alkylating agent of nucleophilic sites on nucleic acid bases, RNA, DNA and protein residues (Rannug, Gothe, Wachtmeister 1976; Osterman-Golkar et al 1977; Barbin et al 1981).

$$
\begin{array}{cc}
\underset{I}{
\begin{array}{c}
\overset{\displaystyle O}{\overset{\displaystyle /\ \backslash}{H-\underset{\underset{Cl}{|}}{C}-\underset{\underset{H}{|}}{C}-H}}
\end{array}
}
&
\underset{II}{
\begin{array}{c}
\underset{Cl}{\overset{H}{\diagdown}}C=C\underset{H}{\overset{H}{\diagup}}
\end{array}
}
\end{array}
$$

Recently it has been shown that the primary _in vivo_
DNA alkylation product of vinyl chloride is the 7-N-(2-oxo-
ethyl) derivative of guanine (III), and it was suggested
that this adduct is responsible for the carcinogenicity of
vinyl chloride (Scherer et al 1981; Laib, Gwinner, Bolt
1981). There is some evidence of an equilibrium between III
and the cyclic hemiacetal IV (Scherer et al 1981). This
would affect the guanine-cytosine hydrogen bonds that involve
O_6 and N_1 of guanine, and could lead to miscoding and repli-
cational and transcriptional errors (Zajdela et al 1980;
Barbin et al 1981; Scherer et al 1981; Spengler, Singer 1981).
In an earlier computational study, we proposed both S_N1 and
S_N2 mechanisms for the formation of the key alkylation
product III (Laurence, Politzer 1984).

In recognition of the crucial importance of the epoxides
in the carcinogenic activities of halogenated olefins, we
have made extensive studies of the reactive properties of a
representative group of epoxides: ethylene oxide (V),
propylene oxide (VI), epichlorohydrin (VII), chlorooxirane
(I), _trans_-dichlorooxirane (VIII) and 1,1-dichlorooxirane
(IX). Since the critical cellular reactions in which we are
interested are believed to involve nucleophilic sites, such
as N_7 of guanine, we have focused specifically upon the reactivities of these epoxides toward nucleophiles, in both S_N1
and S_N2 processes. For earlier discussions of some of these
and related results, see Politzer, Proctor 1982; Laurence,
Politzer 1984; Laurence, Proctor, Politzer 1984; Politzer,
Laurence 1984a.

$$\underset{V}{H_2C \overset{\displaystyle O}{\overset{\diagup\diagdown}{-\!-\!-}} CH_2}$$

$$\underset{VI}{H_2C \overset{\displaystyle O}{\overset{\diagup\diagdown}{-\!-\!-}} CH - CH_3}$$

$$\underset{VII}{H_2C \overset{\displaystyle O}{\overset{\diagup\diagdown}{-\!-\!-}} CH - CH_2Cl}$$

VIII

IX

The present paper will summarize some of our results for all six of these epoxides. We will also expand the list of predicted possible carcinogens, based upon our calculations of the electrostatic potentials of halogenated epoxides.

METHODS AND PROCEDURE

Our approach involves the computation of <u>ab initio</u> SCF molecular orbital wave functions, using the GAUSSIAN 80 program. All geometries are completely optimized at the STO-3G level. We investigate the S_N1 reactivity of a particular bond by computing the energy required to stretch it, in several steps, to an arbitrary final length. The entire structure of the molecule is reoptimized at each step. S_N2 reactivity is studied by allowing an ammonia molecule, chosen as a model nucleophile, to approach and react, in turn, with each epoxide ring carbon. The structure of the whole complex is reoptimized at each of several arbitrary C$\cdots$N distances, the only exception being that the NH$_3$ is assumed to retain its C_{3v} symmetry.

Our starting points for the reactivity investigations to be discussed have been the oxygen-protonated forms of the epoxides. Oxygen protonation is well known to weaken epoxide C-O bonds and facilitate ring-opening (Morrison, Boyd 1973; Politzer <u>et al</u> 1978; Politzer, Estes 1979; Ferrell, Loew 1979; Politzer, Proctor 1982; Laurence, Politzer 1984; Laurence, Proctor, Politzer 1984). Our

assumption that these epoxides are protonated in the environment of interest is based upon the fact that subcellular
regions with high proton activities do exist (Sols, Marco
1970; Welch, Berry 1983). More specifically, certain redox
systems that are believed to produce high local proton activities are contained in the nuclear membrane (Kell 1979;
Welch, Barry 1983), in which occur the enzymatic reactions
involved in DNA replication; one of these is the cytochrome
P-450 system that epoxidizes olefins (Guengerich, Macdonald
1984).

The electrostatic potential that the electrons and
nuclei of a molecule create in the surrounding space is
given rigorously by eq. (1):

$$V(\vec{r}) = \sum_A \frac{Z_A}{|\vec{R}_A - \vec{r}|} - \int \frac{\rho(\vec{r}\,')d\vec{r}\,'}{|\vec{r}\,' - \vec{r}|} \tag{1}$$

Z_A is the charge on nucleus A, located at $\vec{R}_A$, and $\rho(\vec{r}\,')$ is
the electronic density function, which we obtain from the
molecular wave function. $V(\vec{r})$ is a real physical property,
experimentally measurable, which can be interpreted as the
potential of the molecule for interacting with an electrical
charge located at $\vec{r}$. It is an effective guide to the reactive behavior of a molecule (Scrocco, Tomasi 1978; Politzer,
Daiker 1981; Politzer, Truhlar 1981); for example, an
approaching electrophile will tend to go initially to those
regions in which $V(\vec{r})$ is most negative, since those are
where the effects of the molecule's electrons predominate.
In the present work, all electrostatic potentials were
computed with STO-5G basis sets, using the optimized epoxide
structures.

RESULTS AND DISCUSSION

S_N1 Processes

The energy requirement, ΔE_{str}, for stretching each C-O
bond separately from its equilibrium (protonated) value of
approximately 1.50 A to an arbitrarily-selected final 2.20 A

(reoptimized structure) is given in Table 1. In general, these show a consistent pattern. The presence of a −Cl or −CH$_3$ substituent on a ring carbon lowers ΔE_{str} from the 42 − 48 kcal/mole range to about 32 kcal/mole. A second −Cl on the same carbon reduces ΔE_{str} yet further, to 21 kcal/mole. The case of epichlorohydrin is exceptional, and has been discussed in detail elsewhere (Politzer, Laurence 1984a).

The effect of a chlorine substituent in lowering the energy required for stretching the corresponding C-O bond can be interpreted in terms of resonance stabilization of the distorted structure:

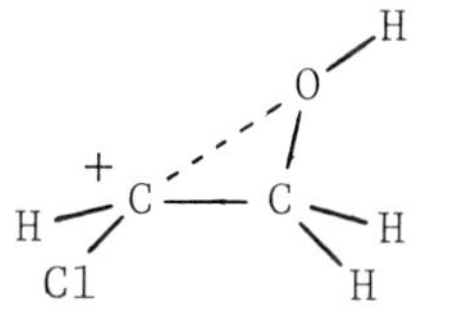

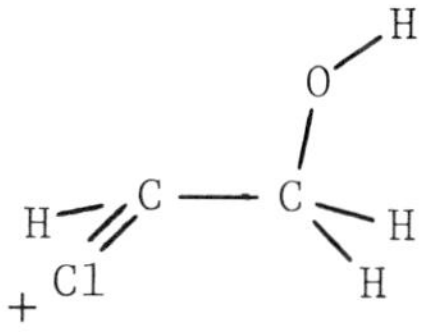

This interpretation is consistent with the observation that stretching this C-O bond is accompanied by a shortening of the other from 1.50 to 1.45 A, very close to the typical alcoholic C-OH bond length of 1.43 A, while the C-Cl distance also decreases, by about 0.06 A, possibly reflecting some degree of double bond character. Having two chlorines on the same carbon, as in 1,1-dichlorooxirane (IX), introduces the possibility of an additional resonance structure analogous to XI, thus stabilizing the distorted system yet further and lowering ΔE_{str}. The effect of a methyl substituent can be explained in a similar manner, invoking hyperconjugation.

S_N2 Processes

The interaction of each epoxide ring carbon, in turn, with an ammonia molecule produces stable intermediate complexes with the general structure of XII:

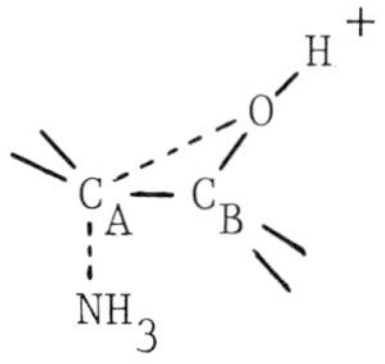

TABLE 1. Calculated electrostatic potentials, bond stretch-[a] ing energies and stabilization energies of ammonia complexes.

Name	Epoxide Structure	V_{min} [b]	ΔE_{str} [b]	ΔE_{stab} [b]
Propylene oxide	$\overset{O}{\overset{/\backslash}{HC - CH_2}}$, CH_3	-53.4	C_1-O: 31.9 C_2-O: 48.5	C_1: -70.1 C_2: -68.0
Ethylene oxide	$\overset{O}{\overset{/\backslash}{H_2C - CH_2}}$	-51.3	C-O: 44.5	C: -71.8
Epichloro- hydrin	$\overset{O}{\overset{/\backslash}{HC - CH_2}}$, CH_2Cl	-43.1	C_1-O: c C_2-O: c	C_1: -75.5 C_2: -77.7
Chloro- oxirane	$\overset{O}{\overset{/\backslash}{HC - CH_2}}$, Cl	-38.1	C_1-O: 32.4 C_2-O: 44.0	C_1: -72.7 C_2: -86.9
1,1-Di- chloro- oxirane	$\overset{O}{\overset{/\backslash}{Cl_2C - CH_2}}$	-26.5	C_1-O: 21.4 C_2-O: 42.1	C_1: -73.6 C_2: -97.0
trans- Dichloro- oxirane	$\overset{O}{\overset{/\backslash}{H - C - C - Cl}}$, Cl H	-23.1	C-O: 30.8	C: -87.8

[a] Some of these results have been presented previously (Laurence, Politzer 1984; Laurence, Proctor, Politzer 1984; Politzer, Laurence 1984a). All values are in kcal/mole.

[b] C_1 and C_2 are the carbons in the epoxide ring. Substituents, such as $-CH_3$ and $-Cl$, are attached to C_1.

[c] See discussion in Politzer, Laurence 1984a.

In this complex, the C_A-O bond length is in the neighborhood of 2.4 A, which represents a substantial opening of the epoxide ring. Both carbons have moved toward tetrahedral configurations, and the atoms bonded to the carbon under attack have undergone an inversion.

The stabilization energies of these complexes, ΔE_{stab}, relative to the protonated epoxide and free ammonia, are presented in Table 1. These show that the interaction with one of the carbons in an epoxide ring is considerably more stable when the other carbon has a chlorine substituent; the effect is yet greater when the second carbon is doubly-chlorinated, as in 1,1-dichlorooxirane (IX). The stabilization energies in such instances are approximately −87 and −97 kcal/mole, respectively, whereas in all other cases they are in the −68 to −78 kcal/mole range. The additional stabilization associated with having a chlorine on the other carbon can also be explained using resonance arguments (Laurence, Politzer 1984; Laurence, Proctor, Politzer 1984):

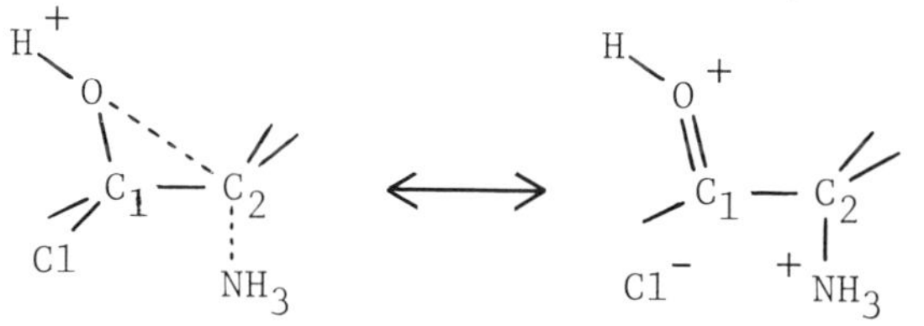

The presence of two chlorines on C_1 makes possible an additional structure analogous to XIV, and thus further increases the stabilizing effect. In agreement with this resonance interpretation, we have found the interaction at C_2 to produce a lengthening of the C_1-Cl bond, while C_1-O becomes shorter.

As mentioned earlier, we have recently proposed both S_N1 and S_N2 mechanisms for the formation of the DNA alkylation product III that has been suggested to be responsible for the carcinogenicity of vinyl chloride (Laurence, Politzer 1984). Our S_N2 mechanism involves the interaction of N_7 of guanine with the non-chlorinated carbon of chlorooxirane (I), resulting in a resonance-stabilized intermediate analogous to the pair XIII − XIV.

Electrostatic Potentials

We have computed the electrostatic potentials of more than thirty halogenated epoxides (Politzer, Laurence 1984a). The most negative value of the potential near the oxygen atom, V_{min}, was shown to correlate well with the proton affinity for protonation of the oxygen, and also with the electron-releasing or electron-withdrawing tendencies of the substituents on the epoxide ring.

This latter property led us to consider the possibility that V_{min} might be an effective quantity to use in developing a quantitative understanding of the reactivities of various epoxides with epoxide hydrase. This is an enzyme that catalyzes the hydrolysis of epoxides. The degree to which it interacts with various epoxides has been thought to depend, qualitatively, upon such factors as the electron-releasing or -withdrawing powers of ring substituents, and also their steric properties (Hanzlik, Walsh 1980). As has just been pointed out, V_{min} is a measure of the former; to take steric effects into account, we used Taft's steric substituent parameter E_s (Taft 1956; Unger, Hansch 1976). We found that there is a good correlation between the abilities of epoxides to inhibit epoxide hydrase and the quantity V_{min}/E_s (Politzer, Laurence 1984b). (Since this inhibition often comes about because the inhibitor is a competing alternate substrate, it reflects the degree of interaction of the molecule with the enzyme.)

We have also discovered a relationship between V_{min} and the carcinogenicities of epoxides. Those that are clearly carcinogenic have relatively strong negative electrostatic potentials near the oxygen, while the weak or inactive ones have less negative V_{min} values. For computations performed at the STO-3G level, the threshold comes at roughly $V_{min} = -30$ kcal/mole (Politzer, Laurence 1984b).

The apparent association of carcinogenicity with a strongly-negative oxygen potential may reflect the importance of protonation. However there are undoubtedly other factors as well that play significant roles in determining the carcinogenic activity of a given olefin or epoxide. These may include the ease of epoxidation (for an olefin), the general reactivity of the epoxide, and the nature of the complex formed with DNA. The epoxide certainly requires some minimum reactivity in order to be carcinogenic; if it is too active, however, it may not reach the cellular site at which the carcinogenic interaction takes place. Such considerations have been discussed earlier, in analyzing possible reasons for the differences in activity between vinyl chloride (active carcinogen) and trans-dichloroethylene (believed to be inactive) (Laurence, Proctor, Politzer 1984).

Even though V_{min} is only one of several factors that are likely to determine carcinogenic activity, the relationship mentioned above does permit us to make certain preliminary assessments of presumptive carcinogenicity. Thus, expanding upon our earlier list (Politzer, Laurence 1984b), we tentatively predict significant carcinogenic activity for: 1-butene oxide, epifluorohydrin, fluorooxirane, 3,3,3-trifluoropropylene oxide, 1,1-difluorooxirane, 3,3-dichloropropylene oxide and trifluorooxirane.

ACKNOWLEDGEMENTS

We express our appreciation to the U. S. Environmental Protection Agency for partial funding of this work under assistance agreement number CR808866-01-0 to Peter Politzer. The contents do not necessarily reflect the views and policies of the Environmental Protection Agency, nor does mention of trade names or commercial products constitute endorsement or recommendation for use. We are also grateful for the financial support provided by the University of New Orleans Computer Research Center.

REFERENCES

Banerjee S, Van Duuren BL (1978). Covalent binding of the carcinogen trichloroethylene to hepatic microsomal proteins and to exogenous DNA14 in vitro. Cancer Res 38:776.
Barbin A, Bartsch H, Leconte P, Radman M (1981). Studies on the miscoding properties of 1,N^6-ethenoadenine, DNA reaction products of vinyl chloride metabolites, during in vitro DNA synthesis. Nuc Acids Res 9:375.
Bartsch H, Malaveille C, Barbin A, Planche G (1979). Mutagenic and alkylating metabolites. Arch Toxicol 41:249.
Ferrell JE, Loew GH (1979). Mechanistic studies of arene oxides and diol epoxide rearrangement and hydrolysis reactions. J Amer Chem Soc 101:1385.

Guengerich FP, Macdonald TL (1984). Chemical mechanisms of catalysis by cytochromes P-450: A unified view. Acc Chem Res 17:9.

Hanzlik RP, Walsh JSA (1980). Halogenated epoxides and related compounds as inhibitors of epoxide hydrase. Arch Biochem Biophys 204:255.

Infante PF (1981). Observations of the site-specific carcinogenicity of vinyl chloride to humans. Environ Health Persp 41:89.

Kell DB (1979). On the functional proton current pathway of electron transport phosphorylation. An electrode view. Biochim Biophys Acta 549:55.

Laib RJ, Gwinner LM, Bolt HM (1981). DNA alkylation by vinyl chloride metabolites: Etheno derivatives of 7-alkylation of guanine? Chem-Biol Interact 37:219.

Laurence PR, Politzer P (1984). Some reactive properties of chlorooxirane, a likely carcinogenic metabolite of vinyl chloride. Internat J Quantum Chem 25:493.

Laurence PR, Proctor TR, Politzer P (1984). Reactive properties of trans-dichlorooxirane in relation to the contrasting carcinogenicities of vinyl chloride and trans-dichloroethylene. Internat J Quantum Chem (in press).

Morrison RT, Boyd RN (1973). "Organic Chemistry", 3rd ed, Boston: Allyn & Bacon, p 562.

Osterman-Golkar S, Hultmark D, Segerback D, Calleman CJ, Gothe R, Ehrenberg L, Wachtmeister CA (1977). Alkylation of DNA and proteins in mice exposed to vinyl chloride. Biochem Biophys Res Commun 76:259.

Politzer P, Daiker KC (1981). Models for chemical reactivity. In Deb BM (ed): "The Force Concept in Chemistry", New York: Van Nostrand-Reinhold, p 294.

Politzer P, Daiker KC, Estes VM, Baughman M (1978). Epoxide-nucleophile interactions: The acid-catalyzed reaction of ethylene oxide with water. Internat J Quantum Chem, Quantum Biol Symp 5:291.

Politzer P, Estes VM (1979). The catalytic effect of hydrogen bonding upon epoxide ring-opening. In Pullman B (ed): "Catalysis in Chemistry and Biochemistry, Theory and Experiment", Dordrecht-Holland: Reidel, p 305.

Politzer P, Laurence PR (1984a). Halogenated hydrocarbon epoxides: Factors underlying biological activity. Internat J Quantum Chem, Quantum Biol Symp 11:(in press).

Politzer P, Laurence PR (1984b). Relationships between the electrostatic potential, epoxide hydrase inhibition and carcinogenicity for some hydrocarbon and halogenated hydrocarbon epoxides. Carcinogenesis (in press).

Politzer P, Proctor TR (1982). Calculated properties of some possible vinyl chloride metabolites. Internat J Quantum Chem 22:1271.

Politzer P, Truhlar DG (1981). (Eds): "Chemical Applications of Atomic and Molecular Electrostatic Potentials", New York: Plenum Press.

Rannug U, Gothe R, Wachtmeister CA (1976). Mutagenicity of chloroethylene oxide, chloroacetaldehyde, 2-chloroethanol and chloroacetic acid, conceivable metabolites of vinyl chloride. Chem-Biol Interact 12:251.

Scherer E, Van Der Laken CJ, Gwinner LM, Laib RJ, Emmelot P (1981). Modification of deoxyguanisine by chloroethylene oxide. Carcinogenesis 2:671.

Scrocco E, Tomasi J (1978). Electronic molecular structure, reactivity and intermolecular forces: An euristic interpretation by means of electrostatic molecular potentials. Adv Quantum Chem 11:115.

Sols A, Marco R (1970). Concentrations of metabolites and binding sites. Implications in metabolic regulation. Current Topics Cell Regulat 2:227.

Spengler S, Singer B (1981). Transcriptional errors and ambiguity resulting from the presence of $1,N^6$-etheno-adenosine or $3,N^4$-ethenocytidine in polyribonucleotides. Nuc Acids Res 9:365.

Taft RW (1956). Separation of polar, steric and resonance effects in reactivity. In Newman MS (ed): "Steric Effects in Organic Chemistry", New York: Wiley, p 556.

Unger SH, Hansch C (1976). Quantitative models of steric effects. Prog Phys Org Chem 12:91.

Van Duuren BL (1975). On the possible mechanism of carcinogenic action of vinyl chloride. Ann NY Acad Sci 246:258.

Welch GR, Berry MN (1983). Long-range energy continua in the living cell: Protochemical considerations. In Frohlich H, Kremer F (eds): "Coherent Excitations in Biological Systems", New York: Springer-Verlag, p 95.

Woo Y-T, Lai D, Arcos JC, Argus MF (1984). "Chemical Induction of Cancer", Vol IIIB, New York: Academic Press, section 5.2.2.1.

Zajdela F, Croisy A, Barbin A, Malaveille C, Tomatis L, Bartsch H (1980). Carcinogenicity of chloroethylene oxide, an ultimate reactive metabolite of vinyl chloride, and bis(chloromethyl)ether after subcutaneous administration and in initiation-promotion experiments in mice. Cancer Res 40:352.

Molecular Basis of Cancer, Part A: Macromolecular Structure, Carcinogens, and Oncogenes, pages 239–248
© 1985 Alan R. Liss, Inc.

THEORETICAL INVESTIGATION OF POSSIBLE INTERMEDIATES IN
CHEMICAL CARCINOGENESIS BY N-NITROSAMINES

Christopher A. Reynolds, and Colin Thomson

National Foundation for Cancer Research Project
Chemistry Department, University of St. Andrews
St. Andrews, Scotland

INTRODUCTION

N-Nitrosamines are an important class of chemical
carcinogens in many different species, and there is good
reason to suspect their involvement in human cancer. They
are not carcinogenic unless metabolically activated, and
show a great deal of organ specificity despite being evenly
distributed throughout the tissues of a particular species;
this is presumably because of variations in the activity of
the metabolising enzymes in different tissues (Pegg 1980).

Understanding of the metabolic pathways is incomplete
since many of the possible intermediates are short lived,
but it is well established that the ultimate carcinogen is
an electrophilic alkylating agent which attacks the DNA,
(Michejda et al, 1982). Theoretical calculations on the
mechanism should be able to shed additional light on the
reaction pathways and possible intermediates, and we review
in this paper our own studies on the decomposition of
N,N-dimethylnitrosamine (DMN) to alkylating species. There
have been other theoretical studies on the metabolism of
DMN, (Andreozzi et al, 1977; Loew et al, 1983), but this
paper considers several new aspects of the problem.

EXPERIMENTAL ASPECTS OF THE DECOMPOSITION

A large body of experimental data, especially in vitro
studies, has shown that oxygen, reduced pyridine nucleotides
and microsomal preparations are necessary for activation of

N-nitrosamines, implicating the microsomal mixed function oxidases and in particular cytochrome P-450. More recent inhibition studies also indicate the involvement of the monoamine oxidases, but the mechanistic implications of this are not clear (Pegg, 1980).

It is usually accepted that the activating step is the oxidation of DMN to the α-hydroxyderivative, which then decomposes to give formaldehyde and methyldiazohydroxide. The latter can give an alkylating agent in several ways. Both formaldehyde and N_2 have been detected by labelling techniques, but it is clear that not all DMN is metabolised via this pathway.

The origin and nature of the alkylating agent is also not certain. Di-n-propyl nitrosamine alkylates N-7 of guanine by an S_N2 mechanism, without rearrangement, but alkylates O-6 of guanine with rearrangement and therefore via an S_N1 reaction (Scribner et al, 1982). However, molecules other than DNA are also alkylated, and it is clear that the reaction pathway may be more complicated than proposed in previous work.

STRATEGY AND METHODS FOR THE THEORETICAL INVESTIGATIONS

The molecules in the proposed decomposition scheme have been studied by ab initio quantum chemical methods, using GAUSSIAN 80 (Binkley et al, 1980), for all energy and gradient calculations, mainly at the RHF/4-21G level of approximation. The geometries of all reactants, inter-mediates and products were fully optimized using the minimization algorithms in GAUSSIAN 80. Transition states were located directly from the minima on either side, where possible, using MINIT (Bell et al, 1984).

In certain cases non-essential methyl groups were replaced by hydrogens, as this speeded up the calculations, and it was found that the energetics for these model reactions were very similar to those for the parent reactions. The influence of solvation on certain reactions was investigated by including one or two molecules of water in the calculations. This approach, although relatively crude, has been shown to be useful in assessing the major effects of solvation (Pullman et al, 1975).

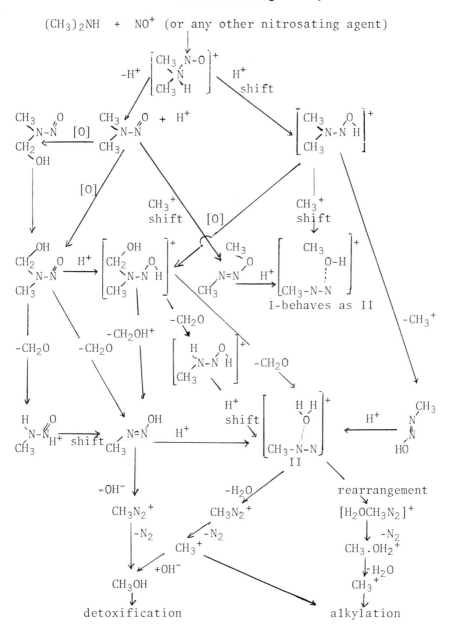

Figure 1: Possible reaction pathways in the production
and decomposition of DMN

RESULTS

The modified reaction scheme suggested by the results of the calculations is given in Figure 1, which also includes some of the energetically unfavourable pathways. This scheme consists of two main parts: a) the activation of DMN and the loss of one methyl group from the amino nitrogen, and b) the formation of the electrophilic alkylating agent. A full discussion of the pathway will be given in a more detailed paper (Reynolds et al. 1984b).

A: Loss of a Methyl Group

Previous work (Reynolds et al, 1984a) has shown that following nitrosation of amines by NO^+, O- protonation can readily occur by a shift of H^+, and furthermore loss of CH_3^+ from protonated DMN is energetically similar to the result for H^+ loss, particularly when solvation is taken into account. In the absence of H_2O direct loss of CH_3^+ is energetically unfavourable

$$\left[\begin{matrix} CH_3 \\ {}^{}\!\!>N\!-\!N {}^{O}\!\!\!\!\!\!\!\searrow_H \\ CH_3 \end{matrix} \right]^{+} \longrightarrow CH_3^+ + {}_{CH_3}\!\!\!\nearrow N\!=\!N {}^{\nearrow O}\!\!\!\!\!\searrow_H \qquad \Delta E = 436 \ kJ \ mol^{-1}$$

but an alternative route involves a shift of CH_3^+ to the oxygen.

Calculations of the energetics for this process for the model monomethylnitrosamine have been carried out.

$$\begin{matrix} CH_3 {}^{O}\!\!\!\!\!\! \\ {}^{}\!\!>N\!-\!N \\ H \end{matrix} \xrightarrow[\displaystyle 294 \ kJ \ mol^{-1}]{\displaystyle \Delta E =} \begin{matrix} H \\ {}^{.\cdot}\!\!>C\!-\!H \\ H\!\!\diagup\!\diagdown \\ H\!-\!N \ \ O \\ {}^{}\!\!\diagdown\!\!N \end{matrix} \xrightarrow[\displaystyle -281 \ kJ \ mol^{-1}]{\displaystyle \Delta E =} \begin{matrix} H_3C\!\!\diagdown \\ {}^{O} \\ N\!-\!N\!\!\diagup \\ H \end{matrix}$$

$$\Delta E = \quad 13 \ kJ \ mol^{-1}$$

and

$$\left[\begin{matrix} CH_3 {}^{O}\!\!\!\!\!\! \\ {}^{}\!\!\diagdown\!N\!-\!N\!\!\nearrow\!\!\searrow_H \\ H \end{matrix} \right]^{+} \longrightarrow \left[\begin{matrix} H_3C \\ {}^{}\!\!\diagdown O\!-\!H \\ {}^{}\!\!\diagup \\ H\!-\!N\!-\!N \end{matrix} \right]^{+} \qquad \Delta E = \quad 7 \ kJ \ mol^{-1}$$

These results not only show the need for activation of the
methyl group by an enzyme, but also give us a standard by
which we can study the effects of activation. The currently
most popular mode of activation involves attack by an
electrophilic O radical (via Cytochrome P-450) on DMN to
give the α-hydroxynitrosamine (Michejda et al, 1982). This
step has been studied in detail previously using MINDO/3
(Loew et al, 1983), using ^{1}S and ^{3}P O atoms as oxidants.
Our ab-initio studies of this step have to date only considered the energetics of the overall process

$$
\underset{H}{\overset{CH_3}{>}} N\text{-}N \overset{O}{\diagup} \;+\; [O] \;\longrightarrow\; \underset{H}{\overset{CH_2OH}{>}} N\text{-}N \overset{O}{\diagup}
$$

for which the results of UHF and ROHF calculations are in
close agreement. $\Delta E = -80$ kJ mol^{-1} and -408 kJ mol^{-1} for
^{1}S O and ^{3}P O respectively. (Corresponding values for
protonated DMN are -89 kJ mol^{-1} and -417 kJ mol^{-1}.)

There is experimental evidence (Swann 1982) that
enzymatic hydroxylation produces the E- isomer, but it is
likely that the decomposition proceeds via the Z- isomer
following a rotation about the N-N bond. Protonation decreases the N-N bond length and raises the barrier to
rotation, and so may be a factor in stabilizing the E- isomer.
The energetics for this interconversion for a model compound
have been calculated, and compared with that of the protonated form.

$$
\underset{H}{\overset{H}{>}} N\text{-}N \overset{O}{\diagup} \quad \xrightarrow[\;81\ \text{kJ mol}^{-1}\;]{\Delta E =} \quad \underset{H}{\overset{H}{>}} N\text{-}N \overset{O}{\diagup} \quad \xrightarrow[\;-81\ \text{kJ mol}^{-1}\;]{\Delta E =} \quad \underset{H}{\overset{H}{>}} N\text{-}N \underset{O}{\diagdown}
$$

$$
\left[\underset{H}{\overset{H}{>}} N\text{-}N \overset{O}{\diagup} {}^{H}\right]^{+} \xrightarrow[244]{\Delta E =} \left[\underset{H}{\overset{H}{>}} N\text{-}N \overset{O}{\diagdown} {}^{H}\right]^{+} \xrightarrow[-244]{\Delta E =} \left[\underset{H}{\overset{H}{>}} N\text{-}N \underset{O}{\diagdown} {}^{H}\right]^{+}
$$

Since protonation has significant effects on the possible
steps in the reaction scheme, we have investigated the
effect of protonation on the decomposition of the hydroxy
compound. Thus ΔE for the loss of CH_2OH^+ is substantially
less than for the loss of CH_3^+ reported above, and a limited
study of hydration was found to reduce ΔE even further. It
is noteworthy that hydroxylation, protonation and hydration
all progressively lengthen the CN bond.

$$\left[\begin{array}{c} CH_2OH \\ \diagdown \\ \quad N\text{-}N \diagup \quad ^O\diagdown_H \\ H \diagup \end{array} \right]^+ \longrightarrow CH_2OH^+ + HNNOH \qquad \Delta E = 206 \text{ kJ mol}^{-1}$$

$$\left[\begin{array}{c} \qquad \ddot{O}H_2 \\ CH_2O\ddot{H} \\ \diagdown \\ \quad \diagup N\text{-}N \diagup ^O\diagdown_H \\ H \diagup \end{array} \right]^+ \longrightarrow H_2COH\ldots\ldots OH_2^+ + HNNOH$$

$$\Delta E = 103 \text{ kJ mol}^{-1}$$

The protonated hydroxy compound may also decompose by one of two concerted processes

$$\left[\begin{array}{c} CH_2OH \\ \diagdown \\ \quad \diagup N\text{-}N \diagup ^O\diagdown_H \\ H \diagup \end{array} \right]^+ \longrightarrow CH_2OH^+ + \left[HNN \diagup ^{OH_2} \right]^+ \qquad \Delta E = \quad 38 \text{ kJ mol}^{-1}$$

$$CH_2OH.NHNOH^+ \longrightarrow CH_2O + H_2NNOH^+ \qquad \Delta E = 107 \text{ kJ mol}^{-1}$$

These concerted reactions are usually considered to involve unprotonated $CH_2OHNHNO$, which may give rise to HNNOH or H_2NNO with an overall energy change of 63 or 52 kJ mol^{-1} respectively. However, to distinguish between these concerted reactions, the relevant transition states need to be located, and this problem is currently being tackled.

B: The formation of the alkylating agent

The species formed in the above steps in the activation are the methyldiazohydroxide, its alkoxide analogue (CH_3NNOCH_3), or their protonated forms (Figure 1).

Considering first the diazohydroxide formed from monomethylnitrosamine, which would arise via an H atom shift, the transition state for the model reaction

$$\begin{array}{c} H \\ \diagdown \\ \quad N\text{-}N \diagup ^{\diagup O} \\ H \diagup \end{array} \xrightarrow[= 188 \text{ kJ mol}^{-1}]{\Delta E} \left[\begin{array}{c} N \\ H\text{-}N \diagup ^{\diagdown} O \\ \quad ''H \diagup \end{array} \right] \xrightarrow[- 185 \text{ kJ mol}^{-1}]{\Delta E} \begin{array}{c} H \\ \quad \diagup O \\ N\text{=}N \diagup \\ H \diagup \end{array}$$

$$\Delta E = \quad 3 \text{ kJ mol}^{-1}$$

has been determined and O-protonation makes little difference
to the barrier or to the structure of the transition state,
although the overall ΔE is negative.

$$\left[\begin{matrix} H \\ \\ H \end{matrix} N-N \begin{matrix} O \\ \\ H \end{matrix} \right]^{+} \xrightarrow[\;200\ kJ\ mol^{-1}\;]{\Delta E\ =} \left[H-N \begin{matrix} N \\ \\ H \end{matrix} O-H \right]^{+} \xrightarrow[\;-269\ kJ\ mol^{-1}\;]{\Delta E\ =} \left[\begin{matrix} H \\ \\ H-N{\equiv}N \end{matrix} O-H \right]^{\ddagger}$$

$$\Delta E\ =\ -69\ kJ\ mol^{-1}$$

Hydration, however, greatly reduces the energy barrier and
changes the saddle point structure.

$$\begin{matrix} H \\ \\ H \end{matrix} O-H \atop N-N{\overset{O}{}} \xrightarrow[\;79\ kJ\ mol^{-1}\;]{\Delta E\ =} \begin{matrix} H \\ O{\cdots}H \\ N{-}N \\ H \end{matrix} O \xrightarrow[\;-70\ kJ\ mol^{-1}\;]{\Delta E\ =} \begin{matrix} H \\ O{\cdots}H \\ N{=}N \\ H \end{matrix} O$$

$$\Delta E\ =\ \ \ 9\ kJ\ mol^{-1}$$

Once the diazohydroxide (or diazoalkoxide) is formed, its
reactions are particularly relevant to the nature of the
alkylating agent.

   Calculations show that O-protonation occurs very
readily, and has a dramatic effect on the structure of the
diazo compound, and furthermore the changes occur without
an energy barrier

$$\underset{CH_3}{}N{=}N{\overset{O-H}{}} + H^{+} \longrightarrow \left[\begin{matrix} H & H \\ \diagdown O \diagup \\ CH_3-\overset{\cdot}{N}-N \end{matrix} \right]^{+} \qquad \Delta E\ =\ -1034\ kJ\ mol^{-1}$$

$$\begin{matrix} CH_3 \\ \diagup \\ N{=}N \\ H \end{matrix} O + H^{+} \longrightarrow \left[\begin{matrix} H_3C & H \\ \diagdown O \diagup \\ H-N-N \end{matrix} \right]^{+} \qquad \Delta E\ =\ -922\ kJ\ mol^{-1}$$

The RNO bond is very long in the above cations ($\sim 2.3\overset{o}{A}$) and
these species are clearly solvated diazonium ions. They
appear to be local minima as the optimization algorithms
have a tendency to locate a lower energy structure

(particularly with the model compounds). The two species must therefore have a small barrier to interconversion.

$$\left[\begin{array}{c} H\diagdown\;\diagup H \\ O \\ \vdots \\ CH_3-N-N \end{array}\right]^+ \longrightarrow \left[\begin{array}{c} H\diagdown\quad\overset{\displaystyle H}{\underset{\displaystyle |}{}} \\ O\cdots C \cdots N\!\equiv\!N \\ H' \quad \diagup\;\vdots \\ \quad H\;\;H \end{array}\right]^+ \qquad \Delta E = -127 \text{ kJ mol}^{-1}$$

An alternative mode of production of CH_3N_2 by separation into ions $CH_3N_2^+$ + OH^- is energetically unfeasible (ΔE = + 912 kJ mol^{-1}) even when hydration is taken into account (ΔE = 477 kJ mol^{-1}).

The diazohydroxides or diazoalkoxides are unlikely to be the alkylating agents themselves since they are surrounded by regions of predominantly negative electrostatic potential. However, the N-hydrated diazonium ions which have a similar structure to the diazonium ion itself could well be the alkylating agent. When this species is converted to the C-hydrated isomer, the CN bond length of $\sim$ 2.9Å indicates it to be more like $CH_3.OH_2^+$. The relevant energies of the possible reactions are given below, showing that $CH_3.OH_2^+$ is the most likely product.

$$CH_3N_2.OH_2^+ \longrightarrow CH_3N_2^+ + H_2O \qquad\qquad \Delta E = \quad 78 \text{ kJ mol}^{-1}$$

$$CH_3N_2.OH_2^+ \longrightarrow CH_3OH_2^+ + N_2 \qquad\qquad \Delta E = -110 \text{ kJ mol}^{-1}$$

$$H_2O.CH_3.N_2^+ \longrightarrow CH_3N_2^+ + H_2O \qquad\qquad \Delta E = \quad 205 \text{ kJ mol}^{-1}$$

$$H_2O.CH_3.N_2^+ \longrightarrow CH_3OH_2^+ + N_2 \qquad\qquad \Delta E = \quad 16 \text{ kJ mol}^{-1}$$

$$CH_3N_2^+ \longrightarrow CH_3^+ + N_2 \qquad\qquad \Delta E = \quad 145 \text{ kJ mol}^{-1}$$

$$CH_3OH_2^+ \longrightarrow CH_3^+ + H_2O \qquad\qquad \Delta E = \quad 334 \text{ kJ mol}^{-1}$$

Both N_2 and CH_3OH have been detected experimentally, the latter probably derived from $CH_3^+OH_2$. Calculations in this laboratory have shown that CH_3^+ is likely to be hydrated by at least four H_2O molecules in its primary hydration shell.

DISCUSSION

The metabolism of N-Nitrosamines requires enzymatic

activation to form the α-hydroxynitrosamine, but our results also indicate that there are additional routes by which an alkylating agent could be formed. The α-hydroxynitrosamine probably decomposes by a concerted mechanism aided by protonation and hydration to give formaldehyde and a diazohydroxide. It seems unlikely that the diazohydroxide itself is involved in the alkylation reaction. Our calculations indicate a more likely possibility: namely, that protonation leads to the formation of an N-hydrated diazonium cation in which N_2 is loosely bound, and its loss leads to a hydrated methyl cation. It is possible that all of these cations could act as alkylating agents in vivo, reacting with the first nucleophile encountered.

One question yet to be answered satisfactorily is how metabolites from nitrosamines oxidised in the endoplasmic reticulum are able to alkylate nuclear DNA in view of their short lifetime. There is evidence for some metabolism in the nucleus (Pegg, 1980), but our results suggest that the metabolites might be divided into two groups: the first, those with limited stability, and a second group formed whenever the diazohydroxide is protonated. This could happen within the nucleus, in particular by interaction of the diazohydroxide with the phosphate groups on DNA, which could result in the generation of the alkylating agent in the correct vicinity to alkylate the DNA bases.

In summary, our calculations show that the influence of protonation on the metabolic intermediates may be of significance in the overall mechanism of action of these important carcinogens.

Acknowledgements

We are indebted to the National Foundation for Cancer Research for a postgraduate research studentship (to C.A.R.), and for continued financial support. We also thank Professor Pople for a copy of Gaussian 80, and the University of St. Andrews Computing Laboratory for the provision of the large amount of computer time necessary for this project.

REFERENCES

Andreozzi P, Klopman G, Hopfinger AJ (1980). Theoretical study of N-nitrosamines and their presumed proximate carcinogens. Cancer Biochem Biophys 4:209.

Bell S, Crighton S (1984). Locating transition states. J Chem Phys 80:2464.

Binkley JS, Whiteside RA, Krishnan R, DeFrees DJ, Schlegel HB, Topiol S, Kahn LR, Pople JA (1980). GAUSSIAN 80, Carnegie-Mellon University.

Loew GH, Poulsen MT, Spangler D, Kirkjian E (1983). Mechanistic structure-activity studies of carcinogenic dialkylnitrosamines. Int J Quant Chem: Quant Biol Symp 10:201.

Michejda CJ, Kroeger-Koepke MB, Koepke SR, Magee PN, Chu C (1982). Nitrogen formation during in vivo and in vitro metabolism of N-nitrosamines. In Magee PN (ed): "Banbury Report 12 Nitrosamines and Human Cancer", Cold Spring Harbour Laboratory, p69.

Pegg AE (1980). Metabolism of N-nitrosodimethylamine. IARC Sci Pull 27:3.

Pullman A, Berthol M, Greoh N (1975). Quantum mechanical studies of environmental effects on biomolecules. An ab-initio study of the hydration of dimethylphosphate. Chem Phys Lett 33:11.

Reynolds CA, Thomson C (1984a). Ab-initio calculations relevant to the mechanism of chemical carcinogenesis: I. The nitrosation of amines. Int J Quant Chem: Quant Biol Symp 11.

Reynolds CA, Thomson C (1984b). To be published.

Scribner JD, Ford GP (1982). N-Propyldiazonium ion alkylates O^6 of guanine with rearrangement, but alkylates N-7 without rearrangement. Cancer Lett 16:51.

Swan PF (1982). Metabolism of nitrosamines: observations on the effect of alcohol on nitrosamine metabolism and on human cancer. In Magee PN (ed): "Banbury Report 12 Nitrosamines and Human Cancer", Cold Spring Harbour Laboratory, p53.

Molecular Basis of Cancer, Part A: Macromolecular
Structure, Carcinogens, and Oncogenes, pages 249–261
© 1985 Alan R. Liss, Inc.

HALOGENATED NUCLEIC ACIDS: BASE PROPERTIES AND
CONFORMATION OF FLUORINATED DERIVATIVES

J.L. Alderfer, R.E. Loomis, M. Sharma,
and G. Hazel

Biophysics Department
Roswell Park Memorial Institute
Buffalo, New York   14263

INTRODUCTION: Base-halogenated nucleic acid constituents
have been of general biological interest since the discovery that they are incorporated into cellular macromolecules
(Dunn, Smith 1954). Fluorinated bases in particular are of
special interest due to their antitumor and fungicidal
properties (Heidelberger, Chaudhuri, Danneberg, Mooren,
Griesbach, Duschinsky, Schnitzer, Pleven, Scheiner 1957;
Bennett 1977). To obtain a more basic understanding of the
physicochemical properties of these nucleic acid analogs, a
comparative study of normal and fluorinated nucleic acid
constituents and homopolynucleotides has been underway
(Alderfer, Loomis, Zielinski 1982; Alderfer, Loomis, Rycyna
1983; Loomis, Alderfer 1984). The present study evaluates
the effects of fluorine substitution on the base moiety
from ultraviolet spectral properties and proton nuclear
magnetic resonance spectroscopy.   The results indicate
marked effects on the pK_a of the base, changes in amount
of base stacking interactions and alterations in the conformation of the ribosylfuranose.

MATERIALS AND METHODS: 5-Fluorouridine and 5-fluorocyti-
dine were kindly provided by Dr. W.E. Scott, Hoffman-
LaRoche. 2-Fluoroadenosine was a gift from Dr. D. Cochran,
Merck Sharp & Dohme.   2-Fluoroinosine was prepared from
fluoroadenosine using adenosine deaminase.   Normal polynucleotides were obtained from commercial sources and
fluorinated polynucleotides were enzymatically synthesized
using polynucleotide phosphorylase (Alderfer, Tazawa,
Tazawa, Ts'o 1974).   Ultraviolet spectra were obtained

TABLE 1

Ultraviolet parameters and pK_a of nucleotides
and derivatives

Compound	$\lambda_{max}(nm)$ [a]	ε_{max}^{mM} [a]	pK_a	Reference
Urd	262	10.1	9.2	b
5FUrd	269	9.2	7.83	c,j
Cyd	271	9.1	4.2	b
5FCyd	281	8.1	2.3	d
Ado	259	15.4	3.4	b
2FAdo	261.5	15.2	2.2[h]	e,f,g
Ino	248.5	12.2	8.8	b
2FIno	244	11.8	4.1	c,i

a. Parameters for base in neutral (unionized) form. b.
Schwarz BioResearch, Inc., Catalog 1967. c. This work. d.
Wempen, Duschinsky, Kaplan, Fox 1961. e. Montgomery, Hew-
son 1960. f. Shigeura, Baxer, Sampson, Meloni 1965. g.
Broom, Amarnath, Vince, Brownell 1979. h. Value is for
2FAdo-5'-P; reference g. i. Michal, Muhlegger, Nelboeck,
Thiessen, Wiemann 1974. j. Berens, Shugar 1963.

using a Cary 14 and Gilford 2600. Proton NMR spectra were
obtained at 200 MHz using a Bruker WP-200.

RESULTS: The effects of fluorine substitution on the
physicochemical properties of nucleic acid bases studied
here depend on the base moiety. The ultraviolet spectral
properties (Table 1) show that introduction of a fluorine
atom results in a red-shift of the absorption maximum and a
decrease of the intensity of that maximum. An obvious exception to this general trend is the blue-shift of FIno.
Another property observed for the fluorine containing
nucleosides is an increased acidity of the base unit (a
reduction of pK_a). Here again FIno appears to be considerably different with a ΔpK_a of 4.7 when the others
are in the range of 1.2-1.9. The effects of the fluorine
substitution on the general shape of the UV absorption
spectrum also vary. For the pyrimidines there are no large
changes (Wempen, Duschinsky, Kaplan, Fox 1961; Berens,
Shugar 1963) while in the purines changes are apparent,

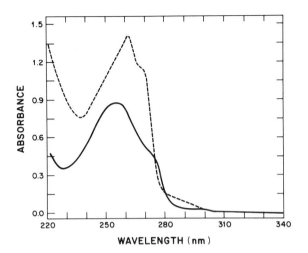

Fig. 1. Ultraviolet spectrum of poly(FA) (———). Spectrum following hydrolysis of poly(FA) (---) with snake venom phosphodiesterase (0.1 M NH₄HCO₃, pH 8.8, 23°C).

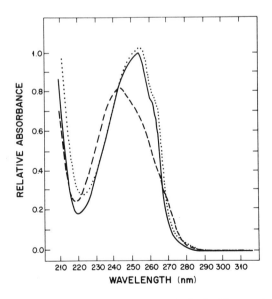

Fig. 2. Ultraviolet spectrum of 2-fluoroinosine at pH 2 (---), pH 7 (———) and pH 12 (····).

TABLE 2

Chemical shifts[a] of polynucleotides

Polymer[b]	°C	H1'	H5	H6	H8
poly(FA)	45	5.622			8.000
	55	5.694			8.071
	65	5.731			8.113
	75	5.756			8.139
poly(C)	35	5.682	5.831	7.808	
	55	5.760	5.908	7.834	
	70	5.825	5.965	7.844	
	85	5.878	6.008	7.840	
poly(FC)	35	5.692		8.017	
	55	5.785		8.026	
	70	5.840		8.017	
	85	5.878		8.002	
poly(U)	30	5.967	5.933	7.883	
(pH6.0)	40	5.967	5.932	7.869	
	50	5.970	5.935	7.855	
	60	5.965	5.932	7.849	
poly(FU)	30	5.978		8.067	
(pH6.0)	40	5.971		8.053	
	50	5.968		8.041	
	60	5.961		8.027	

a. In ppm, with respect to internal TSP.
b. At pH 7, unless otherwise indicated.

especially for FAdo which has a distinct shoulder at 270 nm (Figures 1 and 2).

The chemical shifts of selected hydrogens of various polynucleotides are listed in Table 2 at different temperatures. The most generally observed feature is a downfield-shift with increasing temperature. The most obvious exceptions to this trend are poly(U), poly(FU) and the high temperature chemical shift values for H6 of poly(FC). To obtain a more apparent effect of temperature on polymer structure, the polymer chemical shift is compared to the respective monomer chemical shift at a given temperature. This difference is called the polymerization shift ($\Delta\delta_p$ = $\delta_{polymer}$-$\delta_{monomer}$) and primarily arises when base-base stacking interactions occur in the polymer (Alderfer, Tazawa, Tazawa, Ts'o 1974), as a result of the ring-current anisotropy of the nucleic acid bases (Giessner-Prettre, Pullman 1970). In Figures 3-5 are the temperature dependence of $\Delta\delta_p$ for three sets of polymers. Two features of interest are the magnitude of $\Delta\delta_p$ between different bases and the relative $\Delta\delta_p$ within a fluorinated and non-fluorinated polymer pair. The relative sizes of $\Delta\delta_p$ decrease in the order of adenosine, cytidine, uridine. Also within each base type, the normal base has a larger $\Delta\delta_p$ than the fluorinated base.

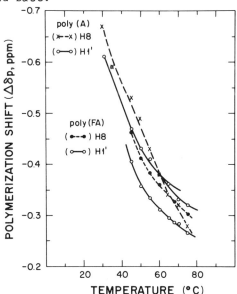

Fig. 3. Temperature dependence of the polymerization shift of poly(A) and poly(FA).

These polynucleotides are also compared with respect to their furanose coupling constant, $J_{H1',H2'}$. The temperature dependence of this value is illustrated in Figures 6 and 7 for the cytosine and adenine polymers, respectively. These data indicate the normal-base polymers have a

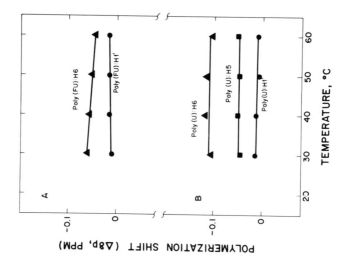

Fig. 5. Temperature dependence of the polymerization shift of poly(U) and poly(FU).

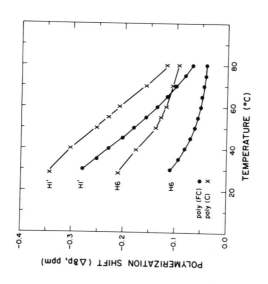

Fig. 4. Temperature dependence of the polymerization shift of poly(C) and poly(FC).

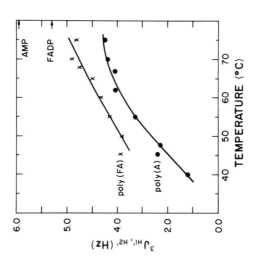

Fig. 7. Temperature dependence of $J_{H1'}$,$H2'$ of poly(A) and poly(FA).

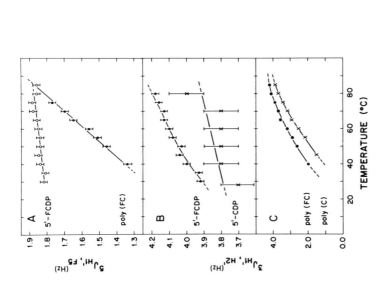

Fig. 6. Temperature dependence of (A) $J_{H1'}$, F5 of 5'-FCDP and poly(FC), (B) $J_{H1'}$,$H2'$ of 5'-CDP and 5'-FCDP and (C) $J_{H1'}$,$H2'$ of poly(C) and poly(FC).

smaller $J_{H1',H2'}$ at a given temperature than the corresponding fluorinated-base polymer. In the cases of poly(U)
and poly(FU), the $J_{H1',H2'}$ are 6.1 and 5.8 Hz respectively, and are temperature independent. A long-range coupling
constant, $J_{H1',F5}$, of poly(FC) is also presented in
Figure 6. This parameter increases markedly with temperature in comparison to the monomer (Figure 6A).

DISCUSSION: The present study is focused on two aspects of
the physicochemical properties of fluorinated nucleic acid
constituents: (1) the effects of fluorine on UV spectral
properties of the base unit, and (2) conformational properties of fluorinated polynucleotides. The effects of fluorine substitution on the UV spectral properties (Table 1)
are generally those observed for fluorinated pyrimidines
(Wempen, Duschinsky, Kaplan, Fox 1961) and fluorinated
purines (Montgomery, Hewson 1960). The UV properties of
FIno do not follow the general trend of bathochromic shifts
and hypochromicity following fluorine substitution at
certain solution conditions. The blue-shift observed in
Ino following fluorine substitution is not without prece-
dent. The sulfur derivative at the C6 position, 2-fluoro-
6-purinethiol-9- β-D-ribofuranose (S^6-FIno), also displays
unusual UV spectroscopic properties (Montgomery, Hewson
1960). At basic conditions (pH 13) the absorption maximum
of S^6-FIno (315 nm) exhibits a slight bathochromic shift
compared to the non-fluorinated 6-thiopurine-9- β-D-ribofuranose (312 nm). The comparably ionized forms of FIno
and Ino have an absorption maximum at 254 and 253 nm,
respectively. At low pH (pH 1) the absorption maximum of
S^6-FIno has an initial value of 326 nm, compared to 322
nm for the non-fluorinated 6-thiopurine ribonucleoside.
However the 326 nm peak of S^6-FIno slowly shifts to an
absorption maximum of 296 nm, a marked blue-shift. By
comparison the absorption maximum of 1-methyl-6(1H)-puri-
methione is at 321 nm while 6-(methylthio)-purine is 294
nm, and both are essentially independent of pH in the range
1-13 (Montgomery, Hewson 1960). These results for S^6-
FIno have been interpreted as the result of an initial
protonation of N1 (λ_{max} 326) followed by a tautomeric
shift from the thione to thiol form, where the sulfur is
protonated (λ_{max} 296). The pKa of S^6-FIno is also
apparently quite low (pKa <7), since the UV λ_{max} at pH
7 and 13 are the same. Considering these data collective-
ly, the blue-shift observed for FIno in the neutral state

(pH <3.5) may be due to the contribution of the enol tauto-meric form.

The proton polymerization shift data in Figures 3 and 4 clearly indicates base-base unstacking of the polymers with increasing temperature. This is not observed with poly(U) and poly(FU), indicating the feeble propensity for base-stacking of uracil. The magnitude of $\Delta\delta_p$ (Figures 3-5) in each set of polymers is reduced for the fluorinated polymer compared to the normal polymer. This is consistent with the idea that the introduction of a fluorine into the base unit reduces polymer base-stacking interactions. It could be argued that these reduced $\Delta\delta_p$ values do not pri-marily reflect changes in amount of base-stacking interac-tions but rather indicate a reduction of ring-current anisotropy which results from introduction of a fluorine. There are two kinds of data which in general support the $\Delta\delta_p$ data. The first is UV hyperchromicity following enzymatic or alkaline hydrolysis of poly(C) and poly(FC) (Folayan, Hutchinson 1974), and poly(A) and poly(FA) (Broom, Amarnath, Vince, Brownell 1979). Poly(C) is con-siderably more hyperchromic than poly(FC) (42 versus 14%), while poly(A) (64%) and poly(FA) (59%) are not significant-ly different. Poly(U) is also reported to be slightly more hyperchromic than poly(FU) (Szer, Shugar 1963).

The second type of data is the temperature dependence of the $J_{H1',H2'}$. The correlation between base-stacking of the ribosyl-polynucleotide and the furanose conformation has been discussed previously (Alderfer, Tazawa, Tazawa, Ts'o 1974). This correlation indicates as the temperature decreases base-stacking increases ($|\Delta\delta_p|$ increases) and the furanose C2'-endo/C3'-endo equilibrium shifts to higher populations of C3'-endo (i.e. $J_{H1',H2'}$ decreases). The $J_{H1',H2'}$ temperature curves (Figures 6 and 7) illustrate at a given temperature, the normal-base polymer has a smaller value than the fluorine-base polymer, indicating a larger C3'-endo population for the normal-base polymer (and more base-stacking). Thus the $J_{H1',H2'}$ data also supports the $\Delta\delta_p$ and hyperchromicity data which show less base-stacking interactions for the fluorinated-polynucleotides. Additional conformational information on poly(FC) is provided by $J_{H1',F5}$ (Figure 6A). The change of $J_{H1',F5}$ with temperature is consistent with a change in sugar-base torsion angle accompanying base-stacking. This change of $J_{H1',F5}$ is not observed in poly(FU).

TABLE 3

UV hypochromicity of uridylic and cytidylic acid polynucleotides

Polymer	h[a]	Reference
poly(U)	15	b
poly(FU)	7	c
poly(ClU)	4	b
poly(BrU)	15	b
poly(IU)	36	b
poly(C)	31	d
poly(FC)	11	e
poly(ClC)	22	f
poly(BrC)	22	g
poly(IC)	32	h

a. Hypochromicity, $h=(1-\varepsilon_{polymer}/\varepsilon_{monomer})$ 100; in some cases hyperchromicity (hyperchromicity=$(A_{monomer}-A_{polymer})100/A_{polymer}$) determined from enzymatic or alkaline degradation was used to calculate h. b. Michelson, Donden, Grunberg-Manago 1962; Massoulie, Michelson, Pochon 1966. c. Szer, Shugar 1963. d. Sarkar, Yang 1965. e. Folayan, Hutchinson 1974. f. Eaton, Hutchinson 1972. g. Howard, Frazier, Miles 1969. h. Michelson, Monny 1967.

    The effects of halogenation on polynucleotide proper-
ties has received considerable attention for several
decades (Michelson, Massoulie, Guschlbauer 1967; Jones
1979). A direct correlation of 5-halogenated uracil and
cytosine residues with respect to single-stranded conformational stability and base-stacking interactions in the
solution and solid states has been suggested (Sternglanz,
Bugg 1975). The experimental evidence supporting this view
for halogenated uracil and cytosine polyribonucleotides
appears tenuous. The hypochromicity data in Table 3 indicates only poly(IU) is substantially stabilized compared to
the non-halogenated polymer. The effect on thermal stability (Tm) of the double-stranded complexes of poly(C) and
halogen analogs with poly(I) has been shown to correlate

well with van der Waals radii of the C5-substituent (Folayan, Hutchinson 1974). Similar correlations of poly(U) and
halogen analogs with poly(A) are not as straightforward,
since double- and/or triple-stranded complexes can form.
It is reported (Massoulie, Michelson, Pochon 1966) that
triple-stranded complexes of chloro-, bromo-, and iodo-
uridylic acid polymers with poly(A) are substantially more
stable than poly(A)·2poly(U), although poly(A)·2poly(FU)
does not realize any stabilization. However, in the case
of poly(FA) (Broom, Amarnath, Vince, Brownell 1979), the
helical complex with poly(U) is significantly destabilized
compared to the poly(A) complex.

In conclusion, our studies have shown that in general
fluorine substitution of these nucleic acid bases induces a
bathochromic shift in λ_{max} and hypochromicity of the ultraviolet spectrum and an increase in acidity of the base.
There are certain exceptions to this observation which may
relate to the tautomeric state of the base. The effect of
fluorine substitution on the polymers studied destabilizes
them relative to the normal polynucleotides with respect to
base-stacking interactions. This destabilization of the
single-stranded form of halogenated uracil and cytosine
polynucleotides appears to be more the rule then exception,
while a stabilization of the helical complexes is generally
observed.

ACKNOWLEDGEMENTS

The authors acknowledge the acquisition of uv data by
Richard Mazurchuk and Akos Tibold. This investigation was
supported by PHS Grant Number CA-25438, awarded by the
National Cancer Institute, DHHS.

REFERENCES

Alderfer JL, Loomis RE, Rycyna RE (1983). Physicochemical
    properties and interactions of fluorinated polynucleo-
    tides. Fed Proc 42:1955.
Alderfer JL, Loomis RE, Zielinski TJ (1982). Fluorinated
    nucleic acid constituents: a carbon-13 nuclear magnetic
    resonance study of adenosine, cytidine, uridine and their
    fluorinated analogues. Biochemistry 21:2738.
Alderfer, JL, Tazawa I, Tazawa S, Ts'o POP (1974). Compar-

ative studies on homopolymers of adenylic acid possessing different C-2' substituents of the furanose. Poly(deoxy-adenylic acid), poly(riboadenylic acid), poly(2'-O-methyladenylic acid), and poly(2'-ethyladenylic acid). Biochemistry 13:1615.

Bennett JE (1977). Flucytosine. Ann Intern Med 86:319.

Berens K, Shugar D (1963). Ultraviolet absorption spectra and structure of halogenated uracils and their glyco-sides. Acta Biochim Polon 10:25.

Broom AD, Amarnath V, Vince R, Brownell J (1979). Poly(2-fluoroadenylic acid). The role of basicity in the sta-bilization of complementary helices. Biochim Biophys Acta 563:508.

Dunn DB, Smith JD (1954). Incorporation of halogenated pyrimidines into the deoxyribonucleic acids of bacterium coli and its bacteriophages. Nature 174:305.

Eaton MAW, Hutchinson DW (1972). Poly(5-chlorocytidylic acid). Biochemistry 11:3162.

Folayan JO, Hutchinson DW (1974). Poly(5-fluorocytidylic acid). Biochim Biophys Acta 340:194.

Giessner-Prettre C, Pullman B (1970). Intermolecular nu-clear shielding values for protons of purines and flavins. J Theor Biol 27:87.

Heidelberger C, Chauduri NK, Danneberg P, Mooren D, Gries-bach L, Duschinsky R, Schnitzer RJ, Pleven E, Scheiner J (1957). Fluorinated pyrimidines, a new class of tumour-inhibitory compounds. Nature 179:663.

Howard FB, Frazier J, Miles HT (1969). Interaction of poly-5-bromocytidylic acid with polyinosinic acid. J Biol Chem 244:1291.

Jones AS (1979). Synthetic analogues of nucleic acids - a review. Int J Biolog Macromolecules 1:194.

Loomis RE, Alderfer JL (1984). Halogenated nucleic acids: effects of 5-fluorouracil on the conformation and proper-ties of a polyribonucleotide and its constituents. Sub-mitted for publication.

Massoulie J, Michelson AM, Pochon F (1966). Polynucleotide analogues. VI. Physical studies on 5-substituted pyrimi-dine polynucleotides. Biochim Biophys Acta 114:16.

Michal G, Muhlegger K, Nelboeck M, Thiessen C, Weimann G (1974). Cyclophosphates VI. Cyclophosphates as sub-strates and effectors of phosphodiesterase. Pharmacol Res Comm 6:203.

Michelson AM, Dondon J, Grunberg-Manago M (1962). The action of polynucleotide phosphorylase on 5-halogen-uridine-5'-pyrophosphates. Biochim Biophys Acta 55:529.

Michelson AM, Massoulie J, Greschlbauer W (1967). Synthetic polynucleotides. In Davidson JN, Cohn WE (eds): "Progress in Nucleic Acid Research and Molecular Biology" Vol 6, New York:Academic Press, p. 83.

Michelson AM, Monny C (1967). Polynucleotide analogues. XII. Poly-5-bromocytidylic acid and poly-5-iodocytidylic acid. Biochim. Biophys Acta 149:88.

Montgomery JA, Hewson K (1960). Synthesis of potential anticancer agents. XX. 2-Fluoropurines. J Amer Chem Soc 82:463.

Sarkar PK, Yang JT (1965). Optical activity of the conformation of polyinosinic acid and several other polynucleotide complexes. Biochemistry 4:1238.

Sternglanz H, Bugg CE (1975). Relationship between the mutagenic and base-stacking properties of halogenated uracil derivatives. The crystal structures of 5-chloro- and 5-bromouracil. Biochim Biophys Acta 378:1.

Szer W, Shugar D (1963). Preparation of poly-5-fluoro-uridylic and the properties of halogenated poly-uridylic acids and their complexes with poly-adenylic acid. Acta Biochim Polon 10:219.

Wempen I, Duschinsky R, Kaplan L, Fox JJ (1961). Thiation of nucleosides. IV. The synthesis of 5-fluoro-2'-deoxycytidine and related compounds. J Amer Chem Soc 83:4755.

Molecular Basis of Cancer, Part A: Macromolecular Structure, Carcinogens, and Oncogenes, pages 263–275
© **1985 Alan R. Liss, Inc.**

QUANTUM CHEMICAL AND OTHER THEORETICAL STUDIES OF CARCIN-
OGENS, THEIR METABOLIC ACTIVATION AND ATTACK ON DNA
CONSTITUENTS

Joyce J. Kaufman, PC Hariharan, WS Koski and
K Balasubramanian*
    Department of Chemistry
    The Johns Hopkins University
    Baltimore, Maryland 21218

ABSTRACT

     We have carried out a variety of different types of
studies on carcinogens: ab-initio quantum chemical, including generation of electrostatic molecular potential contour
(EMPC) maps and graph theoretical generation of polycyclic
aromatic hydrocarbon (PAH) structures and characterization
of the "carcinogenic" bay regions.

     Polycyclic aromatic hydrocarbon (PAH) carcinogens are
activated metabolically from precarcinogen (PAH's) through
proximate carcinogens (PAH epoxides and dihydrodiols) to
ultimate carcinogens (PAH dihydrodiolepoxides) which then
attack DNA constituents. We carried out ab-initio MODPOT/
VRDDO/MERGE calculations on a variety of these molecules
using our own ab-initio programs which incorporate as
options a number of desirable options for ab-initio calculation on large molecules. From these electronic wave
functions, we generated electrostatic molecular potential
contour (EMPC) maps around these molecules. These EMPC
maps indicated predictively the positions at which epoxides would form and the propensity and geometrical preference to form dihydrodiols and dihydrodiolepoxides.
We performed spin and symmetry analyses for attack of O
adding across C=C bonds or inserting in C-H or N-H bonds.
We also carried out ab-initio calculations for attack of
ultimate carcinogens on DNA constituents.

---

* Permanent Address: Department of Chemistry/Arizona State
University/Tempe, Arizona 85287

Using graph theory we generated all possible structures for any arbitrary numbers of aromatic rings and also
set up a graph theoretical characterization of the "carcinogenic" bay region. Most recently, we have incorporated this into a computer program for global prediction
of toxicity.

INTRODUCTION

We have carried out a variety of different types of
studies on carcinogens:
1. Ab-initio quantum chemical calculations
    Kaufman, Popkie, Palalikit, Hariharan, 1978;
    Hariharan, Popkie, Kaufman, 1981; Lowrey,
    Hariharan, Kaufman, 1981) on polycyclic aromatic
    hydrocarbons and their metabolites as well as on
    nitrosamines and their metabolites, including gen-
    eration of electrostatic molecular potential con-
    tour maps (Hariharan, Kaufman, Petrongolo, 1979;
    Hariharan, Kaufman, Petrongolo, 1981) and attack
    of ultimate carcinogens on DNA constituents
    (Hariharan, Popkie, Kaufman, 1979);
2. Spin and symmetry analyses for attack of
    O adding across a C=C double bond or insert-
    ing into C-H or N-H bonds (Kaufman, 1979);
3. Graph theoretical generation of polycyclic
    aromatic hydrocarbon (PAH) structures and
    characterization of the "carcinogenic" bay
    regions (Balasubramanian, Kaufman, Koski,
    Balaban, 1980);
4. Incorporated the above graph theory charac-
    terization of "carcinogenic" bay region into
    our recent computer program for global pre-
    diction of toxicity (Kaufman, Koski, Hariha-
    ran, Crawford, Garmer, Chan-Lizardo, 1983;
    Kaufman, Koski, Hariharan, Garmer, Crawford,
    Chan-Lizardo, Sipos, 1983).

AB-INITIO QUANTUM CHEMICAL CALCULATIONS

Methodology

The ab-initio quantum chemical calculations were carried out with our own fast ab-initio Gaussian programs which, in addition, incorporate as options a number of desirable computational strategies especially for large molecules (Popkie, Kaufman, 1975; Popkie, Kaufman, 1976; Popkie, Kaufman, 1977; Kaufman, Popkie, Hariharan, 1979): ab-initio effective core model potentials (MODPOT) which permit calculations of valence electrons only explicitly, yet accurately, and a charge-conserving integral prescreening evaluation (which we named VRDDO--variable retention of diatomic differential overlap) especially effective for spatially extended molecules; and an efficient MERGE technique, which permits reuse of common skeletal integrals.

The electrostatic potential (Scrocco, Thomasi, 1973; Petrongolo, 1978)

$$V(\vec{R}) = \sum_{\alpha}^{\text{nuclei}} \frac{Z_\alpha}{|\vec{R}_\alpha - \vec{R}|} - \int d\vec{R}_1 \frac{e(\vec{R}_1)}{|\vec{R}_1 - \vec{R}|}$$

has proven a useful tool in characterization of biological and biomedical molecules (Politzer, Truhlar, 1981). The interaction of a unit test positive charge with the potential leads to electrostatic molecular potential contour (EMPC) maps. These EMPC maps in three-dimensional space around a molecule give more detailed information than a population analysis. We had shown that EMPC maps generated from ab-initio quantum chemical wave functions using small, well-balanced atomic basis sets match those from larger well-balanced atomic basis sets (Petrongolo, Preston, Kaufman, 1978). We had also shown that EMPC maps generated from ab-initio MODPOT wave functions matched those generated from wave functions using the full atomic basis set (inner and outer shells) with the same valence basis functions (Kaufman, Hariharan, Tobin, Petrongolo, 1981).

Systems Investigated

Polycyclic aromatic hydrocarbons (PAH's). Polycyclic
aromatic hydrocarbons (PAH's) are activated metabolically
from precarcinogenic (PAH's) through proximate carcinogens
(PAH epoxides and dihydrodiols) to ultimate carcinogens
(PAH dihydrodiolepoxides) which then open thier epoxide
ring and attack DNA (Jerina, Lehr, Jagi, Hernandez, Dansette,
Weslocki, Wood, Chang, Levin, Conney, 1976; Yang, McCourt,
Roller, Gelboin, 1976).

We carried out ab-initio MODPOT/VRDDO/MERGE calculations
for benzo(a)pyrene (BP) (Kaufman, Popkie, Palalikit,
Hariharan, 1978), 3-methylcholanthrene (Kaufman, Popkie,
Hariharan, 1979) and 17 other PAH's and their metabolites
(Balasubramanian, Hariharan, Kaufman, 1981).

As an example for BP and its metabolites, we carried
out the quantum chemical calculations for the following
species including all the possible stereoisomers for each
species:

Benzo(a)pyrene and metabolites by MERGE technique.

From these electronic wave functions we generated the
electrostatic molecular potential contour (EMPC) maps
in three dimensions around BP and its metabolites
(Hariharan, Kaufman, Petrongolo, 1979).

These EMPC maps for BP (or for all of the PAH's themselves) indicated small negative contours in the regions

of all the C=C bonds across which O adds to form the epoxide.
(Figure 2.)

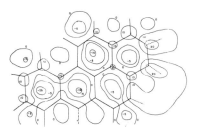

The EMPC maps around the PAH epoxides indicate the direction along which protons will prefer to attack to form PAH
dihydrodiols (Figure 3a and 3b, BP epoxide) [For all the
following EMPC maps only two planes are shown. The conven-
tion is that solid skeletal lines are above the molecular
plane and dotted skeletal lines are below the molecular
plane.]

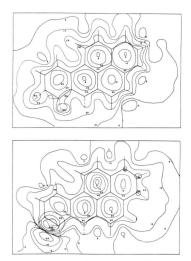

The EMPC maps around the PAH dihydrodiols indicate the
direction of preference for proton attack to form the PAH
dihydrodiolepoxide (Figure 4a and 4b, BP 7,8-dihydrodiol).

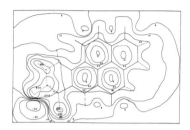
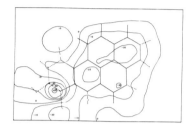

The EMPC maps around the PAH dihydrodiolepoxide again indicate the direction of preference of attack by a proton to form BP 7,8-dihydrodiol-9,10-epoxide (Figures 5a and 5b).

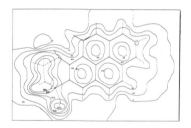
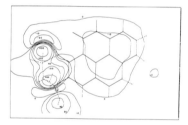

Ultimate carcinogens are electrophilic reagents which attack DNA. It was postulated by experimentalists that this electrophilic species from BP 7,8-dihydrodiol-9,10-epoxide was a ring opened epoxide. The question arose as to how to compare the relative electrophilicities of species with this epoxide ring opened toward C_9 or C_{10}, or, more generally, how to compare relative electrophilicities of congeneric ultimate carcinogens. We suggested as a useful theoretical tool that the farther out in space more positive EMPC maps extend, the more "electrophilic" would be that ultimate carcinogen. This representation of relative electrophilicity has proven useful not only in carcinogenicity but also in a completely different area, the propogation step in cationic polymerization of ring opened cyclic ethers (Tobin, Hariharan, Kaufman, 1981).

$\underline{CH_3^+ + Guanine}$. CH_3^+, believed to arise from metabolic degradation of dimethylnitrosamine, would be one of the simplest ultimate carcinogens. CH_3^+ then attacks DNA constituents. As an initial study we carried out ab-initio single determinant MODPOT/VRDDO/MERGE SCF calculations of CH_3^+ attack on guanine since both CH_3^+ and guanine were closed shell ground electronic state systems (Hariharan, Popkie, Kaufman, 1979) (Figure 6).

However, as the C---O distance became greater than 5.5 a.u., the ab-initio single determinant SCF calculation began to oscillate (although with special damping and extrapolation procedures it was possible to converge the single determinant curve which separated smoothly into CH_3^+ and guanine.

However, the unexpected oscillations led us to investigate closely the fundamental physical phenomena that might be involved in the reaction of CH_3^+ and guanine. There are two types of behavior for ion-molecule reactions of closed shell ground electronic state species $A^+ + B$, depending on the relative ionization potentials of A^+ and B. If the ionization potential of A is less than that of B, then the reaction can proceed along a single potential energy surface from $A^+ + B$ (Figure 7a). However, if the ionization potential of A is greater than that of B, then--even though the reaction starts out on a single potential energy surface from $A^+ + B$--there are at least two lower potential energy surfaces arising from the lower energy asymptote $A + B^+$. (Figure 7b) [See next page for Figures.] This may well explain the difference in carcinogenicity between methylating and ethylating carcinogens, where the ethylating (and higher carcinogens) are more carcinogenic than the methylating carcinogens. For methylating carcinogens--while the reactants start out along the singlet potential energy surface leading from CH_3^+ + DNA constituent--this surface is crossed from below by singlet and triplet surfaces arising from CH_3 + (DNA constituent)$^+$.

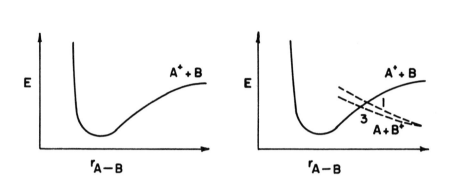

SPIN AND SYMMETRY ANALYSES FOR ATTACK OF O

Carcinogens are activated metabolically partly by adding O across a C=C bond or insertion of O into a C-H or N-H bond. We pointed out (Kaufman, 1979) that if one wanted to compute a proper potential energy surface for the model O + carcinogen it would be necessary

1. To use an ab-initio quantum chemical method since no less-than-ab-initio method (including all zero differential overlap methods) separate properly under any conditions.

2. Further, to use ab-initio MC SCF (multiconfigurational SCF) or CI (configuration interaction) methods since to arrive at the final singlet ground state products

$$\underset{C}{\overset{O}{\underset{|}{\diagup}}}C \diagdown\ ;-\underset{|}{\overset{|}{C}}-O-H \quad or \quad \diagup N-O-H$$

there are six different singlet potential energy surfaces [five arising from O^1Dg + carcinogen and one more potential energy surface arising from O^1Sg + carcinogen]. These six singlet surfaces will mix and must also cross.

The case is even more complicated for attack by O_2 since the asymptotes will involve $O_2(\ ^3\Pi,\ ^1\Delta$ and $^1\Sigma^+)$ + carcinogen.

Our recent methods of ab-initio configuration interaction (CI) calculations and ab-initio coupled cluster calculations with multireference determinants based on localized orbitals for regions of molecules (Kaufman, Hariharan, Chabalowski, Roszak and Laforgue, 1984) hold promise of making such proper ab-initio calculations tractable for attack of O or O_2 on carcinogens.

GRAPH THEORETICAL CHARACTERIZATION OF "CARCINOGENIC" BAY REGIONS

A very pertinent problem in connection with potentially carcinogenic aromatic hydrocarbon effluents from energy production is: "Knowing the number of aromatic rings present, what are all the possible isomeric structures, and which of these isomeric structures have a potentially 'carcinogenic' bay region?"

Using graph theory, we generated all possible structures for any arbitrary numbers of aromatic rings. We also set up a graph theoretical characterization of the "carcinogenic" bay region. For the latter, we derived a new concept of ring adjacency matrices plus a vector connecting the center of each ring having direction including angle. This characterization technique can be overlaid on a search of all ∿ six million unique compounds already identified in Chemical Abstracts to pull out all compounds with potentially "carcinogenic" bay regions (including those with heteroatoms in rings and/or various substituents).

COMPUTER PROGRAM FOR GLOBAL PREDICTION OF TOXICITY

We have recently been involved in formulating and implementing an overall strategy for prediction of toxicity (Kaufman, 1981; Kaufman, Koski, Hariharan, Crawford, Garmer, Chan-Lizardo, 1983; Kaufman, Koski, Hariharan, Garmer, Crawford, Chan-Lizardo, Sipos, 1983) [both for specific series of compounds and for global prediction of toxicity]. The overall program contains the following capabilities:

I. INPUT CHEMICAL STRUCTURE OF MOLECULES IN FORM TO DO EF-
FICIENT SUBTRUCTURE SEARCH - TOPOLOGICAL
II. CREATE 3-DIMENSIONAL GEOMETRY AND OPTIMIZE GEOMETRY OF
MOLECULE IN ORDER TO DO EFFICIENT SUBSTRUCTURE SEARCH -
TOPOGRAPHICAL
III. MOLECULAR AND FRAGMENT PROPERTIES
IV. QUANTUM CHEMICAL CALCULATIONS
   A. CALCULATE QUANTUM CHEMICAL WAVE FUNCTION OF ISOLA-
   TED MOLECULE TO DERIVE THEORETICAL INDICES
   B. CALCULATE QUANTUM CHEMICAL WAVE FUNCTIONS OF INTER-
   ACTING MOLECULES
V. CALCULATE ELECTROSTATIC MOLECULAR POTENTIAL CONTOUR
MAPS
VI. CREATE LIBRARY OF TOXICOPHORES (OR PHARMACOPHORES) FOR
SPECIFIC BIOCHEMICAL TRIGGERING EVENTS
VII. CORRELATION PROCEDURES
VIII.SYSTEMS ANALYSIS, CONTROL THEORY AND CATASTROPHE THEORY
IX. FOR SPECIFIC BIOCHEMICAL TRIGGERING EVENT
   A. CREATE LIBRARY OF CASCADING PHYSIOLOGICAL AND PATH-
   OLOGICAL SIGNS AND SYMPTOMS
   B. INCLUDE CAPABILITY OF BACK-TRACKING FROM OBSERVABLE
   SIGNS AND SYMPTOMS BACK TO TRIGGERING EVENT

The last component, the TOX-MATCH--PHARM-MATCH program,
enables prediction of toxicology and pharmacology from a library of model toxicophores and pharmacophores. For this
purpose, we developed a new method for chemical coding and
retrieval (Kaufman, Koski, Hariharan, Crawford, Garmer, Chan-
Lizardo, 1983; Kaufman, Koski, Hariharan, Garmer, Crawford,
Chan-Lizardo, Sipos, 1983) which is more flexible and powerful than any other method in current use and is ideally
suited for all structure-activity correlations and predictions based on chemical structures. In our chemical coding
technique, among other aspects, atoms are identified by their
atomic number rather than by atomic element symbol. This allows us general searching algorithms based on periodic table
relationships across rows and down columns. For all problems
other than carcinogens, this chemical coding technique uses
as part of its input our generalized topological connectivity
of atoms (atom-by-atom). However, as we showed, polycyclic
aromatic hydrocarbons are more naturally (and much more com-
pactly) described in terms of graph theory, as is the "carcinogenic" bay region (Balasubramanian, Kaufman, Koski,
Balaban, 1980). Thus, we also incorporated our graph theory
coding into our chemical coding scheme for the TOX-MATCH--
PHARM-MATCH program. A comparison of the atom input versus

the graph theory input for benzo(a)pyrene illustrates the great savings in input effort.

ACKNOWLEDGEMENT

The carcinogenesis research was supported in part by the National Cancer Institute under Contract N01-CP-75020. The research on prediction of toxicity was supported by the Office of Naval Research Biophysics under Contract N00014-81-K-0007.

REFERENCES

Balasubramanian K, Hariharan PC, Kaufman JJ. Unpublished Results, The Johns Hopkins University, 1981.

Balasubramanian K, Kaufman JJ, Koski WS, Balaban AT (1980). "Graph Theoretical Characterization and Computer Generation of Certain Carcinogenic Benzenoid Hydrocarbons and Identification of Bay Regions." J Comp Chem 1:149.

Hariharan PC, Kaufman JJ, Petrongolo C (1979). "Electrostatic Molecular Potential Contour Maps Generated from Ab-Initio MODPOT/VRDDO/MERGE Wave Functions of Carcinogenic Benzo(a)pyrene and Its Metabolites." Int J Quantum Chem QBS6:503.

Hariharan PC, Kaufman JJ, Petrongolo C (1981). "Electrostatic Molecular Potential Contour Maps Generated from Ab-Initio MODPOT/VRDDO/MERGE Wave Functions of Carcinogenic 3-Methylcholanthrene and Its Metabolites." Int J Quantum Chem 20:1083.

Hariharan PC, Popkie HE, Kaufman JJ (1979). "Non-Empirical Ab-Initio MODPOT, VRDDO and MODPOT/VRDDO Calculations X. The Attack of the Simplest Carcinogen, CH_3^+, on Guanine by a MERGE Technique and the Fundamental Difference Between Methylating vs Ethylating Ultimate Carcinogens." Int J Quantum Chem S13:255.

Hariharan PC, Popkie HE, Kaufman JJ (1981). "Molecular Calculations with the Nonempirical Ab-Initio MODPOT,VRDDO and MODPOT/VRDDO Procedures. XII. Carcinogenic 3-Methylcholanthrene and Its Metabolites Using a MERGE Technique." Int J Quantum Chem 20:645.

Jerina DM, Lehr PE, Yagi H, Hernandez O, Dansette P, Weslocki PG, Wood AW, Chang PL, Levin W, Conney AH (1976). In DeSeres FJ, Bond JR, Philpot RM (eds): "In-Vitro Activation in Mutagenesis Testing," Amsterdam: Elsevier, p 159.

Kaufman JJ (1979). "Spin, Symmetry and Orbital Filling Re-
strictions Indicate the Necessity for Ab-Initio Configuration Interaction Calculations in Several Fundamental
Chemical Carcinogenesis Problems." Int J Quantum Chem
QBS6:503.

Kaufman JJ (1981). "Strategy for Computer Generated Theoretical and Quantum Chemical Prediction of Toxicity and Toxicology (and Pharmacology in General)." Int J Quantum Chem
QBS8:419.

Kaufman JJ, Hariharan PC, Chabalowski C, Roszak S, Laforgue
A (1984). "Ab-Initio CI and Coupled Cluster Calculations
on Energetic Compounds." Presented at the Sanibel Inter-
national Symposium on Quantum Chemistry, Solid-State
Theory, Many-Body Phenomena, and Computational Quantum
Chemistry, 1984.

Kaufman JJ, Hariharan PC, Tobin FL, Petrongolo C (1981).
Electrostatic Molecular Potential Contour Maps from Ab-
Initio Calculations. 1. Biologically Significant Mole-
cules. 2. Mechanism of Cationic Polymerization. In
Politzer P, Truhlar DG (eds): "Electrostatic Molecular
Potential Contour Maps from Ab-Initio Calculations. 1.
Biologically Significant Molecules. 2. Mechanism of
Cationic Polymerization," New York: Plenum Press, p 335.

Kaufman JJ, Koski WS, Hariharan PC, Crawford J, Garmer DM,
Chan-Lizardo LA (1983). "Prediction of Pharmacology
and Toxicology Based on Model Toxicophores and Pharma-
caphores Using the New TOX-MATCH--PHARM-MATCH Computer
Program." Int J Quantum Chem QBS10:375.

Kaufman JJ, Koski WS, Hariharan PC, Garmer DM, Crawford J,
Chan-Lizardo LA, Sipos EP (1983). "Theoretical and
Quantum Prediction of Toxic Effects." Presented at the
EPA Symposium "Safer Chemicals Through Molecular Design",
Crystal City, VA, September 1983. In Press, Proceedings
of the meetings in Drug Metabolism Review.

Kaufman JJ, Popkie HE, Hariharan PC (1979).   New Optimal
Strategies for Ab-Initio Quantum Chemical Calculations
on Large Drugs, Carcinogenc, Teratogens and Biomolecules.
In Olson EC, Christffersen RE (eds): "Computer Assisted
Drug Design," Washington DC: Am Chem Soc, p 415.

Kaufman JJ, Popkie HE, Palalikit S, Hariharan PC (1978).
"Molecular Calculations with the Ab-Initio Non-Empirical
MODPOT, VRDDO and MODPOT/VRDDO Procedures. IX. Carcin-
ogenic Benzo(a)pyrene and Its Metabolites Using a MERGE
Technique." Int J Quantum Chem 14:793.

Lowrey AH, Hariharan PC, Kaufman JJ (1981). "Molecular Calculations with the Non-Empirical Ab-Initio MODPOT/ VRDDO/MERGE Procedures. XIV. 2,6-Dimethyl-N-Nitroso-Morpholine and its α-OH Isomers: Conformations and Electrostatic Molecular Potential Contour Maps." Int J Quantum Chem QBS8:149.

Petrongolo C (1978). "Quantum Chemical Study of Isolated and Interacting Molecules with biomedical Activity." Gazz Chim Ital 108:445.

Petrongolo C, Preston HJT, Kaufman JJ (1978). "Ab-Initio LCAO-MO-SCF Calculations of the Electrostatic Molecular Potential of Chlorpromazine and Promazine." Int J Quantum Chem 13:457.

Politzer P, Truhlar DG (1981). "Chemical Applications of Atomic and Molecular Electrostatic Potentials. Reactivity, Structure, Scattering and Energetics of Organic, Inorganic and Biological Systems." New York: Plenum Press.

Popkie HE, Kaufman JJ (1975). "Test of Charge Conserving Integral Approximations for a Variable Retention of Diatomic Differential Overlap (VRDDO) Procedure for Semi-Ab-Initio Molecular Orbital Calculations on Large Molecules." Int J Quantum Chem Quantum Biology Symp 2:279.

Popkie HE, Kaufman JJ (1976). "Molecular Calculations with the VRDDO,MODPOT and MODPOT/VRDDO Procedures. I. HF, F_2, HCl, CL_2, Formamide, Pyrrole, Pyridine and Nitrobenzene." Int J Quantum Chem Symp Issue 10:47.

Popkie HE, Kaufman JJ (1977). "Molecular Calculations With the MODPOT, VRDDO and MODPOT/VRDDO Procedures. II. Cyclopentadiene, Benzene, Diazoles and Benzonitrile." J Chem Phys 66:4827.

Scrocco E and Tomasi J (1973). "The Electrostatic Molecular Potential as a Tool for the Interpretation of Molecular Properties." Top Curr Chem 42:95-170.

Tobin FL, Hariharan PC, Kaufman JJ (1981). "Ab-Initio Quantum Chemical Calculations Permit Prediction of Propensities of Substituted Cyclic Ethers to Polymerize." American Chemical Society National Meeting, Atlanta, Georgia.

Yang SK, McCourt DW, Roller PP, Gelboin HV (1976). "Enzymatic Conversion of Benzo(a)Pyrine Leading Predominantly to the Diol-Epoxide R-7,P-8-Dihydroxy-T-9,10-oxy-7,8,9,10-Tetrahydrobenzo(a)pyrene Through a Single Enantiomer of R-7,T-8-Dihydroxy-7,8-Dihydrobenzo(a)Pyrene." Proc Nat Acad Sci 73:2594.

**Molecular Basis of Cancer, Part A: Macromolecular
Structure, Carcinogens, and Oncogenes, pages 277–286**
© **1985 Alan R. Liss, Inc.**

INTRA AND INTERMOLECULAR MODELING STUDIES OF POLYCYCLIC
AROMATIC HYDROCARBONS

A. J. Hopfinger
Department of Medicinal Chemistry
Searle Research & Development
4901 Searle Parkway
Skokie, IL 60077

Researchers have been intrigued by the structure-
mutagenicity/carcinogenicity relationships in polycyclic
aromatic hydrocarbons (PAHs) since data began to become
available in the 1930s. The PAHs have been particularly
attractive to theoretical chemists, and, as a result, many
computational studies have been performed and mechanisms of
action proposed. Lowe and Silverman (1984) have put
together an excellent review, which is to be published
shortly, of these theoretical efforts.

Two investigations on the PAHs are reported here. In
the first study we (Mohammad, Hopfinger and Bickers, 1983)
asked the question "How much information regarding the
mutagenic potency of a PAH can be derived from the parent
structure?" This question was posed in light of the huge
amount of work necessary to identify the metabolic pathway
and resultant "active" metabolite of a PAH. In the second
case (Kikuchi et al, 1983; Nakata et al, 1983) we focused
upon the isomers of the active metabolite of benzo(a)pyrene,
7-8-dihydroxy-9,10-epoxy-7,8,9,10-tetra-hydrobenzo(a)-
pyrene,I, and their interactions with DNA. Two questions
were posed: "Why is the 2-amino group of guanine the
preferred site of alkylation by I, and secondly, why do the
(+) enantiomers form the major adducts?" (60-80% of the
total) (Pulkrabek et al, 1979).

Our approach to answer the first question was to
construct a quantitative structure activity relationship
(QSAR) relating electronic and shape features of 30 PAHs to

their corresponding Ames mutagenic potency. It is to be
emphasized that this QSAR is an empirical model and not
necessarily a representation of the actual mechanism(s) of
action. At best the QSAR can be used to establish
physicochemical criteria that may be globally related to a
mutagenic process.

The data base of PAHs used in the analysis are reported
in Table 1. The mutagenic potency of each compound has been
reported in terms of the lowest concentration, C, of PAH
required to produce an induced mutation (Kaden, Hites &
Thilly, 1979). Mutagenic potency has been expressed as
log (1/C) in the attempt to generate QSARs. The range in C
over the data base is 4-8000µM. The distribution of
concentrations over the data base set is reasonably uniform.

The all valence electron molecular orbital method
MINDO/3 (Bingham, Dewar & Lo, 1975) was used to estimate the
following electronic features of the PAHs:

(i) E_{HOMO}=energy of the highest occupied molecular
   orbital,
(ii) E_{LUMO}=energy of the lowest unoccupied molecular
   orbital,
(iii) $\Delta E=E_{LUMO}-E_{HOMO}$, the energy of excitation, and
(iv) {Q}=electron density distribution.

The calculated electronic properties are quite sensitive
to the valence geometry of PAHs because of the relatively
large size of the molecules. Thus we selected a procedure
for optimizing the geometries of the PAHs using Fletcher's
variable metric method (Fletcher, 1969). In order to keep
the optimization calculations within practical limits, we
first optimized the geometry of a two ring compound, viz.
naphthalene, which then served as a fixed skeleton for a
three ring compound, anthracene. The geometry of anthracene
was then used as a fixed skeleton for the various four ring
compounds such as tetracene, benz(a)anthracene, and so on.
Five, and larger, ring systems were correspondingly built
from appropriate four ring.

Table 1. The physicochemical parameters ΔE and V used to establish equation (1). The observed and predicted (using equation (1) log (1/C) values are also given.

No.	PAH	$C(\mu M)$	$\Delta E(ev)$	$V_0(\text{Å}^3)$	log (1/C) observed	log (1/C) calculated	Difference (Observed-calculated)
1	Benz(a)pyrene	4	7·60	573·4	5·40	4·82	0·58
2	Flourenthen	5	4·95	334·2	5·30	5·47	-0·17
3	Dibenz(a, c)anthracene	13	7·70	533·6	4·89	4·58	0·31
4	7,12-Dimethyl benz(a)anthracene	25	7·70	546·8	4·60	4·64	-0·04
5	7-Methyl benz(a)anthracene	34	7·73	526·8	4·47	4·54	-0·07
6	Picene	36	7·61	533·9	4·44	4·64	-0·20
7	2-Methyl phenanthrene	40	8·10	410·1	4·40	4·01	0·39
8	Triphenylene	44	8·12	430·0	4·36	4·08	0·28
9	Chrysene	45	7·76	520·5	4·35	4·49	-0·14
10	Benz(a)anthracene	65	7·78	520·5	4·19	4·48	-0·29
11	Cyclopenta(c,d)pyrene	73	7·60	430·9	4·14	4·21	-0·07
12	Dibenz(a,h)anthracene	75	8·21	533·6	4·12	4·27	-0·15
13	Quinoline	80	7·19	259·0	4·10	3·80	0·30
14	1-methylphenanthrene	80	8·01	410·1	4·10	3·87	0·23
15	5,6-Benzoquinoline	84	8·17	376·5	4·08	3·63	0·45
16	4-Methyl quinoline	90	8·20	279·0	4·05	3·25	0·80
17	Benz(e)pyrene	90	8·89	507·9	4·05	3·73	0·32
18	Anthraquinone	100	8·28	488·3	4·00	4·03	-0·03
19	3,4-Benzoquinoline	140	8·42	383·2	3·85	3·51	0·34
20	Pyrene	140	7·79	422·8	3·85	4·06	-0·21
21	3-Methyl cholanthrene	190	9·12	546·4	3·72	3·76	-0·04
22	Anthracene	225	8·39	410·8	3·65	3·64	0·01
23	7,8-benzoquinoline	280	8·24	383·7	3·55	3·62	-0·07
24	Flourene	300	8·19	377·3	3·52	3·63	-0·11
25	Phenanthrene	300	8·22	410·1	3·52	3·74	-0·22
26	Tetracene	322	7·85	417·0	3·48	4·00	-0·52
27	Benz(c)phenanthrene	1000	8·29	424·5	3·00	3·75	-0·75
28	Naphthalene	2000	8·60	291·8	2·70	3·05	-0·35
29	Pyridine	6000	9·46	140·5	2·22	2·02	0·20
30	Isoquindine	8000	8·65	258·1	2·10	2·90	-0·80

The only electronic property which significantly enhances the structure activity correlations involving the 30 PAHs is ΔE. This could be taken as evidence that the initial electronic activation of a PAH is part of the rate-determining step governing mutagenic potency.

The quantitative comparison of molecular shapes is based upon a general formalism, called molecular shape analysis, MSA, (Hopfinger, 1980,1981a; Battershell, Malhotra & Hopfinger, 1981) which has been applied to several structure-activity data bases (Hopfinger, 1980,1981a,b; Battershell, Malhotra & Hopfinger, 1981; Hopfinger & Potenzone 1982; Hopfinger, 1983). In this approach one compound in a particular conformation is chosen as a reference standard and each other compound, in some particular conformation, is superimposed and the common overlap steric volume, V_o, computed. V_o serves as the quantitative measure of shape similarity. Normally, all stable intramolecular conformers are used in an analysis as both test samples and as potential reference standards. The significance of statistical fit ultimately dictates the choice in conformation of each compound, the reference standard, and the mode of pairwise overlap. In a recent study (Hopfinger, 1983) the spatially integrated difference in field potential energy of pairs of superimposed molecules was shown to be a superior descriptor to V_o.

Thirty sets of common overlap steric volumes, $\{V_o\}$, were determined using each of the 30 PAHs as a relative shape standard. The most significant correlation was realized, see equation (1) by employing benzo(a)pyrene as the relative shape standard. Other highly mutagenic PAHs, those having $\log(1/C)$ values greater than 4.2, also yielded significant QSARs when used as shape reference standards in computing the V_os.

The optimum regression equation determined in the study is,

$$\log(1/C) = -0.62(\pm 0.09[\ E] + 0.00041(\pm 0.00007) [S_o]^2 + 7.6(\pm 0.8) \tag{1}$$

with $N=30, R=0.876, S=0.375, AE=11\%, F=44.42$ and where $S_o = V_o^{2/3}$. N is the number of compounds, R the correlation coefficient, S the standard deviation, AE the average error in prediction, and F the measure of statistical significance.

The numbers in parentheses are the estimated standard deviations in the regression coefficients.

The specific values of ΔE, V_o, and the computed $\log(1/C)$ values using equation (1) are reported as part of Table 1.

Mutagenicity is inversely proportional to ΔE. This is not too surprising since if it is more difficult to electronically activate a PAH (larger ΔE values), the compound is less likely to ultimately become a mutagenic metabolite. In other words, the more intrinsically stable a PAH, the less prone it will be to metabolic activation. The range in activity governed by ΔE in the data base is 1.43 $\log(1/C)$ units, or about 43% of the total range in observed activity. Thus ΔE, on a statistical basis, plays a major role in specifying mutagenic potency.

It is difficult to assign a definitive geometric meaning to the overlap steric volume term in the regression equation. In general, the shape of a molecule can dictate, at least in part, its biological activity profile. The common overlap steric volume between pairs of molecules, V_o, is a reasonable quantitative means of comparing molecular shapes. Consequently, the assumption can be made and tested that activity should be related to V_o. However, there is no basis for concluding that biological activity measures should necessarily be optimally proportional to V_o and/or V_o under the multi-dimensional linear regression model. Thus the usage of power proportional representations to V_o, like S_o, are both reasonable and justified within the empirical nature of the QSAR representation.

The shape term variance spans 1.64 units in $\log(1/C)$, or about 49% of the total range in observed activity. The most straightforward interpretation of the role of V_o is that a characteristic shape of a PAH is necessary to enhance mutagenic potency. This, in turn, might be related to the steric fit between, say, the binding site(s) of P450s and the PAH. A mechanistic interpretation of the relationship between molecular shape and mutagenic potency, as expressed by equation (1), can be postulated by noting that benzo(a)-pyrene is the shape reference standard molecule and that $\log(1/C)$ is directly proportional to S_o^2. Equation (1) suggests correcting for electronic activation as measured by ΔE, that the more similar in molecular shape a PAH to

benzo(a)pyrene, the greater its intrinsic mutagenic potency.
The additional observation that the more potent mutagenic
PAHs in Table 1, when used as the shape reference standards,
yield more significant QSAR equations than the less potent
PAHs, also supports the concept of a molecular shape
requirement for mutagenic potency. The finding that S_o^2, as
opposed to S_o, is the preferred representation of the shape
descriptor is considered a mathematical artifact of the
analysis.

We now turn to the modeling of the alkylation of the
2-amino group of guanine by enantiomeric isomers of I,
namely 7β,8α–dihydroxy-9α,10α–epoxy-7,8,9,10-tetrahydro-
benzo[a]pyrene (II) and 7β,8α–dihydroxy-9β,10β–epoxy-
7,8,9,10-tetrahydrobenzo[a]pyrene (III) which are shown in
Figure 1. In addition to the enantiomeric isomer
specificity of alkylation mentioned above, a non-covalent
complex formation has been observed between benzo(a)pyrene
and calf thymus DNA (Becker, Straub & Meeham, 1980). This
interaction is postulated to involve intercalation of the
aromatic hydrocarbon between adjacent base pairs. These
observations prompted us to explore the possibility that II
and/or III might intercalate prior to alkylation (Kikuchi et
al, 1983; Nakata et al, 1983). In addition to providing a
physical catalyst for alkylation, intercalation could also
give rise to stereo selectivity to alkylation and account
for the observed isomer reaction preferences.

Intermolecular modeling calculations were carried out by
essentially driving the enantiomeric isomers about and into
a dinucleoside dimer containing guanine. The goal of the
calculations was to find the set of intermolecular energy
minima for each choice in dimer and isomer. The results of
these studies are summarized in Table 2. The intermolecular
variables in Table 2 define the NH_2–guanine transition state
geometry shown in Figure 2. The minimum–energy transition-
state geometry has been computed for isomers of I with
ammonia to be $r=2.0A, \theta_1=110°, \theta_2=80°, \emptyset_1=100°$, and $\emptyset_3=0$ or
$180°$, with $\emptyset_2$ variable (Kikuchi, Hopfinger, & Klopman,
1979). This model system is a reasonable approximation for
I aklylating the 2-amino group of guanine and has been used
to evaluate the reactive potential of the various
intermolecular complexes.

Figure 1 – The enantiomeric isomers of I.
Key: (A) (+) II: (B) (–) II; (C) (+) III: (D) (–) III.

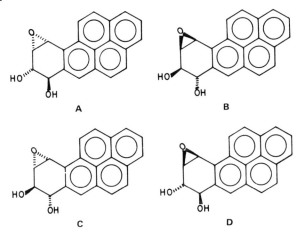

A   B

C   D

Figure 2 – The I-NH$_2$-guanine transition state geometry.

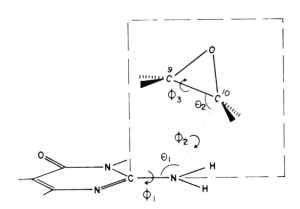

Table 2 –Intercalation Properties of Isomers of I with Dinucleoside Dimers

Dinucleoside Dimer	Isomer	Intercalation Energy, kcal/moles/ complex	Mode[b]	Position of I[a]					
				r, Å	θ_1, °	θ_2, °	ϕ_1, °	ϕ_2, °	ϕ_3, °
$\left(\begin{smallmatrix}C—G\\G—C\end{smallmatrix}\right)$	(+)II	−88.27	d–e	3.7	126	118	97	161	160
	(−)II	−84.00	a–b	7.6	52	112	140	13	−125
		−89.02	e–f	4.2	97	82	80	−77	156
		−88.55	a	5.5	42	126	113	24	−162
	(+)III	−85.94	c	6.8	90	142	143	81	−178
		−85.07	d–e	3.1	123	110	90	168	−148
	(−)III	−88.65	e–f	4.2	100	81	79	−79	151
		−88.12	d	4.8	107	79	126	−179	125
$\left(\begin{smallmatrix}T—A\\C—G\end{smallmatrix}\right)$	(+)II	−89.70	d–e	3.7	104	115	−56	80	175
	(−)II	−82.58	f	4.2	94	78	−123	−167	−154
		−88.79	a	5.2	71	126	−138	−69	−168
		−83.54	d	4.0	63	86	−65	126	145
	(+)III	−86.90	d–e	3.1	111	105	−63	84	176
		−84.43	f	4.2	97	80	−118	−171	−159
	(−)III	−89.00	d	3.9	62	86	−65	126	146
		−80.87	a	5.6	55	139	−145	−48	−173

[a] The transition-state geometric variables.

Intercalation complexes having isomers of I oriented toward the amino group of guanine close to the model transition-state geometry should be particularly reactive. From Table 2 it is seen that the (+) isomers of both II and III have their epoxide groups oriented toward the 2-amino group of guanine, similar to the model transition-state geometry for both dinucleoside dimers. Moreover, these two intercalated stereoisomers also have the minimum distances between the atoms involved in the alkylation process. The distances are 3,7Å and 3.1Å for (+)II and (+)III, respectively. Thus, the (+) enantiomers should be more reactive toward DNA if intercalation is a prereactive step in the alkylation process. This conclusion is consistent with experimental observation (Pulkrabeck et al, 1979).

Stereostick models of the (+)II-[(C-G)(G-C)] intercalation complex are shown in Figure 3. The transition-state orientation of the epoxide group relative to the 2-NH$_2$ of guanine is easily seen.

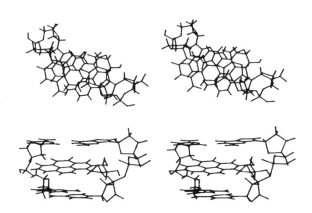

Figure 3 - Stereo-stick models of the (+)II-[(C-G)(G-C)] - intercalation complex in which the epoxide group of II is close to the 2-amino group of guanine and in the transition-state oreientation. The top figures are looking down at the base-pair planes; the bottom figures are looking into the dinucleoside dimer.

All of the computations carried out in these two investigations were done using the CHEMLAB-II computational chemistry software package (Pearlstein, 1983).

Becker, J.F., Straub, K. and Meehan, T.,(1980) "Temperature-Jump Relaxation Rates of Intercalation Complexes Between Benzo(a)pyrene Derivatives and DNA," ASBC/BS Meeting .

Bingham, R.C., Dewar, M.J.S. and Lo, D.H. (1975). J. Am. Chem. Soc. 97,1285.

Fletecher, R. (1969). Optimization, New York; Academic Press.

Hopfinger, A.J. (1980). J. Am. Chem. Soc. 102,7196

Hopfinger, A.J. (1981a). Arch. Biochem. Biophys. 206,153.

Hopfinger, A.J. (1981b). J. Med. Chem. 24,818.

Hopfinger, A.J. & Potenzone, Jr. (1982). Mol.Pharmacol. 21,187.

Hopfinger, A.J. (1983). J. Med. Chem., 26,990.

Kaden, D.A., Hites, R.A. & Thilly, W.G. (1979). Cancer, Res. 39,4152.

Kikuchi, O., Pearlstein, R., Hopfinger, A.J., & Bickers, D.R., (1983). J. Pharm. Sci., 72,800.

Kikuchi, O. Hopfinger, A.J. & Klopman, G., (1979). Cancer Biochem. Biophys., 4,1.

Lowe, J.P. and Silverman, B.D. (1984). Accts. of Chem. Res. in press.

Mohammad, S.N., Hopfinger, A.J., and Bickers, D.R., (1983). J. Theor. Biol. 102,323.

Nakata, Y., Malhotra, D., Hopfinger, A.J., and Bickers, D.R., (1983). J. Pharm. Sci., 72,809.

Pearlstein, R.A. (1983). CHEMLAB-II Users Guide, Molecular Design Ltd., 1122 B. Street, Hayward, CA, 94541.

Pulkrabek, P., Leffler, S., Grunberger, D., and Weinstein. I.B., (1979). Biochemistry, 18,5128.

Molecular Basis of Cancer, Part A: Macromolecular
Structure, Carcinogens, and Oncogenes, pages 287–298
© 1985 Alan R. Liss, Inc.

COMPUTER AUTOMATED EVALUATION AND PREDICTION OF THE IBALL
INDEX OF CARCINOGENICITY OF POLYCYCLIC AROMATIC HYDROCARBONS

Gilles Klopman,
Krishnan Namboodiri and Alexander N. Kalos
Case Western Reserve University
Department of Chemistry
Cleveland, Ohio 44106

The understanding of the mechanism of the metabolism
of chemical compounds resulting in carcinogenesis has been
the subject of many investigations for some time. One class
of compounds that has been extensively investigated is that
of polycyclic aromatic hydrocarbons (PAH's).

Many theoretical approaches have been used to explain
why some members of this class are carcinogenic while others
are not (Wheland 1942; Coulson 1953; Fu, Harvey, Beland
1978). For example, dibenzo[ae]pyrene (I) is carcinogenic,
while its isomer dibenzo[el]pyrene (II) is inactive.

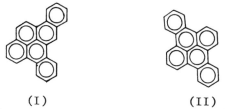

(I)   (II)

One early theory proposed by the Pullmans (Pullman, Pullman
1955; Pullman 1964) to rationalize the differences among
PAH's with respect to their carcinogenic activity, centers
around the existence of two distinct structural regions in
these compounds, the K and L regions:

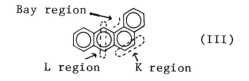

Bay region

(III)

L region   K region

The theory suggests that the presence of a chemically active K region and the absence or concomitant presence of an inactive L region, will render a PAH a carcinogen. Since then, many attempts have been made to quantitate the reactivities of these regions and correlate them with the carcinogenic properties of the compounds in which they are found (Nagata, Fukui, Yonezawa, Tagashira 1955; Mainster, Memory 1967; Herndon 1974;).

However, despite the early success of the K and L region theory in predicting the carcinogenic activity of PAH's, the number of false predictions for many of the PAH's necessitated the development of an alternate explanation. More recent evidence supports the idea that the carcinogenicity of PAH's is related to the existence of an active Bay region (shown in structure III) (Jerina, Lehr 1977). This theory was based on the observation that the metabolites of benz[a]pyrene, (BP), include a Bay region epoxide and that this epoxide is more carcinogenic than benz[a]-pyrene itself (Sims, Grover, Swaisland, Pal, Hewar 1974; Perin-Roussel, Croisy-Delcey, Mispelter, Saguem,Chalvet, Ekert, Fouquet, Jacquignon, Lhoste, Muel, Zajdela 1980; Perin-Roussel, Saguem, Ekert, Zajdela 1983). Since the introduction of the Bay region hypothesis, attempts have been made to identify physicochemical descriptors by which the importance of these structural regions can be expressed (Smith , Berger, Seybold, Serve 1978; Umans, Koruda, Sardella 1980; Poulsen, Lowe 1981).

The present work, based on the "Computer Automated Structure Evaluation" program (CASE), supports the latter theory, and it does so in a unique manner totally independent from the hypothesis and experimental evidence cited above. Specifically, the present methodology identifies relevant structural features of carcinigenic molecules by an "artificial intelligence" recognition process (Klopman 1984). It does not entail the use of Quantum Mechanical nor a priori chosen physicochemical descriptors to explain the carcinogenicity of PAH's: Instead, it utilizes the molecular structure of the compounds in the training set to automatically identify discrete molecular functionalities which are relevant to the carcinogenic activity or inactivity of PAH's. This eliminates the need to arbitrarily choose relevant physicochemical descriptors, which is a necessity for other methods. The CASE program is then used in a predictive mode to classify PAH's as active or inactive with re-

spect to carcinogenicity, based on the molecular fragments
that had been selected during the analysis of the training
set. Furthermore, these descriptors are cast into a regression equation which is used for a quantitative estimation
of the level of carcinogenicity of the objects in the
training set as well as of test cases. In this communication, we have applied the CASE methodology to the Iball
index of carcinogenicity of a series of PAH's.

RESULTS AND DISCUSSION

Classification of Polycyclic Hydrocarbons

The training set (see, Table 1) consisted of 56 polycyclic hydrocarbons, of which 33 were reported to be inactive,
6 marginally active and 17 moderately to extremely active,
in producing epithelial tumors in mice (Arcos, Argus 1968;
Herndon 1974). The experimental carcinogenicity (Iball
Index) is represented in column b of Table 1. The CASE
program identifies the structural fragments that qualify as
descriptors from a statistical analysis of their occurence
in the active and inactive molecules of the training set.
A fragment qualifies as a predictor if it is found in a
distribution that has less than 15% chance of being observed
as a result of a random distribution. The fragments that
qualify under these conditions are considered to be relevant
to activity and are labeled as either activating (biophores)
or inactivating (biophobes), depending on whether they
occur mostly in active or inactive molecules respectively
(Klopman 1984).

The chance that a molecule is a carcinogen is determined
by evaluating the fragments it contains. Thus, to be a carcinogen a molecule, in general, will contain at least one activating fragment and no strongly deactivating ones. The
presence of highly activating and weakly inactivating fragments usually leave the molecule marginally active. The
presence of strongly inactivating and weakly activating fragments generally leads to inactivity. Molecules which have
neither activating nor inactivating fragments are presumed
inactive. Such molecules are reported as having no basis
(NB) available for evaluation. In other words, activity has
to be explicitly demonstrated for a molecule to qualify as
an active one.

Table 1. Carcinogenicity of polycyclic hydrocarbons

Molecule	Presence of important fragments A B C	Carcinogenic activity		
		Probability (a)	Obsd. (b)	Calcd. (c)
1. Naphthalene	2	0%	0	0
2. Anthracene	2	0%	0	0
3. Perylene		NB	0	0
4. Acenaphthene		0%	0	0
5. Fluorene		0%	0	0
6. Pyrene		0%	0	0
7. Benzo(a)pyrene	1	100%	++++	++++
8. diBenzo(el)pyrene		NB	0	0
9. diBenzo(ae)pyrene	1	100%	+++	+++
10. diBenzo(ah)pyrene	2	100%	++++	++++
11. diBenzo(ai)pyrene	2	100%	++++	++++
12. triBenzo(aeh)pyrene	2 2	100%	++	+++
13. triBenzo(aei)pyrene	2	98%	++	++
14. diBenzo(al)pyrene	1 2	100%	++++	+++
15. Naphtho(23a)pyrene	1	100%	++	++
16. Naphtho(23e)pyrene	1	0%	0	0
17. Benzo(e)pyrene		0%	0	0
18. Tetracene	2	3%	0	0
19. Pentacene	2	0%	0	0
20. Phenanthrene		0%	0	0
21. Benzo(a)pentacene	1	0%	0	0
22. Triphenylene		NB	0	0
23. Chrysene		100%	+	0
24. Benzo(c)chrysene	1	100%	++	+
25. Benzo(g)chrysene	2	100%	++	++
26. diBenzo(bk)chrysene	2	0%	0	0
27. diBenzo(gp)chrysene	4	100%	++	++
28. Benzo(b)chrysene	1	27%	0	0
29. Benzo(c)phenanthrene	2	100%	+	+
30. Benzo(a)anthracene	1	7%	+	0
31. diBenzo(ac)anthracene	1	31%	+	0
32. diBenzo(ah)anthracene		24%	++	0
33. diBenzo(aj)anthracene		100%	+	0
34. triBenzo(ach)anthracene		24%	0	0
35. Benzcoronene		99%	0	0
36. Fluoranthene		NB	0	0
37. Benzo(j)fluoranthene	1	100%	+++	+++
38. Benzo(b)fluoranthene	1	87%	+++	+
39. 2,3-Phenylenepyrene		100%	++	++

Table 1 Contd.

Molecule	Presence of important fragments A B C	Carcinogenic activity Probability (a)	Obsd. (b)	Calcd. (c)
40. Benz(ghi)fluoranthene		NB	0	0
41. Benzo(k)fluoranthene	1	31%	++	0
42. diBenzo(bk)fluoranthene	1 1	0%	0	0
43. Naphth(12a)Triphenylene		24%	0	0
44. Picene		0%	0	0
45. diBenz(bg)phenanthrene	1	0%	0	0
46. diBenz(cg)phenanthrene		0%	0	0
47. Benzo(ghi)perylene		NB	++	0
48. diBenz(ac)tetracene	1	10%	+	0
49. diBenz(aj)tetracene		0%	0	0
50. Benzo(a)tetracene	1	1%	0	0
51. Pentaphene	2	0%	0	0
52. Hexaphene	2	0%	0	0
53. Benz(c)pentaphene	1	0%	0	0
54. Anth(12a)Anthracene	2	0%	0	0
55. Anthanthrene		0%	0	0
56. Hexacene	2	0%	0	0

0 : Inactive, + : Marginally active (0–10),
++ : Moderately active (10–30), +++ : Very active(30–60)
++++ : Extremely active(60–100).
NB : No basis available for evaluation; persumed inactive

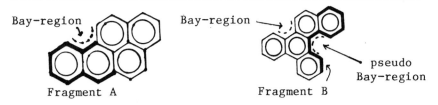

Fragment A   Fragment B

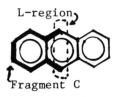

Figure 1. Biophoric and Biophobic Fragments of PAH's

In the present analysis, 49 unique fragments were identified. Out of these 49 fragments, two activating (biophores)
and one inactivating (biophobe) fragments were identified to
be the bare minimum capable of explaining the general trend
of the experimentally observed carcinogenic activity. These
fragments are represented in Fig. 1. Fragments A and B are
present in 8 and 7 molecules respectively, out of a total
number of 23 active molecules in the set. Similarly, fragment C is present in 16 molecules out of a total number of
33 inactive molecules. Fragments A and C are also present in
1 inactive and 5 marginally active molecules respectively.

Based on the number and type of fragments present in a
molecule, its probability of being a carcinogen can now be
estimated.In general, molecules which contain at least one
of the highly significant fragments (such as A or B) are
predicted to be 100% carcinogenic. Thus, all the benzopyrenes which are experimentally found to be very lethal
are also predicted to have 100% chance of being active
(see, Table 1 column a and b). On the other hand, molecules
containing only fragments like C are predicted to be
inactive. For example, naphtho[2,3-e]pyrene is devoid of
any of the activating fragments, it contains fragment C
and is correctly predicted to be inactive. In general most
of the present predictions are well supported by the experimental results (see, Table 1: Column a and b). For the entire set, only five false negatives and one false positive
were found.

There are six cases, in which we find no basis for the
prediction of activity. Out of these, five are known to
be inactive and one active. Thus, the presumption that the
response no basis (NB) to support activity signifies that a
given molecule is inactive, is found to be reasonably well
borne out by experiment.

Among the biophores, fragment A (see, Fig. 1) seems to
be particularly important. It is present in almost all molecules which showed high carcinogenic activity. It is interesting to note that this fragment defines the essential
features of a "bay region". On the other hand, the biophobic
fragment C, indicates the existence of an active "L" region.
The importance of a "pseudo-bay region" and the associated
dihydrol cation formation has recently been recognized in
conjunction with the bay-region hypothesis in polycyclic
aromatic hydrocarbons (Perin-Roussel, Ekert, Barat, Zajdela

1984). In fact, the second most important biophore, fragment
B, defines the essential features of this "pseudo-bay
region" (see, Fig. 1). Thus, even without the a priori
assumption of the currently accepted belief of their
definite involvement in the carcinogenic event, the present
results bear the essence of the bay region theory.

The presence of a fragment descriptor such as C in a
molecule, need not always lead to a predicted inactivity.
Indeed, if an inactivating fragment is in close proximity
to, or embeded in an activating one, a given compound will
most likely be inactive. On the other hand, if the biophobic
site is well separated from the biophoric one, initial
metabolism at the biophobic site need not lead to inactivity.
That is, after such initial metabolism, the molecule can
further undergo oxidative transformation at the biophoric
site, and thus initiate the carcinogenic event. Ideal
examples of such molecules would be various isomers of
naphthalene-substituted benzopyrenes.

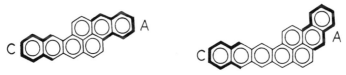

These molecules contain both the fragments (biophore and
biophobe) A and C, but they are well separated by a pyrene
ring. Testing these compounds against our selected fragments,
lead to the prediction that both these molecules are active
(Table 2). However, their experimental activities are not
yet known. Nevertheless, the known carcinogen naphtho-
(2,3-a)pyrene, which contains the inactivating fragment C,
was similarly correctly predicted to be a carcinogen,
because it bears an activating fragment descriptor(E),
remote from the deactivating fragment C.

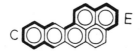

Estimation of Carcinogenic Potencies

It is clear that the statistical significance of the
presence or absence of specific fragment descriptors is a
good criterion for the evaluation of the carcinogenic acti-

Table 2. Carcinogenic activity of test compounds.

	Calculated carcinogenicity		Observed Iball Index
	Herndon	CASE	
1. Benzo(e)pyrene	++++	0	0
2. Picene	+++	0	0
3. Benzo(c)pentaphene	+++	0	0
4. Pentaphene	+++	0	0
5. Naphtho(2,3-e)pyrene	+++	0	0
6. diBenzo(cg)phenanthrene	+++	0	0
7. triBenzo(ach)anthracene	+++	0	0
8. Hexaphene	++++	0	0
9. Benzcoronene	+++	+	0
10. Benzo(b)chrysene	+	0	0
11. diBenzo(bg)phenanthrene	+	0	0
12. diBenzo(aj)tetracene	+	0	0
13. triBenzo(ach)tetracene	+++	0	0
14. diBenzo(al)tetracene	+	0	0
15. diBenzo(ae)fluoranthene		+++	+++
16. Benzene		0	0
17. Naphtho(2,3-h)benz(a)pyrene		+++	?
18. Naphtho(2,3-h)benz(b)pyrene		+++	?
19. Naphtho(1,2-h)benz(a)pyrene		+++	?
20. Naphtho(3,4-h)benz(a)pyrene		++++	?
21. diBenzo(c,fgh)petaphene		++++	?

NB : No basis available for evaluation; presumed inactive
    Herndon 1974 ; Herndon 1974
0 : Inactive, + : Marginally active(0-10),
+++ : Very active(30-60), ++++ : Extremely active(60-100).
Note : Naphthacene = Tetracene; and
       Naphth[2,2-a]naphthacene = Hexaphene

vities of molecules. The next step thus consisted of an attempt to calculate the potencies (Iball indices) using those significant fragment descriptors. However, this is only a secondary objective, since mere reproduction of the numerical values of carcinogenicity does not necessarily contribute any further dimension towards the understanding of the nature of cancer induction or related phenomena (Arcos, Argus 1968 ; Jerina, Lehr 1977 ; Smith, Berger, Seybold, Serve 1978).

The calculation of the activities is based on a multivariate regression analysis of the observed Iball Index of the data base, using as descriptors, the significant fragments obtained from the CASE analysis. The final regression equation included 9 fragment descriptors. These fragments are represented in Table 3. The regression equation resulting from this QSAR study is

$$ICI= -1.6 +26.9(nF1) +36.0(nF2) +54.1(nF3) +6.6(nF4)$$

$$-2.4(nF5) +17.7(nF6) +10.8(nF7) -6.9(nF8) -14.0(nF9),$$

$$N = 56, \ r = 0.89, \ s = 10.1, \ F_{9,46,0.05} = 15.4, \ \sigma = 10$$

where, ICI is the Iball index of carcinogenicity. The descriptors, F1, F2, F3, F4, F6, and F7 are activating fragments, while, F5, F8 and F9 are inactivating. The descriptors, F1 and F4 are the most activating fragments (biophores) A and B and F5 is essentially the inactivating fragment (biophobe) C, discussed earlier. The correlation coefficient between the experimental and the calculated Iball indices is, $r = 0.89$ with a standard deviation of residuals equal to 10. It is to be mentioned that a regression analysis involving the first four descriptors alone, already resulted in a fairly good correlation with a r value of 0.84 and a standard deviation of residuals equal to 14.

The calculated Iball Indices are represented in Table 1 (see, colmns b and c) and are found to agree satisfactorily with the experimetal values. Unlike the early reported QSAR study on polycyclic hydrocarbons (Herndon 1974) there are no false positives in the present calculation.

A slightly high value of the standard deviation (10) was observed in the overall regression analysis. Herndon also reported a deviation of the same magnitude in his QSAR study (Herndon 1974). In the present case, this deviation is mainly attributed to those false negatives described earlier and also to the fact that the calculated carcinogenicity of some benzpyrenes(12,14) and benzo(b)fluoranthene(38) deviated considerably from the observed values.

The CASE program was further used to evaluate the carcinogenicity for a set of 21 polycyclic hydrocarbons (see, Table 2). Herndon (Herndon 1974 ; Herndon 1974) in

Table 3. Fragment descriptors for polycyclic hydrocarbons used in the QSAR analysis.

Fragment	Structure
F1	–C.=C.–CH=CH–CH=CH–C.=CH–C.=CH–
F2	–C.=CH–CH=CH–C.=CH–CH=C.–C.=CH–
F3	–C.=C.–C.=CH–CH=CH–C.=CH–CH=CH–
F4	–CH=CH–C.=C.–C.=CH–CH=CH–CH=
F5	–CH=C.–CH=C.–CH=CH–CH=CH–C.=CH–
F6	–C.=C.–CH=C.–CH=CH–CH=C.–CH=CH–
F7	–C.=CH–C.=CH–CH=CH–CH=C.–C.=CH–
F8	–C.=CH–CH=CH–CH=C.–CH=CH–CH=CH–
F9	–CH=CH–C.=CH–C.=C.–CH=C.–CH=CH–

where C. indicates a carbon atom which is common to two aromatic rings.

---

his QSAR reported the first 14 molecules to be active, based on the K and L region theory. However, the majority of them are observed to be noncarcinogenic. A summary of the results obtained for this set employing the CASE analysis, are given in Table 2 and are found to agree well with the observed values. It is to be noted that the activity of the powerful carcinogen, dibenzo[ae]fluoranthene was correctly predicted. Compounds 13 to 21 in Table 2 had not been included in the training set and were used as test cases. The predicted activities of naphthalene-substituted benzopyrenes are to be verified experimentally.

ACKNOWLEDGEMENT

The authors are grateful to the Environmental Protection Agency for their financial support for this work.

REFERENCES

Arcos JC, Argus MF (1968). Molecular Geometry and carcinogenic activity of aromatic compounds: New Perspectives. Adv Cancer Res 11:305.
Coulson CA (1953). Electronic configuration and carcinogenesis. Adv Cancer Res 1:1.

Fu PF, Harvey RG, Beland FA (1978). Molecular orbital theoretical prediction of the isomeric products formed from
reactions of arene oxides and related metabolites of
polycyclic aromatic hydrocarbons. Tetrahedron 34:857.

Herndon WC (1974). Theory of carcinogenic activity of aromatic hydrocarbons. Trans NY Acad Sci 36:200.

Herndon WC (1974). Quantum theory of aromatic hydrocarbon
carcinogenesis. Int J Quantum Chem: Quantum Biol Symp
1:123.

Jerina DM, Lehr RE (1977). The Bay region theory: a quantum
mechanical approach to aromatic hydrocarbon-induced carcinogenicity. In Ullrich V, Roots I, Hildebrant AG,
Estabrook RW, Conney AH (eds): "Microsomes and Drug Oxidations", Oxford: Pergamon Press, p 709.

Klopman G (1984). Artificial intelligence approach to
structure activity studies. J Am Chem Soc, in press.

Mainster MA, Memory JD (1967). Superdelocalizability Indices
and the Pullman theory of chemical carcinogens. Biochim
Biophys Acta 148:605.

Nagata C, Fukui K, Yonezawa T, Tagashira Y (1955). Electronic structure and carcinogenic activity of aromatic compounds. Cancer Res 15:233.

Perin-Roussel O, Croisy-Delcey M, Mispelter J, Saguem S,
Chalvet O, Ekert B, Fouquet J, Jacquignon P, Lhoste JM,
Muel B, Zajdela FE (1980). Metabolic activation of dibenzo[a,e]fluoranthene, a nonalternant carcinogenic hydrocarbon, in liver homogenates. Cancer Res 40:1742

Perin-Roussel O, Saguem S, Ekert B, Zajdela F (1983). Binding to DNA of bay region and pseudo bay region diol-epoxides of dibenzo[a,e]fluoranthene and comparison with adducts obtained with dibenzo[a,e]fluoranthene or its dihydrodiols in the presence of microsomes. Carcinogenesis
4:27.

Perin-Roussel O, Ekert B, Barat N, Zajdela F (1984). DNA-
protein crosslinks induced by exposure of cultured mouse
fibroblasts to dibenzo[a,e]fluoranthene and its bay and
pseudo-bay region dihydrodiols. Carcinigenesis 5:379.

Poulsen MT, Lowe GH (1981). Quantum mechanical studies of
methyl and fluoro analogs of chrysene: Metabolic activation and correlation with carcinogenic activity. Cancer
Biochem Biophys 5:81.

Pullman A, Pullman B (1955). Electronic Structure and carcinogenic activity of aromatic molecules. Adv Cancer Res
3:117.

Pullman B (1964). Electronic aspects of the interactions
between the carcinogens and possible cellular sites of

their activity. J Cell Comp Physiol 64 Suppl 1:109.

Sims P, Grover PL, Swaisland A, Pal K, Hewar A (1974). Metabolic activation of benzo[a]pyrene proceeds by a diol epoxide. Nature 252:326.

Smith IA, Berger GD, Seybold PG, Serve MP (1978). Relationships between carcinogenicity and theoretical reactivity indices in polycyclic aromatic hydrocarbons. Cancer Res 38:2968.

Umans RS, Koruda M, Sardella DJ (1980). Metabolic activation of polycyclic aromatic carcinogens: A theoretical study. Mol Pharmacol 16:633.

Wheland GW (1942). A quantun mechamical investigation of the orientation of substituents in aromatic molecules. J Am Chem Soc 64:900.

**Molecular Basis of Cancer, Part A: Macromolecular
Structure, Carcinogens, and Oncogenes, pages 299–308**
© **1985 Alan R. Liss, Inc.**

A MOLECULAR MODEL RELATING TO CARCINOGENESIS

Robert C. Hopkins, Ph.D.

Professor of Chemistry
University of Houston - Clear Lake
Houston, Texas   77058

One of the fundamental unsolved questions relevant to
cancer research is how genes are made either accessible or
semi-permanently inactive during cellular differentiation or
development. If the role of certain cellular oncogenes is
to provide essential growth-stimulating functions at appropriate times, what normal processes turn these genes off when
their functions are no longer needed? More importantly,
what types of processes might inadvertently reactivate dor-
mant genes having oncogenic potential? To pursue these
questions, it is assumed that a necessary condition for some
modes of carcinogenesis is the reactivation of one or more
normal cellular genes at an inappropriate time (Comings
1973). Although additional steps may be necessary for cancer progression, the focus of this paper is on gene inactivation and reactivation, and on a molecular mechanism which
may begin to provide answers to these vital questions.

Before proceeding, it is important to consider the information transactions involving DNA which occur during the
first stage of gene expression, RNA transcription. Numerous
proteins and enzymes associated with transcription, including RNA polymerase and various repressor and activator proteins are known to bind to specific recognition sites in the
major groove of double-stranded DNA (Losick, Chamberlin 1976;
Takeda, et al 1983). In brief, the information carried in
the major groove of duplex DNA is essential to the transcription process. Thus, a conceptually powerful route to
inhibition of transcription and subsequent gene expression
would be to block the information in the major groove of DNA
from such recognition processes. One potentially effective

way of making this information inaccessible would be to pair
the DNA duplex with another, highly complementary molecule.
Quite remarkably, this complementary function can be served
almost ideally by a second homologous DNA duplex, as in the
meshing of a gear with one identical to itself.

The pairing of two homologous DNA duplexes to produce a
tetraplex structure has been proposed recently as a mechanism by which semi-permanent gene inactivation and cell differentiation might occur (Hopkins 1984a). This hypothesis
provides a viewpoint for understanding the extreme fidelity
of genome maintenance in eukaryotes (Hopkins 1984b). Furthermore, it a) offers a possible explanation of DNA methylation patterns in higher organisms, b) suggests a fundamental mechanism in the initiation of neoplastic processes, and
c) provides a new structural basis on which the design of
anti-cancer drugs might be approached.

GENE INACTIVATION IN TETRAPLEX DNA

The model assumes that within somatic cells in G_O phase
there exist two complete, homologous copies of the genome as
double-stranded DNA. In regions of the genome which have
been semi-permanently inactivated during cell differentiation or development, the two DNA copies are paired to form
a tetraplex. In regions destined to be accessible for transcription under other types of control, the two DNA duplexes
remain unpaired as a "bubble" within adjacent four-stranded
domains. It is envisioned that the boundaries of each bubble might move in response to the particular combination of
hormones and other chemical messengers present in an individual cell. Thus, the complement of genes exposed as double-
stranded DNA is expected to vary with cell type and time.

Interestingly, a scheme for pairing two homologous base
pairs to form specific hydrogen-bonded tetrads (Löwdin 1963)
and a model of four-stranded Watson-Crick DNA (McGavin 1971;
Fig. 1) have been known for over a decade. However, the
tetraplex models envisaged above are unique in being based
on an alternative family of double-helical models for the
structure of DNA (Hopkins 1981, 1983a). This model family,
Configuration II, preserves the base pairing scheme of the
Watson-Crick models, Configuration I, yet differs in a subtle, fundamental way by having antiparallel chains of the
opposite sense. The left-handed Z-DNA forms are examples of

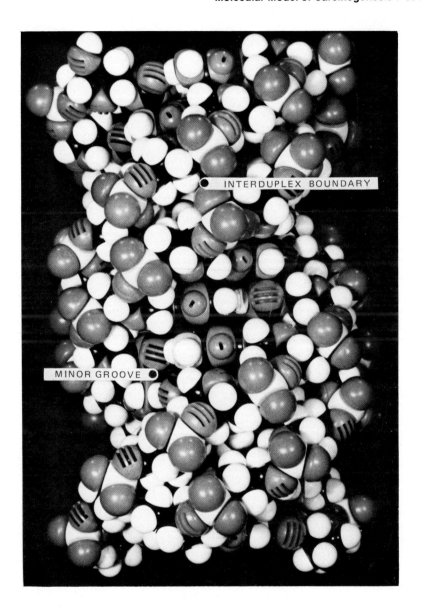

Figure 1. Right-handed tetraplex of two homologously-paired Configuration I (Watson-Crick) duplex models. (CPK model; 11 bp DNA; 3.3Å rise/bp; 10.3 bp/turn; phosphate-phosphate diameter = 21.7Å)

this alternate structural family, but are not members of the topologically distinct Watson-Crick family (Hopkins 1983b).

NEW PERSPECTIVES FROM CONFIGURATION II MODELS

From the Watson-Crick tetraplex model in Fig. 1, it is clear that the encoded information, written as a sequence of polar substituents in the minor groove, is accessible. Thus, a four-stranded Watson-Crick structure offers no visible advantages over duplex DNA for information security or recognition site occlusion. Alternatively, the Configuration II tetraplex models suggest a quite different result.

Figure 2 shows a right-handed Configuration II tetraplex built to dimensions characteristic of the B-form of DNA. Since right- and left-handed Configuration II models can be interconverted by an axial twisting motion (Hopkins 1981, 1983a), a similar left-handed tetraplex (Fig. 3) can also be built with the characteristics of B-DNA (Hopkins 1984a). Study of the actual models reveals that the exterior surfaces of the interduplex boundary regions consist almost entirely of hydrophobic groups. Quite strikingly, the only informational polar group exposed in these structures is the N7 atom of each guanine residue in the interduplex region. The equivalent N7 atom of each adenine residue is blocked by the methyl group at the 5-position of the thymine which lies across the boundary region in the opposing duplex.

Methylation of Cytosine at the 5-position

If the tetraplex structures described above are used in cells to protect encoded information or inhibit its expression, it is proposed that the direct interaction of certain proteins, hormones or other messenger molecules with guanine N7 groups might be a key step in reactivating "tetraplexed" genes. Thus, segments of DNA with particular N7 (receptor) patterns exposed would allow the postulated reactivator molecules to separate the two duplexes, making them accessible for transcription. On the other hand, by methylating cytosine residues in DNA at the 5-position (m^5C), the nucleophilic N7 sites on guanine residues would be blocked. With the N7 recognition sites inaccessible to the exterior of the four-stranded structures, the genes bound inside would be "turned off" in a highly stable manner. Demethylation of

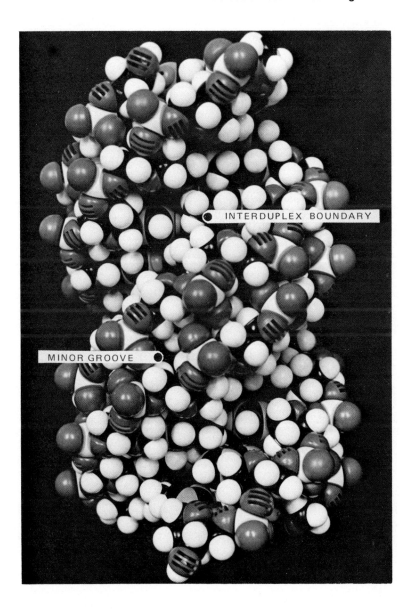

Figure 2.   Right-handed tetraplex of two homologously-paired Configuration II duplex models.   (CPK model; 11 bp DNA; 3.4Å rise/bp; 10.5 bp/turn; P-P diameter = 21.8Å) Reprinted with permission, Gordon and Breach (Hopkins 1984a).

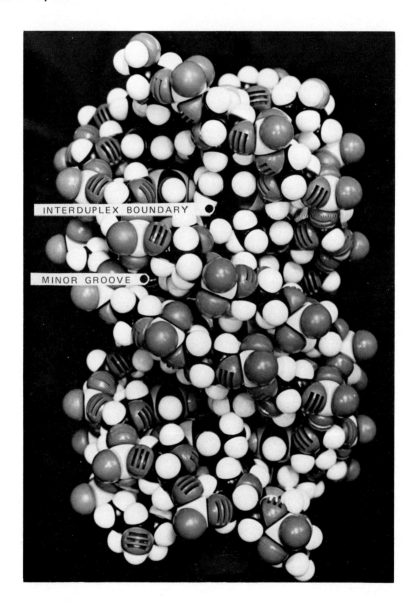

Figure 3. Left-handed tetraplex of two homologously-paired Configuration II duplex models. (CPK model; 11 bp DNA; 3.4Å rise/bp; 10.2 bp/turn; P-P diameter = 22.1Å) Reprinted with permission, Gordon and Breach (Hopkins 1984a).

DNA would initiate reversal of this sequestering process.

Experimental evidence (See reviews by Ehrlich, Wang 1981; Doerfler 1983) is consistent with the above picture:
1. Gene expression appears to be correlated with under-methylation of the gene sequence; DNA methylation tends to be associated with inactive genes.
2. In DNA of higher eukaryotes, m^5C generally is found adjacent to a guanine residue, most commonly in the sequence 5'-CG-3'. This sequence might provide the putative N7 receptor pattern mentioned above.
3. Hormones may stimulate the demethylation of certain DNA sequences, thus reactivating expression of the genes at those loci (Mermod, et al 1983).

The Initiation of Carcinogenesis

As assumed above, the untimely reactivation of certain normal genes or gene combinations may be a critical step in the initiation of cancer. Clearly, not all inappropriately reactivated genes would lead to neoplasia. However, gene products associated with growth stimulation (Sporn, Todaro 1980) might be good candidates for involvement in carcino-genesis. For example, the product of the erbB oncogene from avian erythroblastosis virus may be derived from the gene coding for the epidermal growth factor receptor (Downward, et al 1984), and the sis oncogene product from simian sarcoma virus closely resembles a chain from platelet-derived growth factor (Doolittle, et al 1983). Coincidentally, it has been shown that DNA in some human cancer cells is significantly hypomethylated (Feinberg, Vogelstein 1983).

Perhaps not by chance, processes expected to disrupt a normally "tetraplexed" segment of DNA, making its genes accessible for transcription at an inappropriate time, appear to be similar to those that initiate cancer. Well known active agents such as ionizing radiation, chemical mutagens or clastogens, virus and other pathogens, or physical injury might lead to tetraplex disruption through a) DNA strand breakage, b) removal of protective proteins or polyamines, c) untimely demethylation of DNA segments, d) mutation in one duplex, causing loss of homology needed for tetraplex pairing, or e) mechanical or electronic destabilization of tetraplex structures (e.g., from binding of bulky or reactive molecules at exposed N7 sites). A related situation

can be envisioned whereby some step in the normal cellular
process for inactivating genes is suppressed. For example,
tetraplex formation (and its designated gene inactivation)
could be obstructed by molecules such as alkylating agents
bound in the major groove of an accessible DNA duplex.

Cisplatin-DNA Interaction: An Example

     The molecular mechanism by which the cancer chemothera-
peutic agent cisplatin [cis-diamminodichloroplatinum (II)]
acts remains unclear. However, there is significant evidence in support of the following general conclusions (For
reviews see Roberts, Thomson 1979; Prestayko, et al 1980):
  1. The cis isomer is an active anticancer drug, whereas
     the trans isomer is not.
  2. The mode of action of the drug is through binding with
     DNA, and some aspect of this process inhibits DNA
     replication.
  3. A principal binding site of cisplatin is the N7 atom in
     guanine residues.
  4. Through its bidentate nature, the drug forms both
     inter- and intrastrand crosslinks with DNA; DNA-protein
     crosslinks also form, but are evidently not of major
     therapeutic importance.

     If one assumes that some types of DNA-DNA crosslinks
are the critical lesions for effectiveness of the drug, then
the fact that only the cis isomer is active suggests that
the steric relationship between the leaving groups on the
platinum and the binding sites on the DNA is crucial. From
models of duplex DNA of either Configuration I or II, severe
distortions of the structure would apparently result from
interstrand crosslinks between N7 atoms on guanine residues
in complementary strands. Intrastrand crosslinking between
N7 atoms on adjacent guanine bases in the same strand appears to be sterically possible in either DNA configuration.

     By considering the Configuration II tetraplex models, a
new possibility for interstrand crosslinks becomes evident.
Curiously, an unmethylated 5'-CG-3' sequence in a right-
handed tetraplex (or the sequence 5'-GC-3' in a left-handed
tetraplex) has the N7 atoms of the guanines exposed at about
3.5Å separation in the interduplex boundary region. This
distance is approximately the separation of the two leaving
groups in cisplatin (Roberts, Thomson 1979); see Fig. 4:

Figure 4. Possible interstrand crosslink sites in the interduplex boundary region of Configuration II tetraplexes: a) right-handed, b) left-handed. Only two of the four strands, one from each duplex, are shown in each case.

For replication to occur, the strands of the tetraplex structure would have to separate in some way (Hopkins 1984a, 1984b) in order to provide templates for new DNA synthesis. However, the proposed crosslinks would be expected to maintain the tetraplex, at least locally, thus preventing this process and inhibiting replication. Furthermore, since this type of crosslink would not be possible with duplex DNA, transcription and other normal functions in cells not undergoing replication should be unaffected.

CONCLUDING REMARKS

Configuration II tetraplex models offer new viewpoints in the search for understanding of genome integrity, DNA methylation patterns, carcinogenesis, and DNA-drug interactions. Other encouraging aspects of the Configuration II duplex models have been discussed previously (Hopkins 1984a, 1983a), including binding of the carcinogen 2-acetylaminofluorene to the C8 atom on guanine. This atom is exposed in the new models but is obstructed in the Watson-Crick models. Hopefully, the ideas presented here will provide a unifying thread for interpreting data from diverse areas of research.

I wish to thank Dr. R. E. Dickerson for his generous hospitality during a sabbatical leave in his laboratory at UCLA. Additional thanks are due Star M. Hopkins and Dr. W. Ron Mills for their encouragement and valuable discussions. (Supported by Robert A. Welch Foundation grant E-889)

Comings DE (1973). A general theory of carcinogenesis. Proc Natl Acad Sci USA 70:3324.

Doerfler W (1983). DNA methylation and gene activity. Ann Rev Biochem 52:93.

Doolittle RF, Hunkapiller MW, Hood LE, Devare SG, Robbins KC, Aaronson SA, Antoniades HN (1983). Simian sarcoma virus onc gene, v-sis, is derived from the gene (or genes) encoding platelet-derived growth factor. Science 221:275.

Downward J, Yarden Y, Mayes E, Scrace G, Totty N, Stockwell P, Ullrich A, Schlessinger J, Waterfield MD (1984). Close similarity of epidermal growth factor receptor and v-erb-B oncogene protein sequences. Nature 307:521.

Ehrlich M, Wang RY-H (1981). 5-Methylcytosine in eukaryote DNA. Science 212:1350.

Feinberg AP, Vogelstein B (1983). Hypomethylation distinguishes genes of some human cancers from their normal counterparts. Nature 301:89.

Hopkins RC (1981). Deoxyribonucleic acid structure: a new model. Science 211:289.

Hopkins RC (1983a). Alternative description of the transition between B-DNA and Z-DNA. Cold Spr Harb Symp Quant Biol 47:129.

Hopkins RC (1983b). Transitions between B-DNA and Z-DNA: a dilemma. J Theor Biol 101:327.

Hopkins RC (1984a). Are answers hidden in multistranded nucleic acids? Comments Mol Cell Biophys 2:153.

Hopkins RC (1984b). A checking mechanism for replication fidelity. Biophys J 45:402a.

Losick R, Chamberlin MJ (eds) (1976). "RNA Polymerase", NY: Cold Spring Harbor Laboratory.

Löwdin P-O (1963). Some aspects of DNA replication; incorporation errors and proton transfer. In Pullman B (ed): "Electronic Aspects of Biochemistry", NY: Academic, p 167.

McGavin S (1971). Models of specifically paired like (homologous) nucleic acid structures. J Mol Biol 55:293.

Mermod J-J, Bourgeois S, Defer N, Crépin M (1983). Demethylation and expression of murine mammary tumor proviruses in mouse thymoma cell lines. Proc Natl Acad Sci USA 80:110.

Prestayko AW, Crooke ST, Carter SK (eds) (1980). "Cisplatin: Current Status and New Developments", NY: Academic Press.

Roberts JJ, Thomson AJ (1979). Mechanism of action of antitumor platinum compnds. Prog Nucl Acid Res Mol Biol 22:71.

Sporn MB, Todaro GJ (1980). Autocrine secretion and malignant transformation of cells. New Engl J Med 303:878.

Takeda Y, Ohlendorf DH, Anderson WF, Matthews BW (1983). DNA-binding proteins. Science 221:1020.

**Molecular Basis of Cancer, Part A: Macromolecular
Structure, Carcinogens, and Oncogenes, pages 309-318
© 1985 Alan R. Liss, Inc.**

GRAPH THEORETICAL APPROACH TO STRUCTURE-ACTIVITY STUDIES:
SEARCH FOR OPTIMAL ANTITUMOR COMPOUNDS

Milan Randić

Department of Mathematics and Computer Science,
Drake University, Des Moines, Iowa 50311; and
Ames Laboratory - DOE, Iowa State University,
Ames, Iowa, 50011

ABSTRACT

An approach based on graph theoretical methods for
searching the most potent drug among numerous candidate
structures is outlined. First, we identify the strategic
fragment and describe it by suitable graph theoretical invariants. We have adopted path numbers derived from suit-
ably weighted bonds as basic invariants. Similarity among
structures is quantitatively derived from similarity and
differences in atomic path numbers for the strategic fragment. The approach is illustrated on a selection of antitumor phenyldialkyltriazenes for which $\log(1/C)$ are known.
By starting the search with an unsubstituted parent compound, in few steps we located 1-(4-NHCOCH3-Phenyl)-3,3-di-
alkyltriazene as the most potent drug among those considered.

INTRODUCTION

Advantages and disadvantages of empirical and semiem-
pirical quantitative structure-activity relationship (QSAR)
studies are well known. One can argue about difficulties
and oversimplifications as well as about advantages and opportunities of structure-activity studies. Questions have
been raised about defining relative activities, about separating therapeutic and adverse effects, about obtaining a
different outcome for the same drug in different species.
Notwithstanding the validity of such concerns and the lack
of understanding of underlying mechanisms due to the complexity of biological systems, empirical schemes offer a

useful tool to help to filter out from a collection of
candidate structures less desirable ones, even if they may
not point the most desirable ones (Hansch, Smith, Engle
1975). The graph theoretical approach to be outlined here
appears capable of resolving some of the above concerns.
Graph theory puts emphasis on structural invariants; it
uses only well defined parameters which have a direct structural interpretation, even though the selection of parameters may be ad hoc in nature. One starts with a search
for a mathematical description of a structure which is subsequently used to aid in a comparison of actual structures
and their properties. If among the considered structures
there are one or few with desirable qualities, one can use
these as standards and rank all other structures according
to the degree of similarity with the few selected standards.
One can also screen a large number of hypothetical structures to point to a few that can be expected to show similar (desirable) characteristics. In view of these rather
unique characteristics of the graph theoretical approach
and its complementary character when compared to empirical
QSAR schemes, it is likely that the present approach may
succeed where others failed.

Let's briefly review some past graph theoretical developments that relate to the present approach. The first
question to consider is: Can we characterize a structure
by a single number that will be of use in structure-property
correlations? The connectivity index, suggested by this
author (Randić 1975) proved quite successful in this respect. Use of a pair of parameters is bound to give better
representation of a structure or its properties. Interestingly, Wiener demonstrated this almost forty years ago
(Wiener 1947). Ordered pair, such as the number of paths
of length two and paths of length three (p2,p3) respectively, add an additional novelty. When viewed as coordinates
of a structure on a coordinate grid they lead to a systematic organization of data on isomers, resulting in a Periodic Table of Isomers (Randic, Wilkins 1979). Complete
sequences of path counts (p1,p2,p3,...pk), where pi is the
number of paths of length i in the structure, allows one to
discuss similarity and dissimilarity among structures
(Randić, Wilkins 1979 a). With the premise that similar
structures are likely to show similar properties, one can
in this way make predictions on molecular activity. Several applications include study of dopamines (Wilkins,
Randić 1979), benzomorphans (Randić, Wilkins 1979 b), anti-

malarial phenanthrene carbinols (Randić, Kraus, Jerman-Blažić
1983), and barbiturates (Jerman-Blazic, Randić 1983).

Path sequences appear useful for comparison of structurally similar molecules, particularly isomers and structures having the same heteroatoms in the same positions. One
disadvantage of the characterization by path numbers is that
paths of longer length appear to dominate the comparisons,
merely by being numerically the largest. Thus the approach
gives prominence to structural components that need not be
responsible for molecular properties. A number of improve-
ments are yet to be considered, such as how to account adequately for the presence of heteroatoms, and how to specify
spatial factors. Here we assume these to be constant and
will focus our attention on the importance of local strategic fragments. Local features are very important in a comparative study of compounds because by proper selection of
local regions one can diminish the role of less relevant
parts of the structure which otherwise only obscure comparisons.

OUTLINE OF THE APPROACH

Recently a weighting scheme for path counts has been
suggested in which contributions of longer paths are gradually attenuated (Randić 1984). If weights for individual
bonds are less than one, repeated multiplication of such
factors reduces the role of longer paths dramatically. This
desirable feature can be realized by adopting as the weighting factors the same factors used in the construction of the
connectivity index. In this way one is uniting two very successful schemes: the connectivity index suited for bond ad-
ditivities and path sequences found useful in discussing
structural similarity. The weighting factors are given as
the reciprocal of the square root of the product (m·n), where
m and n indicate the number of nearest neighbors for the bond
considered. The available program ALL PATH for counting
paths of different length (Randić, Spencer, Brissley and
Wilkins 1980) has been modified to incorporate the weighting
factors and produce weighted path count. In Table 1 we show
the result of weighted path counts for the parent structure,
unsubstituted 1-phenyl-3,3-dimethyltriazene(E) and other
selected compounds. The last row in Table 1 gives the total
number of weighted paths, which appears to be a suitable simple label for each compound (Randić, 1984). Here we will
consider corresponding atomic quantities, the atomic labels

derived by summing weighted paths of all lengths for individual atoms. For the unsubstituted parent structure (E)
we show in Table 2 paths sequencies belonging to individual
atoms.

Table 1

Compound	A	B	C	D	E
p(0)	15.00000	16.00000	16.00000	14.00000	11.00000
p(1)	6.84639	7.56819	7.62764	6.75372	5.30940
p(2)	3.36257	3.90644	3.97012	3.40778	2.75341
p(3)	1.43635	1.80433	1.81246	1.57086	1.26642
p(4)	.66644	.83428	.82761	.75407	.58684
p(5)	.35255	.42551	.41353	.39373	.31272
p(6)	.11742	.17717	.15510	.14018	.08242
p(7)	.04366	.07356	.06714	.05817	.03339
p(8)	.01897	.01697	.02847	.02430	.01149
p(9)	.00449	.00500	.00859	.00642	.00040
p(10)	.00086	.00152	.00297	.00163	
p(11)		.00032	.00052		
I.D.	27.84971	30.81334	30.91420	27.11090	21.36012

Table 2

Atom	1	2	3	4	5
p(0)	1.00000	1.00000	1.00000	1.00000	1.00000
p(1)	.57735	1.48803	1.00000	1.00000	1.15470
p(2)	.52578	.22222	.57735	.47222	.62546
p(3)	.12830	.06415	.16666	.38160	.28065
p(4)	.03703	.05555	.08333	.06250	.18232
p(5)	.03207	.02777	.04166	.03125	.05412
p(6)	.01603	.01388	.02083		
p(7)	.00801	.00694	.01041		
p(8)	.00400	.00347			
p(9)	.00200				

Atomic I.D.

	2.33061	2.88204	2.90026	2.91853	3.29727

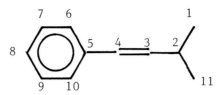

The last row in this table, which is obtained by summing all the entries in the corresponding column, character-
izes atomic environments. We propose to use the above atomic
descriptors (for all atoms that constitute the strategic
fragment) as a collection of structural parameters on which
similarity between similar fragments in other molecules can
be based.

CHARACTERIZATION OF PHENYL-DIALKYLTRIAZENES

To illustrate our approach we will consider a selection
of antitumor 1-(X-phenyl)-3,3-dialkyltriazenes. In all we
have chosen some 20 compounds from a larger group of over 60
studied by QSAR by Hansch and collaborators (Hansch et al.,
1978). Antitumor activity of these compounds was established initially by Rondesvelt and Davis (1957), which allows
us to use experimental values of log (1/C), rather than computed values, which appear less reliable. The selected compounds and log (1/C) values are shown in Table 3. We use
capital letters as compound labels but also, for convenience,
numbering used by Hansch et al., is shown. Compounds not included have halogen atoms, sulphur and other less frequent
functional groups.

In Table 4 we have collected atomic I.D. numbers for
several initial compounds in order to illustrate the degree
of variation of individual atomic path sums. The first five
entries in column (E) are the numbers of the last row of
Table 2 truncated now to three digits. We restricted comparison of atomic path numbers only to atoms common to all
compounds, i.e., fragment phenyl-3,3-dimethyltriazene nucleus,
eleven atoms in all. Major variation in atomic I.D. between
different compounds is caused by substitution at that site,
while minor variations are due to more distant neighbors.
Two compounds differing in their heteroatoms are, at this
stage represented by the same collection of atomic I.D. numbers.

Table 3

Compound		X	R	log(1/C)	I.D.
A	(1)	4-NHCOCH3	CH3	4.04	27.849718
A'	(2)	4-NHCONH2	CH3	3.97	
B	(3)	3-COHN2, 6-OCH3	CH3	3.95	30.813348
C	(4)	4-NHCONH2	CH2CH3	3.87	30.914202
D	(5)	4-NHCOH	CH3	3.85	27.110908
E	(6)	H	CH3	3.85	21.360126
F	(7)	3-CONH2	CH3	3.80	26.940114
G	(8)	4-CH3	CH3	3.76	23.237497
H	(11)	2-COOH	n-C3H7	3.74	30.917926
I	(12)	4-CONH2	CH2CH3	3.66	28.922166
J	(13)	2-COOH	CH3	3.64	26.943244
F'	(18)	m-COCH3	CH3	3.58	
K	(20)	4-CONH2	CH3	3.51	26.939220
L	(26)	3-COOCH3	CH3	3.42	28.894743
M	(27)	3-CH3	CH3	3.40	23.237964
J'	(30)	2-CONH2	CH3	3.31	
N	(32)	2-CONH2, 4-CONH2	CH3	3.27	32.522094
I'	(36)	2-CONH2	CH3	3.26	
O	(37)	2-CONHCH3	CH3	3.25	28.898620
N'	(40)	4-COOH	CH3	3.22	
P	(41)	4-COOCH3	CH3	3.20	28.893635
Q	(42)	4-CONH2	i-C3H7	3.17	30.752253

Table 4

Compound: Atom	A	B	C	D	E	F
1	2.33	2.33	2.40	2.33	2.33	2.33
2	2.88	2.88	3.00	2.88	2.88	2.88
3	2.90	2.92	2.94	2.90	2.90	2.90
4	2.93	2.95	2.95	2.93	2.91	2.92
5	3.34	3.40	3.35	3.34	3.29	3.33
6	3.09	3.13	3.09	3.08	3.03	3.09
7	3.09	3.31	3.09	3.08	3.00	3.28
8	3.35	3.09	3.35	3.34	2.99	3.04
9	3.09	3.10	3.09	3.08	3.00	3.09
10	3.09	3.39	3.09	3.08	3.03	3.06
11	2.33	2.33	2.64	2.33	2.33	2.33

SEARCH FOR THE BEST COMPOUND

From the data in Table 4 we can construct the similarity (or dissimilarity) table by viewing the entries as components of positional vectors in a 11-dimensional space and evaluating Euclidian distance between each pair of structures. For example, we find $D(A,B) = 46.05$ and $D(A,C) = 34.27$, both relatively large quantities indicating limited similarity, while $D(A,D) = 2.33$, $D(C,I) = 9.69$, $D(A,K) = 10.29$ and $D(A,G) = 16.67$, all relatively small, thus indicating considerable structural similarity. A small entry in the similarity table, such as $D(A,D)$ suggests that the activity in D can be traced to active region in A. From the similarity table one can construct the partial order for the structures by selecting the best compounds (here A and B) as standards. In contrast to previous work which was based on path sequences the resulting ranking here would be based on atomic path sums restricted to atoms belonging to a common strategic fragment. Partial ordering of structures is the foundation for our search for the best drug in a collection of candidate structures. All one has to do is to construct path characterization for compounds of interest and construct the similarity table for these compounds with preselected standards. Any small entry in the similarity table (subject to verification on congruency of heteroatoms and spatial conformation) would indicate a potentially useful novel substance. Observe that a small entry (great similarity) only indicates the possibility that two compounds may have similar properties, hence the new compound may surpass the standard in the desired quality. Formally, one may say that if a standard compound has property P, the most similar structure will have property $P \pm \Delta P$. For some properties there will be an enhancement for the desired quality while for other compounds, or for other properties of the same compound there may be attenuation. Only subsequent experiment will show which is the case! With a larger number of such tests one can possibly detect some trends and be more definite about the predictions, but at this stage of the development of the approach all that we can claim is a considerable improvement of the odds that we will eventually detect, among a given collection of compounds, the best ones in relatively few steps.

In order to illustrate the approach we will pretend that we do not know experimental $\log(1/C)$ for the compounds of Table 3 and we will seek the best phenyldialkyltriazene.

Let's start the search by examining unsubstituted 1-phenyl-3,3-dimethyltriazene (E), although one can start with any compound. Experimental log(1/C) of 3.85 is a relatively high value indicating that E has the desired qualities and represents a good standard compound for initiation of the search. Next we determine the similarity between E and the remaining structures using the outlined atomic I.D. numbers for all the 11 atoms of phenyltriazene moiety. In Table 5 we show numerical values for distances between E and a number of compounds. We find structure G to be the most similar to E. Testing of G reveals experimental log(1/C) of 3.76, somewhat smaller, but still of interest. We continue now by searching for a structure which is most similar to G. Several structures are reasonably similar to G: K, D and A. If we were to test all the three compounds we would already at this stage in the search find the best compound. The search would still continue to ensure that indeed A is the optimal compound, as outlined below. Let's instead continue the search with the lead compound K showing the greatest similarity to G. We find as the most similar structures to K to be structures D and A, as can be seen from the corresponding column of Table 5.

Table 5

Compound	E	G	K	D
A	39.48	16.67	10.29	2.23
B	51.94	47.94		46.82
C	52.45	38.22	35.87	34.35
D	37.84	14.73	8.42	–
E	–	23.76	29.61	37.84
F	29.66	31.09	32.66	36.49
G	23.76	–	6.48	14.73
H	59.30	60.94	61.05	64.78
I	45.71	35.08	34.36	35.12
J	29.71	33.04	25.29	39.91
K	29.71	6.48	–	8.42
L	61.57	59.56	58.91	59.31

We have truncated the table by supposing that compounds below some threshold value for log(1/C) would be of no interest. Finally in the following step we are directed from compound D with log(1/C) of 3.85 to compound A with optimal log(1/C) of 4.04. The search ends with structure A because

when we examine similarity between A and all the structures
we find among the best the structures already used in the
search.

CONCLUDING REMARKS

Generally in drug design studies we meet numerous ob-
stacles, particularly that substances of interest may exhibit
detrimental effects which overshadow their beneficial role.
Also we face the dilemma of where to draw the line and restrict examination to a practical and relatively small subset of an enormous possible number of structures bearing the
same substituents. In both these respects the outlined approach can be of assistance. If the beneficial and detrimental effects of a drug are due to different structural details
the outlined approach may delineate and identify local environments associated with each of the two. Then one proceeds
by searching for target compounds that have increased similarity to the beneficial component of the standards and reduced similarity towards unfavorable structural components.
With respect to the second problem one should examine a large
pool of structures. Starting with an acceptable lead compound one arrives at the best structure which corresponds to
a local maximum. The found structure need not represent an
absolute maximum; it is the point of convergence for numerous
structures having the same common strategic fragment. A new
lead compound, if sufficiently different would then lead to
another relative maximum and large territory can be covered
in an efficient way to locate a few most interesting structures.

We may summarize our approach by stating a principle
that underlines the method: "Structures that differ little
in the mathematical properties will differ little also in
their physical, chemical and biological characteristics."
The above principle emphasizes a need for study of mathematical properties of structures. Such properties guide us in
comparisons of structures, facilitate comparisons, make them
possible. They play the role of coordinates in calculus and
analytical geometry; they do not enter the solution as such,
hence their ad hoc nature is not a hinderance but an asset
in the search for alternative routes in comparitive study
of structure-activity relationship.

REFERENCES

Hansch C, Smith RN, Engle R (1974). Quantitative structure-activity relationships in drugs. In "Pharmacological Basis of Cancer Chemotherapy", Williams & Wilkins Co. Baltimore, p.756.

Hatheway GJ, Hansch C, Kim KH, Milstein SR, Schmidt CL, Smith RN (1978). Antitumor 1-(X-aryl)-3,3-dialkyltriazenes. 1. Quantitative structure-activity relationships vs L1210 leukimia in mice. J Med Chem 21:563.

Jerman-Blažič B, Randić M (1983). Modelling molecular structures for computer-assisted studies of drug structure-activity relations. In "Modelling and Simulation", Tassin (France) Vol. 5, p.161.

Randić M (1975). On characterization of molecular branching. J Am Chem Soc 97:6609.

Randić M (1984). On molecular identification numbers. J Chem Inf Comput Sci (in press).

Randić M, Kraus GA, Dzonova-Jerman-Blazic B (1983). Ordering of graphs as an approach to structure-activity studies. Studies Phys Theor Chem 28:192.

Randić M, Wilkins CL (1979). Graph theoretical ordering of structures as a basis for systematic searches for regularities in molecular data. J Phys Chem 83:1525.

Randić M, Wilkins CL (1979 a). Graph theoretical approach to recognition of structural similarity in molecules. J Chem Inf Comput Sci 19:31.

Randić M, Wilkins CL (1979 b). Graph theoretical study of structural similarity in benzomorphans. Int J Quant Chem: Quant Biol Symp 6:55.

Randić M, Brissey GM, Spencer RB, Wilkins CL (1980). Use of self-avoiding paths for characterization of molecular graphs with multiple bonds. Computers & Chem 4:27.

Rondestvedt CS Jr, Davis SJ (1957). 1-Aryl-3,3-dislkyltriazenes as tumor inhibitors. J Org Chem 22:200.

Wiener H (1948). Relation of physical properties of the isomeric alkanes to molecular structure. J Phys Chem 52:1082.

Wilkins CL, Randić M (1979). A graph theoretical approach to structure-property and structure-activity correlations. Theor Chim Acta 58:45.

Molecular Basis of Cancer, Part A: Macromolecular
Structure, Carcinogens, and Oncogenes, pages 319–326
© 1985 Alan R. Liss, Inc.

COMPUTATIONAL CHALLENGES IN MOLECULAR MODELING

Russell J. Athay, Ph.D., Roger S. Davis

Evans & Sutherland Computer Corporation
580 Arapeen Drive
Salt Lake City, Utah

A model is a conceptual tool for understanding some
real world phenomenon. The model can be a set of
equations, a series of procedures, or simply a collection
of data. In recent years many of our models have come to
take the form of computer programs and data bases.
Computer graphics provides a window into this world of
computer based models. Through this window we can begin
not only to see what is happening in our models, but also
to interact with these models, to change them, manipulate
them, and ask "What if?".

Over the last two decades the use of computer graphics
in molecular modeling has grown steadily. The most
notable successes have been in protein crystallography
where computer graphics is now routinely used to solve
structures. At first these tools had limited capacity and
were used cautiously and in parallel with manual methods.
The capabilities of the tools were improved, both at the
hardware level and at the software level, and as
confidence in these tools also improved, the manual
methods were gradually abandoned in favor of the computer
based methods. But progress has continued even further,
so that the current generation of tools not only provides
a easier, faster, and ultimately cheaper way of solving
the old problems, but provides new facilities, for which
there are no manual equivalents, and which allow the
researcher to tackle new problems that could not have been
approached without these tools.

Application of computer graphics to molecular modeling

as by no means been limited to the domain of the protein crystallographer. Especially in the last few years researchers from many different fields have started to apply graphics to a wide variety of molecular modeling applications. The rapid growth of the last few years in drug design, protein engineering, and many other fields has been fueled by better and cheaper hardware, by increasingly sophisticated software, by a growing awareness of the potential benefits, but also by advances in scientific understanding that have allowed scientist to deal with problems at the molecular level.

It is our belief that the age of computer graphics based molecular modeling is just barely dawning. We look for continued and dramatic growth, but we realize that along with these opportunities come challenges which must be met before the potential can be transformed into the actual. The purpose of this paper is to examine some of what we consider to be the fundamental challenges in molecular modeling as viewed from our perspective and background which is in computer science.

Display Technology and Techniques

The fundamental display task in computer graphics is to generate an image on the screen that communicates as much information as possible in a form that is convenient, coherent, and understandable. One can partition this problem into two parts
  o developing display technology
  o effectively using existing technology for a given application.
For the purposes of this paper we will consider display technology as a three dimensional space in which we will label the axes
  o image quality
  o dynamic response
  o display primitives.

Image quality is extremely important. It is not just that poor image quality is annoying, but rather that poor image quality tends to obscure the information content of the picture by introducing artifacts. These artifacts, such as the jaggy lines in a low quality raster picture, introduce a kind of noise that obscures the signal, that is the information content, of the picture. Of course, we realize that the purpose of molecular modeling is not to make pretty pictures, but we maintain that the purposes of molecular modeling are facilitated by high quality images and impeded by poor quality images. There remain important challenges, both at the algorithmic and at the hardware levels, to continue to improve image quality.

The dynamic response of the system is equally important. The purpose of a molecular modeling system is not just to display a static picture of a molecule, but to allow the researcher to interact with it. Part of this interaction involves what one might call "dynamic viewing", that is changing the viewing position, looking around behind the molecule, flying up into the active site, etc. Not only does this motion give a realistic 3D sense to what is, statically, a 2D picture, but it allows one to become familiar with a structure by providing the freedom to explore. Slow, jerky, and unpredictable updates are not only annoying, they distract the operator and impede the ability to interact. It is virtually impossible to do a visual docking in a system that is updating only once every few seconds. Again in this area, there are important challenges. Part of the challenge is to simply to make hardware faster, smaller, and cheaper, and VLSI and other emerging technologies will facilitate some of this development, but expanding the range of display primitives to include solids while still maintaining useful update rates and image quality may well require development of new algorithms which make effective use of parallel processing.

The display primitives provide the basic building blocks from which an application must build its display. Most vector systems are limited to lines and points, but have good image quality and dynamic update. Raster systems usually provide some sort of "solid" (perhaps simply a 2D area), but tend to have poorer image quality for lines and points and slower updates. There are specialized types of raster systems which are used for simulators of various types. These provide very high quality images with fast update rates. However, they are both expensive and specialized (i.e. even if one could afford one for molecules it wouldn't work very well because it makes assumptions about the scene that is to be displayed that aren't true for molecules).

The emerging raster technology promises to expand the basic building blocks to include useful three dimensional solid primitives like planes, spheres, sculptured surfaces, etc. But it is important to sort out the claims and demonstrations from the realities. In particular, there are lots of tricks for generating real time solid image pictures. There is nothing wrong with a trick as long as one realizes that it is a device that works only in certain cases, what those cases are, and how they apply to the problem at hand. In evaluating a system, it is important to chart the full space. That is, one needs to know the image quality and dynamic performance for each of the display primitives and for combinations of them.

In fact, the greatest advances in display technology over the next few years are likely to be in the area of expanding the display primitives. The real challenge is not so much to be able to claim to display this or that primitive, but to build a unified, coherent system that maintains image quality, dynamic update rates, and a useful set of display primitives.

Of course, how effective your molecular modeling system is in the display area is dependent not only on the display technology provided by your hardware, but also on the effectiveness with which your software uses that technology to generate pictures. The use of lines to represent bonds in wire frame models is the obvious, and effective starting place. This representation provides good feedback on atomic positions and the overall shape of the molecule. It is not very good, however, for revealing details of the molecular surface such as one might like to see in the active site of a protein. Lines can also be used effectively to display contours, of electron density for example. It has become particularly popular to contour in three planes to build "cage" densities. Lines can also be used to represent force fields or other properties of the molecule that are a function of position.

When one thinks of surface displays, the attention usually changes to the raster systems. Special algorithms have been developed to generate CPK type pictures and someday there may well be special hardware that is capable of updating these pictures dynamically. The only problem with these pictures, other than that they don`t move, is that they are a little too solid. That is, the solid plastic sphere type representation hides too much of what is going on inside of, or on the other side of, the molecule. In fact, one would like transparent spheres, with carefully controllable and controlled transparency. Front and back clipping planes, which are very useful in line drawing systems, would also be necessary in a solid image system.

However, static raster pictures do not provide the only alterative for displaying surface information. This is a case where those developing application software have made effective use of the existing technology by using dots distributed across the surface. These dots may be placed on the solvent accessible surface with the Connelly algorithm, or may simply be on the Van der Waals surfaces as in work done at UCSF. Especially when used in conjunction with clipping planes and viewed dynamically, these dot surfaces are very effective indeed in conveying the shape and position of the surface.

One area where application systems differ widely in their effectiveness is in their use of color. Color can be used to carry all sorts of information such as atom type, hydrophilic properties, charge distribution, or local energy parameters. Used effectively, color can focus the user's attention and convey vital information, but used ineffectively it can simply be a gimmick.

There is another feature of most existing display systems which appears to not to be utilized as well or as often as it might be. This is the use of the dynamic capabilities of the system not only to provided viewing and positional feedback, but also to animate sequences of events. There are some notable exceptions which appear to show the great promise in this area. As the sophistication of our molecular modeling grows to the point that we begin to model the dynamic behavior as well as the static properties of a molecule we need to make more effective use of the dynamic capabilities already provided by much of the existing hardware.

User Interface

One of the primary challenges that faces anyone attempting to develop molecular modeling tools is to develop a user interface which is easy to learn and use.

Much can be, and has been, said about user interfaces. It is a sign both of the difficulty of the area and of neglect that many of the programs we buy for $100 for our home computers have infinitely better user interfaces than some of those for which we may pay over 1000 times that much. Most molecular modeling systems are still used mainly by specialists. This is partly due to the newness and the developing nature of the field, but it is partly due to needlessly obscure and difficult user interfaces.

This in neither the time nor the place for an extended lecture on user interfaces, so we will simply list some of the features that we have come to feel are necessary in a good interface:

The user interface is an integral part of the system rather than a facade that can be added or fixed up latter. This is because the user interface involves not only the mechanics of interacting with the system, which are often easy to change, but more importantly the conceptual basis for interaction. Lack of conceptual clarity almost always pervades the entire system so that attempting to paste on a new user interface does little to remove the confusion.

Flexibility is vital. Most systems will have users with widely different experience, uses, and backgrounds. For a novice user who can`t type, a system that requires commands to be typed in with no help or prompts is almost completely useless, while a system that guides someone through detailed menus with detailed instructions at every stage can be exasperating for an expert user who has done all this a hundred times before. The user interface should meet the needs of both types of users by adapting to the skill, background, and wishes of the user.

Use of screen information. Most graphic systems provide a display in which some representation of the current state of the model is displayed and provide a mechanism for allowing elements of the display to be picked. The operands for many operations are rendered somehow on the screen, but far too many systems force the user to type in the name of something rather than picking it off the screen.

o Simplicity, in software engineering as in science, is elegance.

Data Base Management

To someone just getting started in molecular modeling, the hardware might seem like the most valuable part of the system, the software next, and finally the loose set of files that make up the data. Within a very few years, however, not only is that priority likely to reverse itself completely, but the management of that data base is likely to become one of the most important and difficult problems.

Commercial data base management systems provide some assistance in this area, but are, on the whole, no more suitable for molecular modeling than they are for CAD/CAM. Again, this is not the place for a data base lecture, but we cannot omit it as one of the primary challenges in molecular modeling. If we loose control of our data bases, our systems will be useless, but if we maintain organization and control, the accumulation of information in the data base will become one of the prime assets of our companies or research groups.

System Integration

We have listed several aspects of a molecular modeling system and indicated the associated challenges that we see from the perspective of computer science. There are other aspects of the problem where the challenges are primarily chemical, medicinal, biological, or mathematical. However, the greatest challenge of all is to integrate the various pieces, the graphics hardware, the general purpose computing system, perhaps special energy calculation hardware, user interfaces, data base management systems, and a variety of application programs into a coherent, useful, usable system.

In time the evolution pressures of the survival of the fittest will sort out the companies and research organizations with the best tools to meet the challenges of the future. If the development of these tools is organized and rational rather than random, the chances of success go up dramatically.

Our long term goal is to develop integrated molecular modeling workstations. These will fit in your office, cost less than half your unburdened yearly salary, and provide a wide variety of computation and display tools as well as access to a huge data base. And because you are scientists and scientists, thank goodness, cannot bear to leave things as they are, the system will be "open" and many of you will be adding your own programs to try new methods or to make something work better.

This won't happen tomorrow, or next year. Whether it happens in a timely fashion and whether we are successful vendors or you are able to adapt to and contribute to new methods is dependent on how well we each meet and conquer the the computational and scientific challenges that we currently face in molecular modeling.

Molecular Basis of Cancer, Part A: Macromolecular
Structure, Carcinogens, and Oncogenes, pages 327–339
© 1985 Alan R. Liss, Inc.

THE MCS-MODEL OF CHEMICAL INITIATION OF CANCER

László v. Szentpály

Institut für Theoretische Chemie, Universität
Stuttgart, Pfaffenwaldring 55
D-7000 Stuttgart 80, Germany

A.   INTRODUCTION

"Any comprehensive theory of carcinogenesis must
take into account the likelihood of molecular structural
effects at each stage of enzymatic activation, detoxification, nucleic acid binding, repair and replication"
(Harvey 1981). In contrast to full theory, models
concentrate upon the most important and characteristic
steps in the process of tumor formation. Considering the
complex initiation of cancer (review: Sims and Grover
1981), it is not surprising that correlations of carcinogenic potency with a single theoretical variable are
unsatisfactory (Jerina and Lehr 1977, Smith et al. 1978,
Osborne 1979). But even multilinear regressions on
theoretical indices (Herndon 1974; Umans et al. 1979)
show a serious number of exceptions, namely false positives. As pointed out recently (Szentpály 1984), the
indices used so far were inadequate, and it is necessary
to differentiate between cations and radicals in order
to improve the correlation.

The MCS-model of chemical carcinogenesis (Szentpály
1984) seeks to quantify three important influences on
carcinogenicity:
M: the initial epoxidation of the M-region, in
competition with reactions at other centers of the PAH;
C: carbocation intermediates in the M-region epoxide

hydration and/or the reaction of the bay-region diol epoxide with DNA;
S: a size and solubility dependence.

The MCS-model assumes that the carcinogenicity of a polycyclic aromatic hydrocarbon (PAH) is mainly determined by the electronic properties of the PAH and its metabolites formed during the initiation process, and that the promotion is not specifically influenced by the carcinogen.

The separate components of this model have been discussed before (Borgen et al. 1973, Jerina and Daly 1974, Sims and Grover 1974, Herndon 1974, Smith et al. 1978, Loew et al. 1979) but
a) they have not been combined into a synoptic form,
b) the formation of carbocations has not been calculated correctly, except by Loew et al.,
c) the reactions competing with the activating metabolism have not received enough attention, except those at the L-region (Pullman 1954, Herndon 1974),
d) the influence of the molecular size has been discussed (Arcos and Argus 1968, Herndon 1974, Scribner et al. 1980) but has been combined with theoretical indices only by Herndon.

The MCS-model could be tested using quantum chemical approximations with explicit inclusion of electron interaction, e.g. the PPP- (Pariser and Parr 1953; Pople 1953) and INDO-methods (Pople et al. 1967) accounting for the differences between radicals and ions. However, the simplest model that is appropriate should be tried first, otherwise one would loose chemical intuition. For neutral molecules, the HMO- and perturbational PMO-indices (Dewar 1952, 1969; Dewar and Dougherty 1975) show general trends in reactivity at practically no computational expense. Such indices have also been quite popular in obtaining a fast prescreening of carcinogenic PAHs (e.g. Jerina and Lehr 1977; Smith et al. 1978; Umans et al. 1979). The trouble is that they fail to describe PAH-ions (Dewar 1969). The simplest way to include electron repulsion and to deal with PAH-ions is given by the ω-technique (Wheland and Mann 1949; Streitwieser 1961). As shown recently, PMO can be extended to PMO-ω by a perturbational ω-type electron repulsion term (Szentpály 1984). PMO-ω-calculations still *require only a pencil and the back of an envelope.*

B.   *THE INDICES USED WITH THE MCS-MODEL*

1.   *The Metabolic Index M*

In choosing a proper reactivity index describing epoxidation, one has to accept a biomimetic model for the enzymatic action. Two mechanisms have been under discussion: a concerted oxidation across a C=C bond, or a nonconcerted addition beginning at the more reactive carbon atom (Cvetanovic 1970; Klein and Scheer 1970; Keay and Hamilton 1976). There has been increasing evidence (Groves et al. 1978; Hanzlik and Shearer 1978; Pudzianowski and Loew 1983) that epoxidation is nonconcerted. Therefore, the rate of epoxidation at the M-region is negatively correlated to N_m, the smaller of the Dewar reactivity numbers (Dewar 1969) in this region, defined as

$$N_m = 2 \, (c_{o,m-1} + c_{o,m+1}) \qquad\qquad (1)$$

$c_{o,m-1}$ *and* $c_{o,m+1}$ *being the nonbonding MO coefficients at atoms m-1 and m+1 if the π-system is interrupted at atom m. These coefficients are obtained by pencil and paper (Longuet-Higgins 1950) as illustrated for two positions of benzo(g)chrysene in fig. 1.*

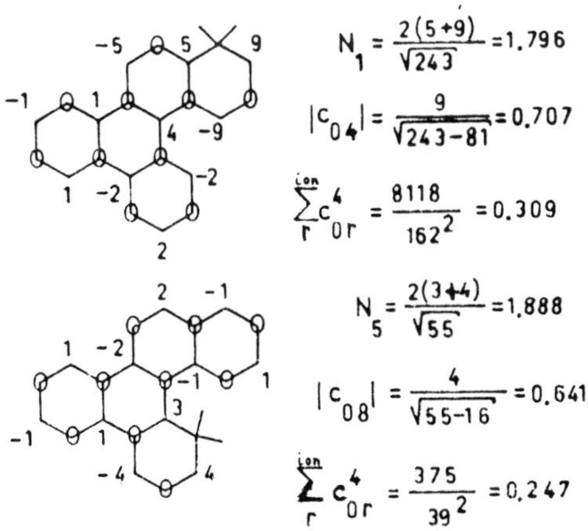

$$N_1 = \frac{2(5+9)}{\sqrt{243}} = 1.796$$

$$|c_{04}| = \frac{9}{\sqrt{243-81}} = 0.707$$

$$\sum_{r}^{ion} c_{0r}^4 = \frac{8118}{162^2} = 0.309$$

$$N_5 = \frac{2(3+4)}{\sqrt{55}} = 1.888$$

$$|c_{08}| = \frac{4}{\sqrt{55-16}} = 0.641$$

$$\sum_{r}^{ion} c_{0r}^4 = \frac{375}{39^2} = 0.247$$

Fig. 1. *Pencil and paper calculation of* $N_m, |c_{ob}|$ *and* $\sum_{r}^{or} c_r^4$ *for different steps in the metabolism of benzo(g)-chrysene.*

There are different centers and regions where disactiva-
ting reactions compete with the initial epoxidation. It
is assumed, that the fastest competing reaction predomin-
ates and the others are unimportant, thus the smallest
reactivity number N_C will be compared with N_m. These
numbers are combined into a *single* metabolic index M

$$M = (N_m - N_C)^2. \tag{2}$$

With $N_C \leq N_m$, the definition is unequivocal. The analytic
form of M seems both simple and satisfactory, since it
simulates an exponential relation at a limited range. An
exponential relation would require some hidden parameters
because we lack detailed knowledge of the transition
structures and don't know their connection to carcinogenic potencies.

2.   The Carbocation Formation

    Carbocation intermediates occur either during the
M-region epoxide hydration, or in the ultimate reaction
with DNA, or in both reactions. Topological considerations (Szentpály 1984) show, that corresponding M-region
and bay-region carbocations have strongly related charge
distributions. With cationic intermediates, the rate of
ring opening at a given M-region epoxide is closely
correlated to that at the corresponding bay-region diol
epoxide. At the level of approximation chosen, we can
answer the question, whether carbocation intermediates
occur during the initiation of chemically induced
tumors. However, it cannot be decided, during which
metabolic step(s) they are formed. It is necessary and
sufficient to calculate the formation of one of the
related carbocations, otherwise we would introduce
linear dependencies in the regression analysis.

    In the PMO-ω-method, the reaction of an epoxide or
a diolepoxide to a carbocation intermediate is associated
with a resonance-energy $E_{R,\omega}$ of the "arylmethyl-ion" additional to that of the aromatic system of the educt.

$$E_{R,\omega} = E_D + E_{C,\omega} \tag{3}$$

E_D is the delocalization energy arising without explicit
electron interaction. According to Dewar's thermocylic
argument (Dewar and Dougherty 1975)

$$E_D \cong 2(1- |c_{ob}|)\beta \qquad (4)$$

c_{ob} is the NBMO amplitude at the atom where the oxirane ring is opened. The Hückel delocalization energy has been approximated by a similar formula (Mason 1958).

$$E_D = (1.50 - 1.03 |c_{ob}|)\beta \qquad (5)$$

Two examples of how to calculate $|c_{ob}|$ are shown in fig. 1.

   The second term E_C has been called charge dispersal energy (Pople and Brickstock 1954, Mason 1958) because there is a lower probability to find the π-electrons on the same atom of a carbocation than in any of the classical structures describing it. In the PMO-ω-method, the corresponding stabilization energy is obtained by changing the Hückel parameter α_r by an amount $\omega\beta q_r$, where q_r is the net charge on atom r and ω is a parameter. For odd PAH cations, we have $q_r=c_{or}^2$ (Longuet-Higgins 1950), and $(1-q_r)=Q_r$ is the total electronic charge. To the first order, the extra stabilization energy of a carbocation is given by

$$E_{C,\omega} = \omega\beta \sum_r (1-q_r)q_r = \omega\beta(1-\sum_r c_{or}^4) \qquad (6)$$

The summation goes over all atoms of the π-system and $\sum_r q_r = 1$. There is a close linear correlation between $E_{C,\omega}$ and E_C obtained by a simplified PPP-method (Pople and Brickstock 1954), the latter is approximated (Szent-pály 1984) in kcal/mol units by

$$E_C = -41.71 + 56.64 \sum_r c_{or}^4 \qquad (7)$$

The calculation of $\sum_r c_{or}^4$ is indicated in fig. 1. The change in π-energy during the formation of a carbocation is obtained with $\beta=-20$kcal/mol as

$$-C=E_D+E_C=-20.0(1.50-1.03 |c_{ob}|)-41.7+56.6 \sum_r c_{or}^4 \qquad (8)$$

   The change in σ-energy during the carbocation formation is regarded as independent of the parent molecule, since such changes are well described by the localized bond model (Dewar 1969).

3.   A. Size Criterion

In determining the importance of molecular size for carcinogenicity, at least two facts have to be considered:

a)   Generally, there is an optimum size on any receptor. Although the enzyme systems involved in carcinogenic activation of PAHs show very broad substrate-specificities (Guenther and Oesch 1981) there must be increasing steric hindrance from some size on. The influence of an optimum size for intercalation of carcinogens in DNA remains to be discussed.

b)   There is an at least two-fold crossing of polar-nonpolar interfaces during the metabolic activation to an ultimate carcinogen: first, the PAH must enter into the microsomal endomembrane system in order to reach the monooxygenase enzyme system, second, the dihydrodiolepoxide must leave the lipid phase to get transferred through a hydrophilic medium to the cell nucleus. A more lipophilic substance enters easier into the membrane, but it is more difficult for its diolepoxide to return into the hydrophilic medium that surrounds the cell nucleus. The inverse is true for less lipophilic PAHs.

The connection between size and molecular partitioning across polar-nonpolar interfaces is obtained by the following argument. The lipophilicity of aromatic molecules is linearly proportional to $\sum_r S_r$, the sum of electrophilic superdelocalizabilities (Fukui et al. 1954), whereas hydrophilicity is proportional to $\sum_r |q_r|$, the sum of absolute charges on the atoms. They are related by a multilinear regression (Rogers, Cammarata 1969) to the partition coefficient P

$$\ln P_{calc.} = 0.667 \sum_r S_r - 2.540 \sum_r |q_r| + 0.478 \qquad (9)$$

For neutral PAHs, i.e. $q_r = 0$, there is only a poor correlation between carcinogenic potency and $\sum_r S_r$ (Smith et al. 1978), which is not surprising considering a single variable only. The data disclose, however, a strong correlation between $\sum_r S_r$ and the size, i.e. the number n of carbon atoms. This supports the statement (Herndon 1974) that an entropy term can be defined by either solubility or size.

The optimum molecular size is taken as an empirical parameter and seems to be between 20 and 24 carbon atoms. The size criterion is chosen as:

$$\Delta = \left| n-20 \right|^3 \tag{10}$$

This is a modification of Herndon's size criterion. Δ cannot be a dominating parameter, since there are many PAH molecules with $n \cong 20$ which are definitely non-carcinogenic, e.g. pentacene. Prior to quantitative discussion, this is an evidence that the intrinsic activity, i.e. the activity once the carcinogen has reached its site(s) of action, will be governed by the molecular electronic structure. Considering the broad specificities of the enzyme systems, Δ should not contain a strong bias towards large carcinogenic potency with n=20. Therefore, it is not surprising to find the exponent 3.

C.   RESULTS, DISCUSSION AND PREDICTIONS

The MCS model is tested in a multilinear regression analysis on the carcinogenic potencies of 26 PAHs given in table 1. The analysis is not limited to bay-region containing molecules, and similar samples have been considered to be representative of this class of compounds (Herndon 1974; Smith et al. 1978; Osborne 1979). Fluoranthene is included as an example for nonalternant PAHs that are calculated as proposed by Herndon (Herndon 1972). The "false positives" of earlier theoretical work (Herndon 1974, Osborne 1979) are discussed separately.

The three independent variables M (2), C (8) and Δ (10) are assumed as linearly related to the experimental Iball papilloma index I (Iball 1939; Arcos and Argus 1968). The latter is proportional to the fraction of subject animals that show carcinogenic response divided by the mean latent period. The Iball index can be trusted within a range of $\pm$ 10 (Herndon 1983). A multilinear regression analysis yields the equation

$$I_{calc} = -80.47M + 8.244C - 0.0739\Delta - 331.7 \tag{11}$$

The multiple correlation coefficient is $r=0.961$ and the standard error is $S=\pm\,6.8$. The accuracy could and should not be any better considering the uncertainty ± 10 of the experimental Iball index. The weight of the individual variables, documented by partial F-tests (Draper and Smith 1981), is as follows: the variable C expressing the carbocation formation is by far the most important ($F=261$), it is followed by the metabolic index M ($F=72$), the size criterion Δ is the least significant ($F=48$) (Szentpály 1984).

With $C=\left|E_D+E_C\right|$ as the prime variable, it is of interest to check the importance of the ω-correction E_C within this variable. Without E_C, i.e. on a Hückel level that would be appropriate for radicals instead of cat-ions, the quality of correlation drops drastically to $r=0.824$ and $SE=+14.1$ (Szentpály 1984). The partial F-value of $\left|E_D\right|$ is $F=46$ only.

This analysis of variances represents a strong evidence for carbocations as intermediates either in the ultimate reaction with DNA, or in the M-region epoxide hydration, or in both. As discussed in section B.2, it cannot be decided whether the first or second oxirane ring opening is more important for the carcinogenesis and this renders the bay-hypothesis somewhat nebulous.

In addition to the prime importance of C in a quantitative correlation, the metabolic index M is essential to explain the lack of carcinogenic potency of polyacenes and phenes. In these series, C increases with linear annelation, and this would lead to very potent molecules, were it not for the detoxification at the centers of the L-region. The Dewar number N_C at the most reactive competitive center decreases much more rapidly than N_m at the M-region, consequently, the first epoxida-tion is becoming less probable with increasing linear annelation. Thus, one important class of false positives (Osborne 1979) disappears due to the combination of C and M (Szentpály 1984).

Benzo(g)chrysene is the only exception so far, where the limitation to two competing reactions breaks down. As shown in fig. 1, two initial epoxidations are competing with each other, and the theoretically faster leads to a less carcinogenic carbocation than the slower one. It is difficult to describe such a situation by simple reactivity indices. As a compromise, averaged N_m and C are used c. f. table 1.

The size criterion becomes effective for $n \leq 14$ and $n \geq 26$. Its small partial F-value indicates

a) the broad and overlapping size-specificities of the enzyme systems involved,

b) the dominance of the electronic structure, once the carcinogen has reached its site(s) of action.

Nevertheless, the size criterion is believed to be conceptionally important in any model of carcinogenic action. The present small F-value may be related to the limited size-range of molecules for which Iball indices are available. The size criterion may also absorb the influence of other size dependent steps that could occur after the initiation of cancer, e.g. during the DNA-repair.

The noncarcinogenic molecules 27–33 (table 1) have been reported as unexplained false positives with $I \cong 40$ in earlier calculations (Herndon 1974; Umans et al. 1979). According to the MCS-model, these molecules are calculated with $I \leq 8$, picene being the sole exception with $I=17$. By its electronic structure, picene is at least as potent as chrysene ($I=5$), this is also concluded from INDO-calculations (Loew et al. 1979). It is suggested that the experiments be repeated and reevaluated.

Dibenzo(a,l)pyrene has not been included in the regression, because the experimental values $33 \leq I_{obs} \leq 82$ (Arcos and Argus 1968; Lacassagne et al. 1968) need reinterpretation. The supposed dibenzo(a,l)pyrene that gave $I_{obs} \cong 33$ was later identified as dibenzo(a,e)fluoranthene (Lavit-Lamy and Buu-Hoi 1966). On the other hand, $I_{obs} \cong 82$ is a sarcoma index obtained by subcutaneous injections. The significance of the sarcoma index is rather doubtful, at least as long as the tumor locations are not specified (Theiss 1982). Thus the unequivocal experimental determination of the potency of dibenzo(a,l)-pyrene has still to be done. The MCS-model predicts $I_{calc}=33\pm15$, where $2.074 \cdot s_p^2=14.8 \cong 15$ represents the 95% tolerance interval for individual future observations.

Table 1. Metabolic indices M, carbocation indices C, size factors Δ, observed and calculated Iball indices I of polycyclic aromatic hydrocarbons.

hydrocarbon	M	C	Δ	I^*_{obs}	I_{calc}
1 benzo(e)pyrene	0.125	42.4	0	2	8
2 benzo(a)pyrene	0.155	49.6	0	72	65
3 dibenzo(e,l)pyrene	0.040	42.1	64	0	7
4 naphtho(2,3-a)pyrene	0.151	44.7	64	27	20
5 dibenzo(a,e)pyrene	0.106	46.8	64	50	41
6 dibenzo(a,h)pyrene	0.186	50.1	64	68	62
7 dibenzo(a,i)pyrene	0.176	52.2	64	74	80
8 tribenzo(a,e,h)pyrene	0.111	48.0	512	~20	17
9 tribenzo(a,e,i)pyrene	0.121	48.8	512	17	23
10 tetracene	0.151	40.1	8	0	-14
11 pentacene	0.252	42.9	8	0	1
12 hexacene	0.294	45.5	216	0 ?	4
13 phenanthrene	0.004	41.1	216	0	-9
14 benzo(a)anthracene	0.235	43.8	8	7	10
15 benzo(a)tetracene	0.500	45.9	8	0	5
16 benzo(a)pentacene	0.771	49.3	216	0	-4
17 triphenylene	0.000	40.8	8	0	-4

Table 1. continued

hydrocarbon	M	C	Δ	I_{obs}	I_{calc}
18 chrysene	0.017	41.7	8	5	10
19 benzo(c)chrysene	0.012	41.7	8	~10	10
20 benzo(g)chrysene	0.021**	42.2**	8	18	14
21 benzo(c)phenanthrene	0.002	39.8	8	4	-4
22 dibenzo(a,c)anthracene	0.246	42.9	8	3	2
23 dibenzo(a,j)anthracene	0.167	43.7	8	4 ?	15
24 dibenzo(a,h)anthracene	0.101	44.6	8	26	27
25 tribenzo(a,c,h)anthracene	0.069	43.4	216	0 ?	5
26 fluoranthene	0.027	41.5	8	0	8
27 pentaphene	0.077	40.8	8	0	-3
28 benzo(c)pentaphene	0.226	44.7	216	0	4
29 hexaphene	0.274	42.2	216	0	-22
30 picene	0.019	42.5	8	0 ?	17
31 dibenzo(c,g)phenanthrene	0.008	41.4	8	0	8
32 naphtho(2,3-e)pyrene	0.041	38.8	64	0	-20
33 benzocoronene	0.046	43.1	512	0	-18
34 dibenzo(a,l)pyrene	0.128	46.1	64	see text	33
35 dibenzo(g,p)chrysene	0.000	44.4	216	unknown	18
36 dibenzo(a,j)tetracene	0.321	46.8	216	unknown	12

* experimental values taken from Arcos and Argus, (1968)

** mean values, as explained in text

Positive Iball indices are predicted by the MCS-model for dibenzo(g,p)chrysene $I_{calc} = 18 \pm 15$ and dibenzo(a,j)-tetracene $I_{calc} = 12 \pm 15$.

Acknowledgements: Discussions with Drs. Fraschio, Herndon, Lutz, Párkányi, Peter, Preuss, Stoll, Tews and Zander are gratefully acknowledged.

References:

Arcos JC, Argus MF (1968). Advan. Cancer Res. 11: 305.

Borgen A, Darvey H, Castagnoli N, Crocker TT, Rasmussen RE, Wang IY (1973). J. Med. Chem. 16:502.

Cvetanovic RJ (1970). J. Phys. Chem. 74:2730.

Dewar MJS (1952). J. Am. Chem. Soc. 74:3341, 3357

Dewar MJS (1969). "The Molecular Orbital Theory of Organic Chemistry". New York: McGraw-Hill.

Dewar MJS, Dougherty, RC (1975). "The PMO Theory of Organic Chemistry". New York:Plenum.

Draper NR, Smith H (1981). "Applied Regression Analysis". New York:Wiley.

Fukui K, Yonezawa T, Nagata C (1954). Bull. Chem. Soc. Japan 27:423.

Groves JT, McClusky GA, White RE, Coon MJ (1978). Biochem. Biophys. Res. Commun. 81:154.

Guenther TM, Oesch F (1981). In Gelboin HV, Ts'o POP (eds): "Polycyclic Hydrocarbons and Cancer". Vol. 3. New York: Acad. Press, p. 182.

Hanzlik RP, Shearer GO (1978). Biochem. Pharmacol. 27: 1141.

Harvey RG (1981). Acc. Chem. Res. 14:218.

Herndon WC (1972). Tetrahedron 28:3675.

Herndon WC (1974). Int. J. Quantum Chem.: Biol. Symp. 1:123.

Herndon WC (1983). private communication

Iball J (1939). Am. J. Cancer 35:188.

Jerina DM, Daly JW (1974). Science 185:573.

Jerina DM, Lehr RE (1977). In Ullrich V, Roots I, Hildebrandt AG, Estabrook RW, Conney AH (eds): "Microsomes and Drug Oxidations". Oxford: Pergamon, p. 709.

Keay RE, Hamilton GA (1976). J. Am. Chem. Soc. 98:6578.

Klein R, Scheer MD (1970). J. Phys. Chem. 74:2732.

Lacassagne A, Buu-Hoi NP, Zajdela F, Vingiello FA (1968). Naturwissenschaften 55:43.

Lavit-Lamy D, Buu-Hoi NP (1966). Chem. Commun. 1966:92.
Loew GH, Sudhindra BS, Ferrell JE (1979). Chem. Biol.
    Interact. 26:75.
Longuet-Higgins HS (1950). J. Chem. Phys. 18:265,275,283.
Mason SF (1958). J. Chem. Soc. 1958:808.
Osborne MR (1979). Cancer Res. 39:4760.
Pariser R, Parr RG (1953). J. Chem. Phys. 21:466,767.
Pople JA (1953). Trans. Farad. Soc. 49:1375.
Pople JA, Brickstock A (1954). Trans. Farad. Soc. 50:901.
Pople JA, Beveridge DL, Dobosh PA (1967). J. Chem. Phys.
    47:2026.
Pudzianowski AT, Loew GH (1983). Int. J. Quantum Chem.
    23:1257.
Pullman A (1954). Bull. Soc. Chim. France 1954:595.
Rogers KS, Cammarata A (1969). J. Med. Chem. 12:692.
Scribner NK, Woodworth B, Ford PG, Scribner JD (1980).
    Carcinogenesis 1:715.
Sims P, Grover PL (1974). Advan. Cancer Res. 20:165.
Sims P, Grover PL (1981). In Gelboin HV, Ts'o POP (eds)
    "Polycyclic Hydrocarbons and Cancer". Vol. 3. New
    York: Acad. Press, p. 117.
Smith IA, Berger GD, Seybold PG, Servé MP (1978).
    Cancer Res. 38:2968.
Streitwieser A (1961). "Molecular Orbital Theory for
    Organic Chemists". New York:Wiley, p. 115
Szentpály Lv (1984). J. Am. Chem. Soc., in press.
Theiss JC (1982). Regul. Toxicol. Pharmacol. 2:213.
Umans RS, Koruda M, Sardella DJ (1979). Molec.
    Pharmacol. 16:633.
Wheland GW, Mann DE (1949). J. Chem. Phys. 17:264.

III. ONCOGENES
A. RELATION TO MUTAGENS, CARCINOGENS, AND ACTIVATION MECHANISMS

Molecular Basis of Cancer, Part A: Macromolecular Structure, Carcinogens, and Oncogenes, pages 343–356
© 1985 Alan R. Liss, Inc.

PHYSICAL MECHANISMS OF THE ACTIVATION OF ONCOGENES THROUGH CARCINOGENS

János J. Ladik

Chair for Theoretical Chemistry, Friedrich-Alexander-University Erlangen-Nürnberg, Egerlandstr. 3, D-8520 Erlangen, FRG and Laboratory of the National Foundation for Cancer Research at the Chair for Theoretical Chemistry, University Erlangen-Nürnberg

Abstract. - In the last years about twenty human oncogenes have been discovered. It is shown that their main activation mechanisms: 1. through non Watson-Crick-type point mutation, 2. through activation by LTR binding to the end of an oncogene and 3. through transposition of an oncogene to another chromosome need an external agent.

The principal mechanisms of short- and long-range effects of chemical carcinogens are reviewed. A possible very effective mechanism for long-range effects of chemical carcinogenesis through generation of conformational solitons in DNA are discussed in detail.

1. INTRODUCTION

After the discovery of oncoviruses and oncogenes in plants and animals in the last few years about twenty human oncogenes have been discovered. These oncogenes show three basic biochemical mechanisms (besides a less extent of methylation of cytosine molecules in them than in other genes and the repetition of the oncogene in another part of DNA). In one case a simple base substitution (the codon GGC has been changed to GTC) transforms a protooncogene to an active oncogene which causes human EJ bladder carcinoma (Santos, Tronick, Aaronson, Pulciani, Barbacid 1982; Tabin, Bradley, Bargmann, Weinberg, Papageorge, Scolnick, Dhar, Lowy, Chang 1982). The change which has been determined through the sequencing of important part of the gene in normal and tumor cells (Pincus 1984) corresponds to a single glycine-valine substitution in position 12 of the protein coded by this gene. The oncoprotein coded by this gene has been sequenced and with the aid of empirical potential energy calculations it has been shown (Yuasa, Srivasta, Dunn, Thim, Reddy, Aaronson 1983) that the substitution of glycine by the more bulky valine at position 12 causes a kink of the handed-ness of the original protein helix. This most probably inactivates this enzyme (or changes its function) which obviously changes the regulation of the cells in which this has occurred.

Another example for a single base substitution causing the transformation of a protooncogene to an active oncogene is the CAG $\longrightarrow$ CTG codon transition (Yuasa, Srivasta, Dunn, Thim, Reddy, Aaronson 1983). This point mutation corres-ponds to a substitution of leucine for glutamine in the 61 position of the protein coded by the protooncogene. The transformed gene (oncogene) was detected in a human lung carcinoma-derived cell line, Hs 242 (Yuasa, Srivasta, Dunn, Thim, Reddy, Aaronson 1983) but proved to be transformed from the same protooncogene which can be activated also through the GGC $\longrightarrow$ GTC point mutation (but at position 12 instead of 61) (Yuasa, Srivasta, Dunn, Thim, Reddy, Aaronson 1983). One should further observe that in both cases at final end an amino acid with the branched isopropyl group is substituted into the protein instead of the original amino acid leading to the probable inactivation of an enzyme although in the second case leucine is not larger than glutamine.

In the second case a gene occurring in normal cells becomes overactivated (without any change in the sequence) by the binding to its end a new control element (the so-called long terminal repeat (LTR)). The slicing out of LTR (which is of viral origin) from another part of DNA and its insertion to DNA at the end of the oncogene happens in an enzymatic way (Chang, Furth, Scolnick,Lowy 1982). The over-production of the protein (which can reach 10^3 times of its original amount) coded by the overactivated oncogene (by binding to it the LTR) obviously changes again so much the regulation of the cells that this can lead again to a malignant transformation (Chang, Furth, Scolnick, Lowy 1982).

The third mechanism is similar to the second one. In

this case a whole normally functioning gene gets sliced out
from one chromosome region (mostly from chromosome 8) and
becomes inserted into another "more active" chromosomal
region (mostly to chromosome 14) (Rechavi, Givol, Canaani
1982). This DNA transposition (performed with the help of
appropriate enzymes) causes again the overproduction of the
protein coded by this gene. Thus results again in such
changes of cell regulation (Rechavi, Givol. Canaani 1982)
which causes at the final end the development of a tumor.

In the case of $\begin{array}{ccc} G & G \\ \downarrow \\ G & \rightarrow T \\ C & C \end{array}$ and $\begin{array}{ccc} C & C \\ A & \rightarrow T \\ G & G \end{array}$ point mutation (first
mechanism) one has to observe that there is no way to get a
$G \longrightarrow T$ or an $A \longrightarrow T$ base substitution in the same strand
of DNA with the help of the usual Watson-Crick-Löwdin
tautomeric shift-mutation mechanisms (Watson, Crick 1953;
Watson 1968; Löwdin 1963). A possibility to obtain a $G \longrightarrow T$
transition would be through depurination of G (Weinstein),
but this mechanism is not established in this case. On the
other hand if during a duplication procedure in the complementary strand of DNA instead of C an A molecule is built
in (A can form two hydrogen bonds with G), in the consequent
duplication instead of G the nucleotide base T can be incorporated into the original strand. (The same is true in
the second case, before which an $A \longrightarrow G$ point mutation has
to occur which can take place via the usual tautomeric shift).

Under normal conditions the described procedure is
not possible, because both G and A are purine bases and
therefore for a G-A base pair there would not be enough
space in the double helical structure of B DNA. On the other
hand if the double helix becomes through the binding of a
chemical carcinogen (especially through the binding of a
bulky one) in the neighborhood of the critical $\begin{array}{ccc} G & A \\ C & G \end{array}$
codons distorted enough, the formation of the unusual G-A
base pair can be easily visualized.

2. BRIEF REVIEW OF POSSIBLE SHORT-RANGE AND LONG-RANGE EFFECTS OF CARCINOGENS

In a previous paper (Ladik, Suhai, Seel 1978) assuming
already then the existence of human oncogenes we have

reviewed the most probable local as well as long-range effects
caused by carcinogen binding to DNA and/or proteins. Besides
changes in charge distribution of the DNA constituents (including charge transfer) and changes of the vibrations in the
neighborhood of the carcinogen binding (as well as breaking
of bonds or forming of new bonds) first of all <u>conformational</u>
<u>changes</u> caused by binding of carcinogens can be expected
(Ladik, Suhai, Seel 1978). In this way though the

$$\begin{array}{ccc} G & G & C & C \\ G \rightarrow T & A \rightarrow T \\ C & C, G & G \end{array}$$

cancer causing point mutation cannot be explained by the
usual tautomeric shifts in the base pair, it is still understandable on the basis of <u>local</u> (short-range) <u>effects</u> caused
by carcinogen binding.

This is, however, not the case for the second and third
above mentioned mechanisms. The transposition of LTR sequence
in DNA (2. mechanism) or the transposition of a whole gene
to another chromosome is explained on the biochemical level
by enzyme action (Chang, Furth, Scolnick, Lowy (1982;
Rechavi, Givol, Canaani 1982). To understand, however, on the
physical and physico-chemical level how the binding of
another DNA sequence (the LTR) to the end of a gene
influences strongly its regulation, one has to suppose that
DNA-protein interactions are influenced by the sequences
of the neighboring DNA segments. (The overactivation of the
oncogene means most probably that it is blocked by a protein
in a smaller fraction of time, than under normal conditions.)
In the same way for the transposition of longer DNA sequences
(at mechanism 2 of LTR, at mechanism 3 of a whole gene) into
another location one has to assume that the DNA-protein
interactions of these DNA segments have been weakened in an
extent (the DNA segments become deblocked) that the necessary
enzymatic reactions could take place. Since the experiments
described in ref.-s (Chang, Furth, Scolnick, Lowy 1982;
Rechavi, Givol, Canaani 1982) have been performed with whole
cancer cells and the corresponding normal cells, they do not
contain any information for the start of these processes.

The most plausible assumption is also in the cases of
mechanisms 2 and 3 that they were initiated by carcinogens
and/or radiations which have besides local also long-range
effects. In (Ladik, Suhai, Seel 1978) a number of possibilities for long-range effects of carcinogen binding on DNA-
protein interactions have been reviewed. (Change of the
strength of DNA-protein interactions in a longer sequence

caused by charge transfer which can influence strongly the
polarization and dispersion forces between the two chains,
long-range effect of carcinogen binding on the tertiary
structure which results again in a change of DNA-protein
interaction, additional aperiodicity caused by carcinogen
binding influencing DNA-protein interaction, etc. (for
details see (Ladik, Suhai, Seel 1978)).

3. PROBABLE ROLE OF CONFORMATIONAL SOLITONS CAUSED BY CARCINOGENS

In the present paper we should like to elaborate on a
possibility only shortly mentioned in (Ladik, Suhai, Seel
1978): long-range effects of carcinogens through formation
of solitons in DNA. Let us assume that a bulky carcinogen,
like the epoxydiol ultimate of 3,4-benzopyrene is bound to
a nucleotide base. Certainly, in the neighborhood of the
attached carcinogen the structure of DNA, first of all the
positions of the stacked base pairs will become strongly
changed. With this conformational distortion a change in the
electronic interaction due to the stacking of the base
pairs is strongly dependent on the relative position of the
superimposed base pairs. In this way a non-linear change
(conformational change coupled with electronic structure
change) takes place at the site and neighborhood of the
carcinogen binding (see Fig. 1).

In vitro a covalently bound ultimate carcinogen would
remain attached to DNA for an indefinitely long time. Not
this is the case, however, in vivo where for instance repair
enzymes can remove the carcinogen wihtin a few hours
(Weinstein). Until the carcinogen sits at its binding site
the above described non-linear change will remain localized
to the neighborhood of this site. After the removal of the
carcinogen however, it seems rather probable that the
system will not relax immediately (the original conformation
will not be restored instantanously) because for this bulky
molecular constituents of DNA (together with the water and
ion structure surrounding them) have to be moved. On the
other hand it is well known 1.) solitary waves have several
orders of magnitudes longer life times than simple electronic excitations and 2.) they can travel in an extended
system (Davydov, Kislusha 1973). Therefore, one can postulate that after the removal of a carcinogen from DNA the
non-linear (but previously local) change caused by its

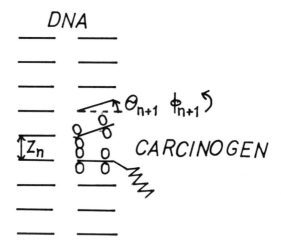

Fig. 1. Distortion of a DNA stack due to the binding of a bulky carcinogen to a nucleotide base. Z_n denotes the change of the stacking distance at the n-th unit, the tilting angle θ_{n+1} is measuring the deviation of the plane of the n+1-th nucleotide base from its original position (perpendicular to the latter unit from the equilibrium value of rotation around the helix axis (36^0 in DNA B).

binding can travel through rather large distances along the chain (see Fig. 2) causing a long-range effect which may effect a larger segment of DNA and its interaction with a protein molecule.

To test this hypothesis one can start by writing down a Hamiltonian for the soliton. Generalizing the theory of Su, Schrieffer and Heeger (SSH) (Su, Schrieffer, Heeger 1980) which was developed for the non-linear change caused by a kink in polyacetylene, we can write

$$\tilde{H} = \tilde{H}_{el} + \tilde{H}_{conf} + \tilde{H}_{el-conf} \tag{1}$$

Here we take as first (and rough approximation for the description of the overlapping π electrons of the stacked basis $\tilde{H}_{el}$ in the form (Hückel type, or tight-binding

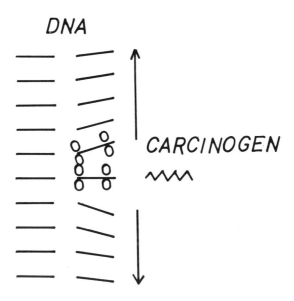

Fig. 2. After the removal of the carcinogen the originally pinned down non-linear change in the DNA stack starts to travel either upwards or downwards.

approximation)

$$\widetilde{\hat{H}}_{el} = -t_o \sum_{n,s,\alpha} (\hat{C}^+_{n+1,s,\alpha}\hat{C}_{n,s,\alpha} + \hat{C}^+_{n,s,\alpha}\hat{C}_{n+1,s,\alpha}) \quad (2)$$

where n is the site index (which base), $s(\pm 1/2)$ stands for the spin and $\alpha = 1,2$ indicates the strand in the DNA double helix. Further the $\hat{C}^+$-s and $\hat{C}$-s are creation and annihilation operators, respectively, and t_0 is the hopping integral for the undistorted chain. One should point out immediately that $\hat{H}_{el}$ is incomplete because it does not contain electron-electron interaction terms.

To describe the conformational changes of the stacked bases one has to introduce three variables (in contrary of the one variable of the polyacetylene case (Su, Schrieffer, Heeger 1980)). We can denote by $Z_{n,\alpha}$ the shift from its equilibrium position along the Z axis (the main axis of the double helix) of the n-th base in the α-th chain (if Z_n is positive Z_{n+1} will also be positive, Z_{n-1} and Z_{n-2} will be, however, negative (see Fig. 1.)) and by $\phi_{n,\alpha}$ (following Krumhansl and Alexander 1957) the rotation of this base (again measured from its equilibrium position) in the plane perpendicular to the Z axis. Finally, the angle $\theta_{n,\alpha}$ measures the tilting of the base (thus θ is the angle between the plane of the displaced base and the plane perpendicular to the Z axis) (see Fig. 2.). Assuming that the motion of the base described by these three variables can still be treated in the harmonic approximation we can write

$$\widetilde{H}_{conf} = 1/2 \sum_{n,\alpha} \left[K_1 (Z_{n+1,\alpha} - Z_{n,\alpha})^2 + K_2(\phi_{n+1,\alpha} - \phi_{n,\alpha})^2 \right.$$

$$\left. + K_3(\theta_{n+1,\alpha} - \theta_{n,\alpha})^2 + M_{n,\alpha}(\dot{Z}^2_{n,\alpha} + \dot{\phi}^2_{n,\alpha} + \dot{\theta}^2_{n,\alpha}) \right] \quad (3)$$

Here K_1, K_2 and K_3 are the force constants belonging to the three variables Z, ϕ and θ and $M_{n,\alpha}$ is the mass of the n-th base in the α-th strand.

Finally, for the coupling of the conformational change with the electronic structure change we have to introduce the modified hopping integral $t_{n+1,\alpha;n,\alpha}$ as

$$\widetilde{t}_{n+1,\alpha;n,\alpha} = t_o - \left[\beta_1(Z_{n+1,\alpha} - Z_{n,\alpha}) + \beta_2(\phi_{n+1,\alpha} - \right.$$

$$\left. - \phi_{n,\alpha}) + \beta_3(\theta_{n+1,\alpha} - \theta_{n,\alpha}) \right] \quad (4)$$

where β_1, β_2 and β_3 are the electron-base displacement (phonon) coupling constants. One should point out that equ. (4) is a straightforward generalization of equ. (2.2) of SSH. Using the expression (Chang, Furth, Scolnick, Lowy 1982) we can write for the non-linear electron-displacement coupling term

$$\widetilde{\widetilde{H}}_{el-conf} = \sum_{n,s,\alpha} (\widetilde{t}_{n+1,\alpha;n,\alpha} - t_o)(\hat{C}^+_{n+1,s,\alpha}\hat{C}_{n,s,\alpha} +$$

$$+ \hat{C}^+_{n,s,\alpha}\hat{C}_{n+1,s,\alpha}) \quad (5)$$

Following SSH (Su, Schrieffer, Heeger 1980) and Krumhansl and Alexander (Krumhansl, Alexander 1957), respectively, one can substitute the Hamiltonian (1) with definitions (2) - (5) (after taking the expectation value of the electron-operators with the many electron reference function which gives one) into the classical equations of motion of Hamilton. For actual numerical calculations one has to choose a set of K_i and β_i (i = 1,2,3) values or one can try to determine them on the basis of quantum mechanical potential surface calculations and by computing the corresponding electron-phonon matrix elements.

However, in reality, the three variables describing the change of the positions of nucleotide bases are not independent but have to be coupled. Further an at least approximate treatment of the electron-electron interaction is indispensable. Therefore we have to rewrite our Hamiltonian (1) as

$$\hat{H} = \tilde{\hat{H}} + \hat{H}' \tag{6}$$

where

$$\hat{H}' = \hat{H}'_{el} + \hat{H}'_{conf} + \hat{H}'_{el-conf} \tag{7}$$

Here

$$\hat{H}'_{el} = \sum_{n,m} \gamma_{n,m} (\hat{n}_n - 1)(\hat{n}_m - 1) \tag{8}$$

where

$$\hat{n}_m = \hat{C}_m^+ \hat{C}_m$$

is the number operator at site m. Equ. (8) describes the electron-electron interaction in the well known Pariser-Parr-Pople (PPP) approximation (for the $\gamma_{n,m}$ integrals the well known Mataga-Nishimoto expression could be taken) (Mataga, Nishimoto 1957). Further H'_{conf} can be written as

$$\hat{H}'_{conf} = 1/2 \sum_{n,\alpha} \big[X_1 (Z_{n+1,\alpha} - Z_{n,\alpha})(\phi_{n+1,\alpha} - \phi_{n,\alpha}) +$$
$$+ X_2 (Z_{n+1,\alpha} - Z_{n,\alpha})(\theta_{n+1,\alpha} - \theta_{n,\alpha}) +$$
$$+ X_3 (\phi_{n+1,\alpha} - \phi_{n,\alpha})(\theta_{n+1,\alpha} - \theta_{n,\alpha}) \tag{9}$$

where X_1, X_2 and X_3 are coupling constants between the different coordinates describing the distortion of the original position of a nucleotide base (these coupling constants could be computed also from the corresponding potential surface). Finally, $H'_{el-conf}$ can be easily constructed, if one substitutes into equ. (5) instead of $t_{n+1,\alpha;n,\alpha}$

$$t_{n+1,\alpha;n,\alpha} = \tilde{t}_{n+1,\alpha;n,\alpha} + t'_{n+1,\alpha;n,\alpha} \tag{10}$$

with

$$t'_{n+1,\alpha;n,\alpha} = -\left\{ \left[\tilde{\mathcal{S}}_1(\phi_{n+1,\alpha} - \phi_{n,\alpha}) + \tilde{\mathcal{S}}_2(\theta_{n+1,\alpha} - \theta_{n,\alpha}) \right] \right.$$

$$\left. (z_{n+1,\alpha} - z_{n,\alpha}) + \tilde{\mathcal{S}}_3(\phi_{n+1,\alpha} - \phi_{n,\alpha})(\theta_{n+1,\alpha} - \theta_{n,\alpha}) \right\} \tag{11}$$

The additional electron-phonon coupling constants could be calculated again with the help of quantum mechanically computed electronic wave functions of the stack (band structures) using again a potential hypersurface to determine the wave functions of these coupled vibrations. Presently, however, to obtain an orientation one can treat these coupling constants as parameters substituting different values for them.

One should point out that writing down equ.-s (1) - (11) we have tacitly assumed a periodic stack. In real aperiodic DNA with the four nucleotide bases one has to work with parameters $t_0^{r,s}$, $K_i^{r,s}$, $\beta_i^{r,s}$, $X_i^{r,s}$ and $\mathcal{S}_i^{r,s}$, respectively ($i = 1,2,3$, $r = A,T,G,C$ and independently $s = A,T,G,C$). This means that due to the aperiodicity in DNA we have instead of 7 7.16 = 112 different parameters in the case of an SSH Hamiltonian (Su, Schrieffer, Heeger 1980) and instead of 13 13.16 = 208 parameters in the case of the more full Hamiltonian defined by equ.-s (6) - (11). It is obvious that one cannot solve the dynamical equation with 208 different parameters. On the other hand one could investigate the much simpler polyacetylene kink problem (which has in the SSH approximation only 3 parameters) assuming two different constitutents (a CH unit and say a CF unit). In this case the number of necessary parameters is only 3 x 4 = 12. In this way one could study how much the disorder influences the life time (or even existence) of a solitary wave. If one would find that the changes due to the disorder are not very large, one could conclude that the results obtained for periodic DNA stack are <u>qualitatively</u>

correct also in the case of aperiodic DNA.

To solve the dynamical problem at least classically one can follow the numerical iterative procedure of Su and Heeger (Su, Heeger 1980) and of Su (Su 1982) respectively. The adaption of this procedure to our problem in the case of the simple SSH type Hamiltonian ($\hat{H}$) as well as of the more complete Hamiltonian $\hat{H}$ (defined by equ.-s (6) - (11) is described in another paper (Ladik, Cizek 1984).

Applying this procedure to the polyacetylene problem of 50 CH units with one kink, it turned out that only by a special choice of the paramter values to, K and β it was possible to obtain a true soliton solution (with an infinite life time)(Mataga, Nishimoto 1957).

One should point out, however, that the simple SSH-type Hamiltonian (equ.-s (1) - (5)) does not include couplings between the three different distortion variables of a DNA stack. Therefore the dynamical treatment of this Hamiltonian would describe three independent distortion problems which differ from each other only in the values of the parameters. For this reason the existing polyacetylene kink program can be easily used to study the time dependence of these distortions of a DNA stack.

If one wants to describe, however, the dynamic behaviour of the more realistic system defined by the Hamiltonian given through equ.-s (6) - (11) one needs a somewhat more complicated program system. The development of this is in progress.

The solutions of the classical equations of motion will then provide the time evolution of the solitary wave generated at the site of carcinogen binding. In this way one can learn about the life time and the range of the travelling of the non-linear distortion caused by carcinogen binding and subsequent releasing as a function of the parameter values. Most probably with a realistic estimate of the parameter values one would not obtain a soliton in a strict sense (infinite life time) but rather probably a solitary wave δ which has a long enough life time to travel along the stack causing long-range interference with the DNA protein interactions. In this way possibly it can initiate the activation of an oncogene. Obviously such results will have besides their physical significance a profound biolological importance.

Finally, it should be mentioned that in our model we have neglected 1.) distortions of the nucleotide bases themselves (we have treated them as rigid units), 2.) the role of vibrations and 3.) in contrary to Krumhansl and Alexander (Krumhansl, Alexander 1957) the coupling of the distortions of the stacked bases with the changes in the conformation of the sugar rings (the sugar puckering), 4.) non-linear terms in the motion of the bases and the sugar rings and 5.) the coupling to the environment (water molecules and ions). One hopes with time to find comparatively simple ways to model these effects also, but taking all them into account in one step would make the problem hopelessly complicated.

4. CONCLUSIONS

As the pattern of human oncogenes emerges more and more the theoretician comes to the conclusion that a much closer cooperation between different disciplines (molecular biologists, biochemists, experimental physical chemists and physicists as well as theoreticians) is needed to understand the different mechanisms of oncogene activation deeply enough to be able to counteract or more probably prevent (i.e. decrease the probability) the initiation of cell transformations. For instance the example of the G   G point

$$\begin{array}{c} G \\ C \end{array} \rightarrow \begin{array}{c} T \\ C \end{array}$$

---

§ If a solitary wave passing along a DNA stack has a lasting effect (for instance breaking hydrogen bonds between the base pairs or between the polynucleotide and a polypeptide chain) it would quickly loose its energy. Therefore, such dissipative solitary waves would have a very short life time. On the other hand the water and ion environment of DNA can easily serve as an energy reservoir slowing down in this way in a large degree the energy dissipation of the solitary wave. Thus the life time of a solitary wave travelling along a DNA stack which is embedded in its environment can become considerably larger.

mutation in a protooncogene and the subsequent determination of the structure of the corresponding oncogene protein with the help of combined experimental and theoretical methods, shows that besides counteracting carcinogen action/cancer initiation by chemicals at the DNA level there is a possibility also by influencing the changed protein. Further in the cases of overproduction of the same protein due to oncogene overactivation one could think of ways to inactivate these proteins.

Finally, if one looks at the oncogenes in a more general context, one cannot help to suspect, that they form only the tip of the iceberg. One would expect that we have genes in our organisms which are especially sensitive to bacterial and viral DNA attacks causing different other diseases. In this way with time one could order besides the oncogenes also genes to at least of a part of other diseases. From this it is only one step further to assume the existence of <u>gerontogenes</u> that is normal genes in our different cells which - if changed by mutations or if over- or underactivated - are first of all responsible for the aging process.

ACKNOWLEDGMENTS

The author would like to express his gratitude for the very fruitful discussions to Professors F. Martino, J. Cizek and I.B. Weinstein on the different aspects of the problems described here. The financial support of the "Fond der Chemischen Industrie" is gratefully acknowledged.

REFERENCES

Chang EH, Furth ME, Scolnick EM, Lowy DR (1982). Tumorigenic transformation of mammalian cells induced by a normal human gene homologous to the oncogene of Harvey murine sarcoma virus. Nature 297:479.

Davydov SA, Kislukha NI (1976). Solitons in one-dimensional molecular chains. Phys stat sol (b) 75:735

Krumhansl JA, Alexander DM (1983). Nonlinear dynamics and conformational excitations in biomolecular materials. In Clementi E, Sarma RH (eds): "Structure and Dynamics: Nucleic Acids and Proteins," New York: Plenum, p 61.

Ladik J, Suhai S, Seel M (1978). The electronic structure of biopolymers and possible mechanisms of chemical carcinogenesis. Int J Quant Chem QBS 5:35.

Ladik J, Cizek J (1984). Probable physical mechanisms of the activation of oncogenes through carcinogens. Int J Quant Chem (in press).

Löwdin P-O (1963). Proton tunneling in DNA and its biological implications. Rev Mod Phys 35:724.

Martino F, Wang CL, Ladik J (to be published).

Mataga N, Nishimoto K (1957). Electronic structure and spectra of nitrogen heterocycles. Z Phys Chem (Frankfurt) 13:140.

Pincus M (1984). Lecture at the NFCR Workshop "Oncogenes and Oncogenic Polypeptides" New York, and at this conference.

Rechavi E, Givol D, Canaani E (1982). Activation of a cellular oncogene by DNA rearrangements: Possible involvement of an IS-like element. Nature 300:607.

Santos E, Tronick SR, Aaronson SA, Pulciani S, Barbacid M (1982). T24 human bladder carcinoma oncogene is an activated form of the normal human homologue of BALB- and Harvey-MSV transforming genes. Nature 298:343.

Su WP, Heeger AJ (1980). Proc Natl Ac Sci 77:5626.

Su WP, Schrieffer JR, Heeger AJ (1980). Soliton excitations in polyacetylene. Phys Rev B 22:2099.

Su WP (1982). In "Molecular Crystals Liquid Crystals" Proceedings of the International Conference on Low Dimensional Conductors, Boulder, Colorado, vol. 83.

Tabin CJ, Bradley SM, Bargmann CT, Weinberg RH, Papageorge AG, Scolnick EM, Dhar R, Lowy DR, Chang EH (1982). Mechanism of activation of a human oncogene. Nature 300:143.

Watson JD, Crick FHC (1953). Nature 171:964.

Watson JD (1968). "The Double Helix." New York: Atheneum.

Weinstein IB (personal communication).

Yuasa Y, Srivasta SK, Dunn CY, Thim JS, Reddy P, Aaronson SA (1983). Acquisition of transforming properties by alternative point mutations within c-bas/has human proto-oncogene. Nature 303:775.

Molecular Basis of Cancer, Part A: Macromolecular Structure, Carcinogens, and Oncogenes, pages 357–368
© **1985 Alan R. Liss, Inc.**

MUTATIONAL ACTIVATION OF PROTO-ONCOGENES

Robert Rein, Masayuki Shibata, Thomas Kieber-Emmons, Theresa J. Zielinski
Unit of Theoretical Biology, Roswell Park Memorial Institute, 666 Elm Street Buffalo, New York 14263

Cellular homologues of transforming viral ras genes have been found in a variety of carcinoma cell lines. These transforming genes presumably arise by somatic mutational activation of the respective cellular ras genes. DNA sequence analyses have suggested that a single nucleotide change in the codon corresponding to position 12 in the encoded gene products is sufficient to confer transforming properties on the ras (p21) gene product. This activation process has been associated with tumor induction mediated by alkylation of nucleic acid bases (Weinberg 1983; Sukumar et al. 1983; Santos et al. 1984).

Table 1 summarizes the observed mutations within codon 12 of various ras genes. In the upper half of the Table is the c-K-ras proto oncogene nucleotide sequence followed by the various point mutations leading to activation in human cell lines (Santos et al. 1984) and a viral cell line (Nakano et al. 1984). In the lower half of the Table the same information is given for the Harvey-ras gene (Tabin et al. 1982; Reddy et al. 1982; Sukumar et al. 1983). The common feature of these mutations is that the glycine in position 12 is replaced by some other amino acids. The underlying mutations, also indicated in Table 1, include two transversions and one transition. These require the mispairings shown in the last column of the Table.

The objective of this study is to examine the mechanism of these mutations by identifying the nature, structure, and energetics of the respective intermediates both under spontaneous and carcinogen induced conditions. The two mechanisms to be considered for the observed mutations involve the use of minor tautomeric forms of the bases or non Watson-Crick hydrogen bonding schemes with backbone deformation.

TABLE 1
OBSERVED POINT MUTATIONS IN ras p21

		Triplet	Amino Acid	Mutation	Mispair
c-K-ras	Gly GGAGCTGGTGGCGTA[a]				
human cellular oncogenes		GTT	Val	G:C→T:A	G:A or C:T[a]
		TTGT	Cys	G:C→T:A	G:A or C:T[a]
		TCGT	Arg	G:C→C:G	G:G or C:C[a]
v-k-ras		TAGT	Ser	G:C→A:T	G:T or C:A[b]
H-ras-1	Gly GGCGCTGGAGGCGTG[c]				
NMU induced v-has		GAA	Glu	G:C→A:T	G:T or C:A[c]
		TAGA	Arg	G:C→A:T	G:T or C:A[c]
c-Ha-ras	Gly GGCGCCGGCGGCGGT[d]				
EJ-T24		GTC	Val	G:C→T:A	G:A or C:T[d]

a) Santos et al. 1984; b) Nakanao et al. 1984; c) Sukumar et al. 1983; d) Reddy et al. 1982.

PRINCIPLES OF THE ANALYSIS

For a passive polymerase replication model, mutational frequencies can be expressed in terms of thermodynamic parameters by the following expression:

$$\text{Misinsertion Frequency} = \frac{\{B_m\}^O}{\{B_c\}^O} \, \text{EXP} \, \frac{-(\Delta G_m^O - \Delta G_c^O)}{RT}$$

where $\{B_c\}^O$ and $\{B_m\}^O$ are the complementary and noncomplementary dNTP (deoxynucleotide triphosphate) concentration and ΔG_c^O and ΔG_m^O are the respective free energies of formation of the complementary and noncomplementary base

pairs. The details of obtaining the required free energies
have been published elsewhere (Rein et al. 1983). In
brief, the energy components consist of tautomeric energies
(MINDO/3), backbone deformation energies and interaction
energies (molecular mechanics). The free energies obtained
were used to calculate misinsertion frequencies which were
then compared to experimentally available data to determine which mispairing scheme was most probable. This data
is reproduced in Table 2 (Rein et al. 1983).

TABLE 2
CALCULATED AND EXPERIMENTAL MISINSERTION FREQUENCIES
BY MISPAIRS

		MISINSERTION FREQUENCIES		
		CALCULATED		EXPERIMENTAL
MUTATION	MISPAIR	TAUTOMERIC PAIR^c	WOBBLE PAIR	
AT→GC	G:T	1.6×10^{-2} (G:T*) 1.9×10^{-6} (G*:T)	1.8×10^{-3}	6.8×10^{-6} a) 8.3×10^{-3} b)
AT→CG	A:G	4.1×10^{-22} (Asyn:G**)	9.5×10^{-6}	5.6×10^{-7} a) 1.1×10^{-5} b)
AT→GC	A:C	6.1×10^{-11} (A:C*) 5.0×10^{-8} (A*:C)	5.7×10^{-7}	9.0×10^{-8} a) 2.2×10^{-5} b)

The calculations are performed with the duplex sequence
dGMC where M indicates a mispair. a) Sinha and Haimes
1981; b) Fersht et al. 1982; c) * and ** minor tautomers.

SPONTANEOUS ACTIVATION OF PROTO-ONCOGENES

First the transition G:C→A:T, for which the possible
mispairs are G:T or C:A, is considered. Table 3 shows the
mispair frequencies obtained as described above. It can
be seen that the lowest energy pathway involves the
tautomer mechanism with thymine in its enol form followed
by the G:T wobble pair. All C:A mispairs are much less
likely. It is safe to conclude that the G:C→A:T spontaneous transition occurs via a G:T mispairing intermediate
and the probability of the process is between 10^{-4} to 10^{-5}.
In fact, G:T wobble pairs have been observed in RNA's
(Sundaralingam 1977) as well as in synthetic oligonucleotides (Patel et al. 1982).

TABLE 3
SPONTANEOUS MISINSERTION FREQUENCIES

MUTATION	TAUTOMERIC PAIR		WOBBLE PAIR	
G:C→A:T	G*:T	1×10^{-10}	G:T	1×10^{-5}
	G:T*	1×10^{-4}		
G:C→A:T	C:A*	4×10^{-10}	C:A	5×10^{-9}
	C*:A	9×10^{-9}		
G:C→T:A	G**:Asyn	6×10^{-18}	G:Asyn	8×10^{-8}

Calculations are for the dGMC duplex. *Indicates minor
tautomer. G** Imino-enol form of guanine tautomer.

Purine-purine pairs have been considered as the intermediate mispairs leading to transversion mutations. Two
mechanisms, that using a syn purine with an anti purine
pair in normal tautomeric forms (Garduno et al. 1977) and
the one involving a minor tautomer (Topal and Fresco 1976)
have been proposed. The G:A pairs of this type are examined
as possible intermediates for the G:C→T:A transversions
and the results are also shown in Table 3. The mispair
containing the normal tautomer (G) is much more stable
than the tautomeric alternative (G**). The probability
of this transversion is of the order of 10^{-7}. Finally,
the G:C→C:G transversion can occur through a G:G or a
C:C mispair. Preliminary results for the G:G mispair are
obtained in the following manner. For the syn-anti
equilibrium, the experimental data on dGTP was taken from
the literature (Stolarski et al. 1984) and the interaction
energy was calculated for the template with a base flanking
environment corresponding to the one observed in the
activated oncogene sequence. To avoid the steric contact
between the N_2 amino group of guanine and the phosphate
group, the glycosidic angle was rotated by 200 degrees
from its normal angular B-DNA value as suggested by Taylor
et al. (1983). No optimization was performed. To obtain
misinsertion frequencies, the energy difference between
the complementary and the noncomplementary complexes were
calculated for the dGTP in the syn conformation, but no
competition was assumed when a guanine in the syn conformation was formed on the template strand. All calculations are performed with the B-DNA geometry and the
results are shown in Table 4 and Figure 1. The frequencies
presented show that the most likely intermediate is the
Gsyn:G mispair with a frequency of the order of 10^{-4}. The

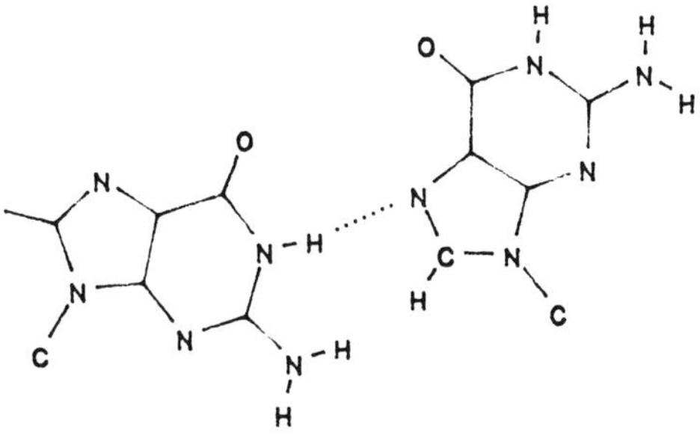

G   Gsyn

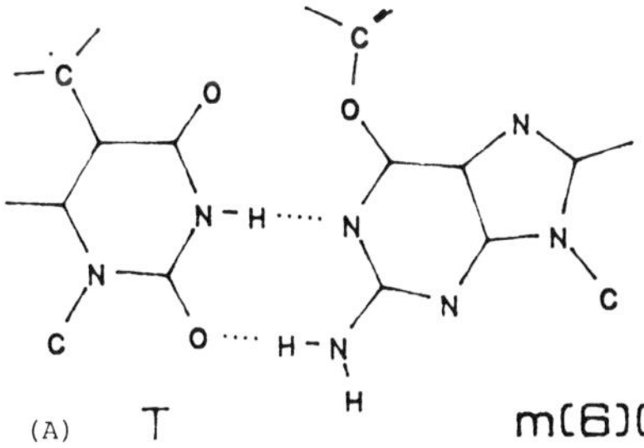

(A) T   m(6)G 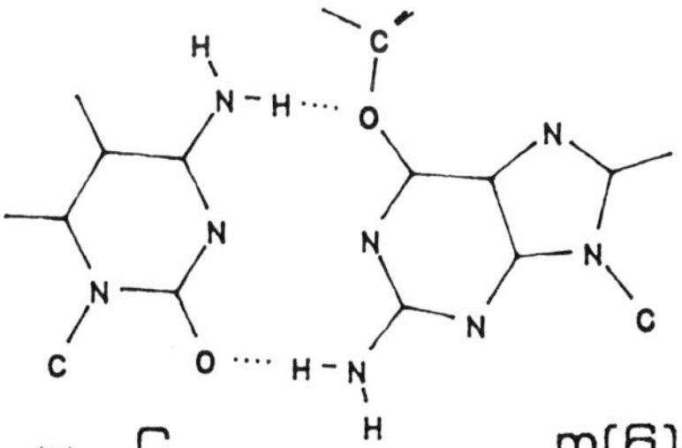   (B) C   m(6)G

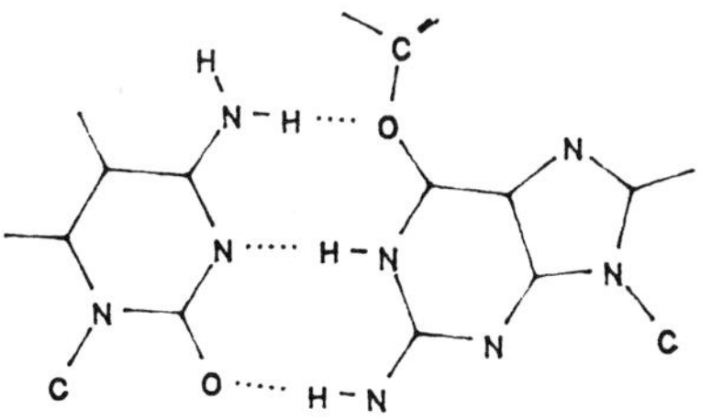

(C) C   m(6)G *

involvement of a minor tautomer can be rejected because of
the very unfavorable energetics of tautomer formation.

TABLE 4

G:C→C:G TRANSVERSION WITH G:G MISPAIR

A) Total Energy of the Template Strand Involving Syn/Anti
   Isomers (kcal/mol).

Template	$\downarrow \begin{array}{c} T \\ G \\ G \end{array}$	$\downarrow \begin{array}{c} T \\ Gsyn \\ G \end{array}$
Interaction Energy	-51.2	-45.5

B) Syn⇌Anti Equilibria

	ΔE^{o} (kcal/mol)	K_{eq}
Ganti ⇌ Gsyn (Template)	5.71	7×10^{-5} a)
Ganti ⇌ Gsyn (dGTP)	.72	3×10^{-1} b)

C) Mispair   Insertion Frequency
   Template : Primer

	Insertion Frequency
Gsyn:G	7×10^{-5}
G:Gsyn	1×10^{-7}
G**:Gsyn	2×10^{-17}

**Indicates the imino-enol form of guanine. a) This work;
b) Stolarski et al. 1984.

INDUCED MUTATION

Only for the case of NMU has the mutated codon been
identified and shown to involve the G:C→A:T transition
with the possible O^6methylguanine (m^{6}G):T intermediate
(Sukumar et al. 1983). The possible mispairing schemes of
the m^{6}G with the bases T and C are shown in Figure 2. The
energetics involved in the G:C→A:T transition are shown in
Table 5 and Table 6 using the B-DNA geometry without
optimization. The conclusion from this is that structure
(a) shown in Figure 2 is the most likely intermediate.

The Pur:Pur pairs involving a syn conformer were considered for the spontaneous transversions in the previous
section. Similarly, the m^{6}G:G pairs can be accommodated
into the B-DNA helical environment without causing any

steric hindrance (results not shown). The formation of Pur(syn):Pur(anti) pairs can be facilitated by the covalent modification of purine bases by some carcinogens. If the N_2 position of guanine is substituted by a bulky group, the steric hindrance created in the minor groove may force the nucleotide to covert to a syn conformation (Taylor et al. 1983). Thus, A:C→C:G and G:C→T:A transversions may involve several different processes. The biological significance of the carcinogen induced mutation will be discussed in a later section.

TABLE 5
TAUTOMERIC EQUILBRIUM OF O^6-METHYLGUANINE (KCAL/MOL)

	ΔE^a	$\Delta H^O_{sol}{}^b$	$\Delta G^O_{calc}{}^c$
$m^6G \rightleftarrows m^6G*$	8.12	-0.83	7.29

a) Intrinsic tautomerization energy using MINDO/3 with full geometry optimization; b) Difference in solvent effect calculated by the reaction field method. The dipole moments used were 2.69D(m^6G) and 3.32D(m^6G*); c) Estimated theoretical tautomerization energy in solution.

TABLE 6

A.   ENERGETICS FOR O^6-METHYLGUANINE INDUCED
G:C→A:T TRANSITION (KCAL/MOL)

	$\begin{array}{c}\text{G:C} \uparrow \\ m^6\text{G:T} \\ \text{A:T} \downarrow\end{array}$	$\begin{array}{c}\text{G:C} \uparrow \\ m^6\text{G:C} \\ \text{A:T} \downarrow\end{array}$	$\begin{array}{c}\text{G:C} \uparrow \\ m^6\text{G*:C} \\ \text{A:T} \downarrow\end{array}$
INTERACTION ENERGY	-123.77	-119.5	-122.1
TAUTOMERIZATION ENERGY	-----	----	7.3
TOTAL	-123.77	-119.5	-114.8

B.   COMPARISON OF EXPERIMENTALLY OBSERVED dm^6GTP

Ratio	EXPERIMENT[a]		THEORY
$\dfrac{m^6G:C}{m^6G:T}$	1/20	1/50	1/1200

a) Toorchen and Topal (1983).

MUTAGENESIS BY O^6-METHYLGUANINE

The promutagenic potential of m^6G due to a change in the hydrogen bonding capability introduced by the methlyation at the O^6 position was proposed by Loveless (1969). In fact, it was shown in an in vitro assay with E. coli DNA polymerase I measuring the incorporation of complementary and noncomplementary dNTPs, using a methylated template, that a specific misincorporation of dTMP but not dAMP occurred (Abbott and Saffhill 1979). The incorporation of dm^6GTP during replication in vitro by "klenow" E. coli pol I over an opposite T template residue was also found by Toorchen and Topal (1983). However, the relative affinity of m^6G to T over C is not conclusive. Abbott and Saffhill (1979) showed that the misincorporation rate of dTMP corresponds to approximately one error for every three m^6G residues present when equal amount of precursors are available. On the other hand, the m^6dGTP was found to incorporate with more than a 20 fold preference for T over C by Toorchen and Topal (1983). The hydrogen bonding energy for m^6G:T and m^6G:C pairs using different theoretical methods were reported by Psoda et al. (1981) and by Poltev et al. (1981). Both results indicate that the m^6G:T pair is more stable than the m^6G:C pair in the B-DNA geometry. However, Poltev et al. (1981) also showed that the m^6G:C pair can attain more stable hydrogen bonding if one allows some wobbling.

Our results in Table 6 are consistent with previous calculations of the B-DNA conformation but from our experience with previous studies, the m^6G:C wobble pair is quite feasible. It should be noted that recent experiments indicate that m^6G can pair with all four nucleic acid bases in synthetic oligonucleotides and the m^6G:C had the lowest melting point (Gaffney et al. 1984).

BIOLOGICAL SIGNIFICANCE

The creation of intermediate mispairs allows for the calculation of insertion probabilities. In order to incorporate a mispair into DNA duplex, the mispair must escape any proofreading process. The induced process would also be controlled by the extent of repair of the lesion. SOS repair synthesis can in fact enhance not only the incorporated mispair, but actually the mutational processes. It is noteworthy that the involvement of SOS repair can lead to transversions occurring via the independent mechanism of depurination. Since the effects of these processes are not quantitatively understood, it is not yet possible to make any accurate estimate of the probabilities of ras gene activation. However, some speculative considerations are possible.

Studies on the quantitation of DNA damage by alkylating agents suggest that the damage occurs once in 5×10^6 bases, with O^6-methylation exhibiting 7% - 9% of the reaction yield (Singer 1979). It is important to realize that it may not be the extent of alkylation on O^6 of G which is specifically important in carcinogenesis but rather the removal of the premutational lesion from a given cell population. The lack of enzymatic excision of O^6-alkyl-G has been correlated with the tumorigenic potential of a mammalian cell (Pegg 1977). The defectiveness of alkylation repair enzyme activities in malignant cells have been noted. Evidence for an enzyme that does not depurinate but instead dealkylates O^6-alkyl-G has been demonstrated for mammalian systems (Pegg 1978). Half life estimates for alkyl-base derivatives differ greatly in various biological systems, with O^6-alkyl-G ranging from 6-240 hours (Singer 1979). It is this persistence or stability of O^6-alkyl-G which can be correlated with tumorigenic potential (Pegg 1977). As a result, a factor of two orders of magnitude may be applied to the occurrance rate for lesion formation, giving as an estimate 10^{-4} or once in 10,000 bases. This factor is not imposed for the spontaneous process. Estimates range for the spontaneous process from 10^{-6} to 10^{-11}.

Presuming that the probability of a ras gene being activated is 10^{-6} and presuming that there are approximately 10^{13} cells per 100 kg individual, the population of ras activated cells is $(10^{13} \times 10^{-6} \times 10^{-4}) 10^3$ cells. Accounting for a reduction of 20% due to lethal lesions (Shooter and Howsel 1973) upon methylation, this amounts to 800 activated ras cells. If the requirement that a ras gene is activated in a stem cell is imposed, then the number of activated cells per stem cell population would at best be a few. This provides some insight as to the time course of tumor development by a single dose (Sukumar et al. 1984) of alkylating agent.

In summary, the prospect of intrinsic activation of ras genes by spontaneous processes is less likely than by

induced processes. Several factors affect the relative
rates. These include: 1) the exposure of the target organ
to a mutagen after the mutagen has been appropriately metabolically activated; 2) the effectiveness of repair of pre-
mutation lesions; 3) the effectiveness of repair during the
replicative process (spontaneous mispairs appear to be more
easily corrected); and 4) the effectiveness of post replicative repair such as SOS repair. Typically, the concentration dependence for tumor promotion (Santos et al.
1984) or cell survival (Shooter and Howse 1975) has been
in the millimolar range. Because of such large doses, some
damage to the cellular repair system may be expected. As a
result of the above discussion, it is not clear whether the
activation of the ras gene precludes such damage. Therefore,
it appears to be prudent to conduct experiments which aim
to show causative relations between oncogene activation
and tumor promotion utilizing much lower concentrations of
alkylating agents.

ACKNOWLEDGEMENTS

These studies were conducted pursuant to a contract with
the National Foundation for Cancer Research and partially by
a grant from NASA #NSG-7305. TJZ affiliated with the Department of Chemistry, Niagara University, Niagara University
New York, 14109. The authors would like to thank Deborah
Raye for her assistance in the preparation of this manuscript.

REFERENCES

Abbott PJ, Saffhill R (1979). DNA synthesis with methlyated
  poly (dC-dG) templates. Biochim Biophys Acta 562:51.
Fersht AR, Knill-Jones JW, Tsui WC (1982). Kinetic Basis
  of spontaneous mutation. J Mol Biol 156:37.
Gaffney BL, Marky LA, Jones RA (1984). DNA fragments
  containing d(O^6Me)G: synthesis and physical studies.
  Proceedings of the Conference on the Molecular Basis of
  Cancer.
Garduno R, Rein R, Egan JT, Coeckelenberg Y, MacElroy RD
  (1977). Purine-purine base pairs and the origin of transversion type mutation. Int J Quantum Chem QBS 4:197.
Loveless, A (1969). Possible relevance of O^6alkylation
  of deoxyguanosine to the mutagenicity and carcinogenicity
  of nitrosamines and nitrosamides. Nature 223:206.
Nakano H, Yamamoto F, Neville G, Evans D, Mizuno T, Perucho

M (1984). Proc Natl Acad Sci USA 81:71.

Patel DJ, Kozlowski SA, Marky LA, Rice JA, Broka C, Dallas J, Itakura K, Breslauer KJ (1982). Structure, dynamics, and energetics of deoxyguanosine thymine wobble base pair formation in the self-complementary d(CGTGAATTCGCG) duplex in solution. Biochem 21:437.

Pegg AE (1978). Enzymatic removal of O^6-methylguanine from DNA by mammalian cell extracts. Biochem Biophys Res 84:166.

Pegg AE (1977). Formation and metabolism of alkylated nucleosides: possible role in carcinogenesis by nitroso compounds and alkylating agents. Adv Cancer Res 25:195.

Poltev VI, Shulyupina NV, Bruskov VI (1981). Molecular mechanisms of errors in nucleic acid biosynthesis induced by alkylation of nitrogenous bases. Mol Biol (Russ) 15:1286.

Psoda A, Kierdaszuk B, Pohorille A, Geller M, Kusmierek JT, Shugar D (1981). Interaction of the mutagenic base analogs O^6-methylguanine and N^4-hydroxycytosine with potentially complementary bases. Int J Quantum Chem 20:543.

Reddy EP, Reynolds RK, Santos E, Barbacid M (1982). A point mutation is responsible for the acquisition of trans-forming properties by the T24 human bladder carcinoma oncogene. Nature 300:149.

Rein R, Shibata M, Garduno-Juarez R, Kieber-Emmons T (1983). Structure of mispairs leading to substitution mutations. In Clementi E, Sarma RH (eds): "Structure and Dynamics: Nucleic Acids and Proteins", New York: Adenine Press, p 269.

Santos E, Martin-Zanca D, Reddy EP, Pierotti MA, Della Porta G, Barbacid M (1984). Malignant activation of a k-ras oncogene in lung carcinoma but not in normal tissue of the same patient. Science 223:661.

Shooter KV, Howse R (1975). The inactivation of bacteriophage R17 by ethylating agents: the lethal lesions. Chem Biol Interaction 11:563.

Singer B (1979). N-nitroso alkylating agents: formation and persistence of alkyl derivatives in mammalian nucleic acids as contributing factors in carcinogenesis. JNCI 62:1329.

Sinha NK, Haimes MD (1981). Molecular mechanisms of sub-stitution mutagenesis. J Biol Chem 256:10671.

Stolarski R, Hagberg C-E, Shugar D (1984). Studies on the dynamic syn-anti equilbrium in purine nucleosides and nucleotides with the aid of ^{1}H and ^{13}C NMR spectroscopy. Eur J Biochem 138:187.

Sukumar S, Notario V, Martin-Zanca D, Barbacid M (1983).
Induction of mammary carcinomas in rats by nitroso-
methylurea involves malignant activation of H-<u>ras</u>-1 locus
by single point mutations. Nature 306:658.

Sundaralingam M (1977). Non-Watson-Crick base pairs in
ribonucleic acids. Int J Quantum Chem QBS 4:11.

Tabin CJ, Bradley SM, Bargmann CI, Weinberg RA, Papageorge
AG, Scolnick EM, Dhar R, Lowy DR, Chang EH (1982).
Mechanism of activation of a human oncogene. Nature 300:
143.

Taylor ER, Miller KJ, Bleyer AJ (1983). Interactions of
molecules with nucleic acids X. Covalent intercalative
binding of the carcinogenic DPDE I(+) to kinked DNA.
J Biomol Structure Dynamics 1:883.

Toorchen D, Topal MD (1983). Mechanisms of chemical mutagenesis and carcinogenesis: effects of DNA replication
on methylation at the O^6-guanine position of dGTP.
Carcinogenesis 4:1591.

Topal MD, Fresco JR (1976). Complementary base pairing and
the origin of substitution mutations. Nature 263:285.

Weinberg RA (1983). Alteration of the geneomes of tumor
cells. Cancer 52:1971.

**Molecular Basis of Cancer, Part A: Macromolecular
Structure, Carcinogens, and Oncogenes, pages 369–377
© 1985 Alan R. Liss, Inc.**

DNA FRAGMENTS CONTAINING d(O[6]Me)G: SYNTHESIS AND PHYSICAL
STUDIES

Barbara L. Gaffney, Luis A. Marky, and
Roger A. Jones
Department of Chemistry, Rutgers, The State
University of New Jersey, New Brunswick, NJ 08903

The formation of O[6] alkyl guanine derivatives in DNA is
thought to constitute the principal carcinogenic lesion
produced by alkylating agents (Cairns 1981). The existence
of specific repair enzymes has been demonstrated, and, moreover, low levels of repair activity have been correlated with
tissue specific tumorigenicity (Swenberg 1984). The molecular
basis for these effects is thought to reside in the promutagenic nature of the O[6]-alkylguanine base.

The introduction of an O[6] alkyl group to the guanine
ring makes obvious changes in its electronic structure. Not
only is a somewhat bulky alkyl group present, but the important N[1] proton is absent. Thus two of the three sites of

normal G:C H-bonding are disrupted. This has led to the
hypothesis that O^6 alkyl guanine should pair like adenine,
rather than guanine, and therefore misincorporate thymidine
upon replication (Loveless 1969). A substantial amount of
biochemical evidence has accumulated in support of this
hypothesis (Grunberger, Singer 1983). However, physical
evidence of H-bonding between O^6-alkylguanine and thymine
residues has not emerged. Both an IR study of the bases
themselves (Psoda 1981) and a UV study of homopolymers
(Mehta, Ludlum 1976) failed to find evidence for any specific
interaction.

In an effort to elucidate the effects of O^6 alkylation
on DNA structure, and to clarify the base pairing properties
of O^6 alkyl guanine, we have embarked on a program of defined
chemical synthesis coupled with physical characterization of
oligonucleotides containing O^6 alkyl guanine. We now wish
to report the synthesis and preliminary characterization of
the set of molecules d[CGNGAATTC(O^6Me)GCG], where N = A, C,
G, or T. These molecules are self complementary and are
designed such that the duplex form has the d(O^6Me)G lesion
on one strand well separated from that on the other strand.

OMe

d(CGNGAATTCGCG)
d(GCGCTTAAGNGC)

OMe

This would seem to be a better biological model than the two
hexanucleoside pentaphosphates we have previously reported,
d[CGC(O^6Me)GCG] and d[CGT(O^6Me)GCG], in which the d(O^6Me)G
lesions are close together in the duplex (Kuzmich, Marky,
Jones 1983).

The O^6-methyl-2'-deoxyguanosine used in these syntheses
was prepared by the route we have reported previously
(Gaffney, Jones 1982). The N = C and N = A sequences were
synthesized by the phosphate triester method outlined in
Table 1. In this approach dinucleotide blocks were used for
elongation. In addition to the standard protecting groups,
each guanine residue was also O^6 protected with the 4-nitro-
phenylethyl group, as we have recently reported (Gaffney,
Marky, Jones 1984; Kuzmich, Marky, Jones 1983).

TABLE 1

SYNTHESIS OF CGCGAATTC(O^{6}Me)GCG AND CGAGAATTC(O^{6}Me)GCG
BY A PHOSPHATE TRIESTER METHOD ON POLYSTYRENE

CONDENSATION CYCLE

1. DETRITYLATE: either 2% benzene sulfonic acid in CH_2Cl_2:
    CH_3OH (70:30), 4 x 45 sec, quench with pyridine; or 1 M
    $ZnBr_2$ in CH_2Cl_2:iPrOH (85:15), 2 x 30 min, quench with
    0.5 M TEAA in DMF; wash 3 x CH_2Cl_2:iPrOH, 3 x CH_2Cl_2,
    3 x (CH_3OH, then CH_2Cl_2), 3 x Et_2O.
2. DRY: 3 x evaporation of pyridine.
3. CONDENSE: 5 eq next phosphorylated dinucleotide, 3 eq
    TPS-Cl, 9 eq N-methylimidazole, 2 hr; wash 3 x pyridine,
    3 x CH_2Cl_2, 3 x CH_2Cl_2:CH_3OH (70:30), 3 x (CH_3OH, then
    CH_2Cl_2), 3 x CH_2Cl_2, 3 x Et_2O.
4. CAP: 10% Ac_2O, 1% methylimidazole in pyridine, wash as
    in step 3.

DEPROTECTION AND PURIFICATION

1. DBU in pyridine: β-elimination of guanine O^6 protecting
    group.
2. 2-Nitrobenzaldoxime: phosphate deprotection.
3. DBU with CH_3OH: cleavage from resin and amine
    deprotection.
4. HPLC (reversed phase).
5. 80% HOAc: detritylation.
6. HPLC (anion and reversed phase).

The N = G and N = T sequences were prepared by the
phosphite triester method outlined in Table 2. In this
approach deoxynucleoside methyldiisopropylaminophosphor-
amidites were used for elongation. The synthetic details
will be reported elsewhere.

TABLE 2
SYNTHESIS OF CGTGAATTC(O^6Me)GCG AND CGGGAATTC(O^6Me)GCG
BY A PHOSPHITE TRIESTER METHOD ON SILICA

CONDENSATION CYCLE
1. DETRITYLATE: 2% CCl_3CO_2H in CH_2Cl_2, 4 x 30 sec; quench
    pyridine; or 1 M $ZnBr_2$ in CH_2Cl_2:iPrOH (85:15), 2 x 30
    min; quench 0.5 M TEAA in DMF; wash 3 x CH_2Cl_2,
    3 x CH_3CN.
2. DRY: N_2, 20 min.
3. CONDENSE: 10-20 eq next phosphoramidite and 30-60 eq
    tetrazole in CH_3CN, 20 min; wash 3 x CH_3CN, 1 x lutidine:
    THF:H_2O (2:2:1).
4. OXIDIZE: 0.2 M I_2 in lutidine: THF:H_2O (2:2:1), 1 min;
    wash 3 x CH_3CN.
5. CAP: 10% Ac_2O, 1% methylimidazole in pyridine; wash
    3 x CH_3CN, 3 x CH_2Cl_2.

DEPROTECTION AND PURIFICATION
1. THIOPHENOXIDE, 45 min - phosphate deprotection.
2. NH_4OH, 16 hours r.t. - cleavage from support and partial
    amine deprotection.
3. DBU/CH_3OH, 3 days - complete amine deprotection.
4. HPLC (reversed phase).
5. 80% HOAc: detritylation.
6. HPLC (reversed phase).

After deprotection each of these four sequences was
purified to homogeneity by reversed phase hplc (Figure 1).
In addition, each sequence was enzymatically degraded to its
constituent deoxynucleosides (also shown in Figure 1). We
have reported that ammonolysis of d(O^6Me)G to 2-amino-2'-
deoxyadenosine may occur during deprotection (Kuzmich, Marky,
Jones 1983). We have now found that thiophenoxide ion is
able to slowly demethylate d(O^6Me)G, giving back deoxyguanosine. Extreme care during deprotection and rigorous
chromatographic purification and analysis under the highest
resolution conditions possible are essential if a homogeneous
product is to be obtained.

Figure 2 shows a plot of Tm^{-1} vs ln concentration for
the four molecules described above. The "parent"
d[CGCGAATTCGCG] and the "mismatch" sequence d[CGTGAATTCGCG]
(Patel, Pardi, Itakura 1982) are included for purposes of
comparison. The molecules containing d(O^6Me)G each show a

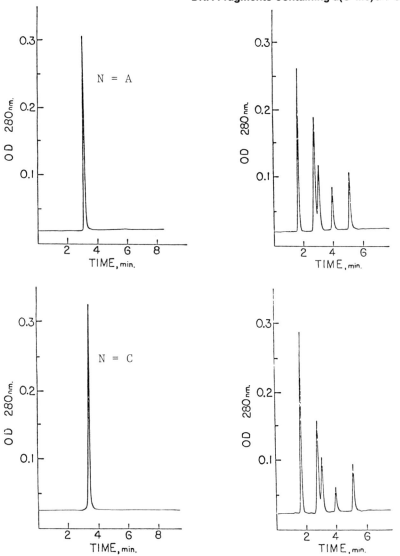

Figure 1. HPLC of the molecules d[CGNGAATTC(O⁶Me)GCG] after
purification (left), using a gradient of 12–30% CH₃CN:
0.1 M TEAA in 5 min at 4 mL/min on a μ Bondapak C₁₈ cartridge
in a Waters Z-Module; and after degradation with venom

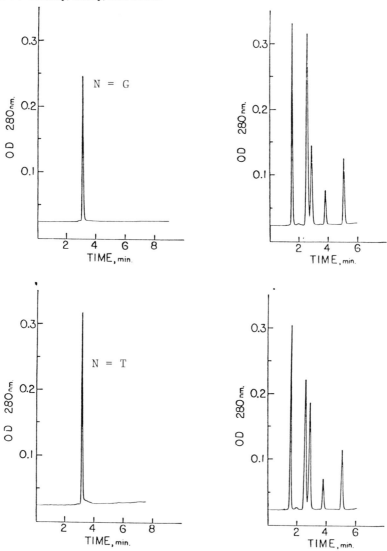

phosphodiesterase and alkaline phosphatase (right), using a gradient of 6-20%, where the deoxynucleosides elute in the order: dC, dG, T, dA, d(O⁶Me)G, in the expected ratios.

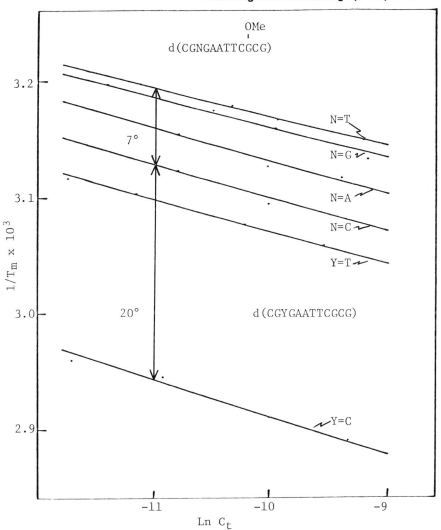

Figure 2. Plot of inverse melting temperature vs ln of concentration.

T_m more than 20° below that of the unmodified "parent" sequence; in fact, they are even lower melting than is the "mismatch" sequence. Moreover, the lowest T_m is seen with the N = T molecule, the sequence with the d(O^6Me)G opposite thymidine. However, the T_m observed for a molecule is the result of a complex aggregate of interactions, of which pairing may not be the most significant. Other interactions, particularly stacking, may well be the determining factor in the T_m data shown. Thus the more favorable stacking expected in the N = G and N = A sequences, coupled with the weaker stacking expected in the N = T sequence, may simply obscure the effects of pairing. In addition, there is the possibility of wobble pairing between the O^6 methyl guanine and cytosine residues in the N = C sequence and between guanine and thymine in the "mismatch" sequence (Patel, Pardi, Itakura 1982).

Thus the significance of the relative stabilities reported here will not be clear until some of these other factors can be separated out. This we hope to begin to accomplish through nmr studies as well as through further syntheses. However, for the present, clear evidence for the existence of any base pairing involving O^6 alkyl guanine remains elusive.

Cairns J (1981). The origin of human cancers. Nature (London) 289:353.
Gaffney BL, Jones RA (1982). Synthesis of O^6-alkylated deoxyguanosine nucleosides. Tetrahedron Lett 23:2253.
Gaffney BL, Marky LA, Jones RA (1984). The influence of the purine 2-amino group on DNA conformation and stability. 2. Synthesis and physical characterization of d[CGT(2-NH_2)ACG], d[CGU(2-NH_2)ACG], and d[CGT(2-NH_2)AT(2-NH_2)ACG]. Tetrahedron 40:3.
Grunberger D, Singer B (1983). "Molecular Biology of Mutagens and Carcinogens." New York: Plenum.
Kuzmich S, Marky LA, Jones RA (1983). Specifically alkylated DNA fragments. Synthesis and physical characterization of d[CGC(O^6Me)GCG] and d[CGT(O^6Me)GCG]. Nucleic Acids Res 10:3393.
Loveless A (1969). Possible relevance of O-6 alkylation of deoxyguanosine to the mutagenicity and carcinogenicity of nitrosamines and nitrosamides. Nature (London) 223:206.
Mehta JR, Ludlum DB (1976). Synthesis and properties of poly(O^6-methylguanylic acid) and poly(O^6-ethylguanylic acid). Biochemistry 15:4329.

Patel DJ, Pardi A, Itakura K (1982). DNA conformation, dynamics, and interactions in solution. Science 216:581.

Psoda A, Kierdaszuk B, Pohorille A, Geller M, Kusmierek JT, Shugar D (1981). Interaction of the mutagenic base analogs O^6-methylguanine and N^4-methylcytosine with potentially complementary bases. J Quantum Chem 20:543.

Swenberg JA, Lewis JG, Bedell MA, Billings KC, Dyroff MC, Lindamood C (1984). "Biochemical Basis of Chemical Carcinogenesis." New York: Raven, pp 287-292.

Molecular Basis of Cancer, Part A: Macromolecular Structure, Carcinogens, and Oncogenes, pages 379–388
© 1985 Alan R. Liss, Inc.

A MULTI-PATH THEORY OF CHEMICAL CARCINOGENESIS IN THE RAT MAMMARY GLAND

L. David Meeker, Professor of Mathematics
Henry J. Thompson, Associate Professor of Animal and Nutritional Sciences

University of New Hampshire Durham, NH   03824

INTRODUCTION

An accumulating body of evidence suggests that activation of cellular oncogenes is an essential component of carcinogenesis (Cooper 1982; Astrin and Rothberg 1983). Recent reports of oncogene "cooperation" propose oncogene activation as the "basic step" of the multistep process of chemical carcinogenesis (Land, Parada and Weinberg 1983). It is natural to conjecture that the activation of cellular oncogenes provides the biological mechanism for the "hits" which have played such a prominent role in mathematical theories of carcinogenesis (Crump et al 1976; Whittemore and Keller 1978; Brown and Koziol 1983). This paper explores this hypothesis within the context of an important experimental breast cancer system. Our purpose in this investigation is two-fold. In addition to an exploration of the limits of a well-known mathematical theory of carcinogenesis, we seek to develop a tool which will help us to address a question of considerable importance in our search for effective agents for the chemoprevention of breast cancer. Specifically:

Is the diversity we observe in the chemically induced mammary cancer population of our experiments - diversity in response to chemopreventive agents; in cancer latency; in ability to stimulate angiogenesis; and in hormone dependence - simply due to the random influence of the macro- and micro-environment of the developing clone on the mechanism(s) of cancer promotion and progression; or is it, at least in part, determined by initiatory events at the level of the cellular genome?

To investigate these issues the mathematical model we propose seeks to relate gross, but easily observable, properties of the induced cancer population (e.g., dose response and tumor latency) to the, essentially, unobservable events of cancer initiation.

Based on this model our analysis indicates that, even in this carefully controlled laboratory system, the induced cancer population displays a heterogeneity which is incompatible with the concept of an underlying uniform "m-hit" carcinogenic process. Rather, our mathematical investigations and interpretation of the experimental data lead us to propose that: (1) the genome of the target cells of the rat mammary gland contains multiple oncogenes; (2) the genome contains a distinguished cellular oncogene, *c-onc-1* whose activation is necessary, but, in general, not sufficient for transformation; (3) that the activation of additional oncogenes (of the same or different types) increases the probability of transformation and, following transformation, increases the rate of progression of the resulting malignant clone to a detectable cancer; and (4) different patterns of oncogene activation among transformed cells underlies much of the diversity we observe within the induced cancer population.

The model, from which these proposals stem, contains the "m-hit theory" of carcinogenesis as a special case. While the latter implies a homogeneous population of induced cancers, the more general model predicts a heterogeneous population composed of subpopulations with distinguishable characteristics which form stochastically stable proportions of the whole. The terms "multi-path theory" and "multi-path model" (MP-theory, MP-model) are intended to suggest this distinguishing feature of the theory.

MNU INDUCTION OF MAMMARY CANCERS IN THE RAT

The induction of mammary cancers in Sprague Dawley rats by a single exposure to the direct carcinogen 1-methyl-1-nitrosourea (MNU) (Gullino *et al* 1975; Thompson and Meeker 1983) is widely used in investigations of breast cancer. MNU is a direct carcinogen which has a very short half-life in tissues (less than 5 minutes (Swan and Magee 1968)) and provides a close approximation to a true "spike" dose of carcinogen. The induced tumors are easily detected by palpation without sacrificing the animals. It is a highly reproducible experimental tumor system and is especially amenable to mathematical analysis.

MULTI-PATH THEORY

The model of neoplastic transformation, tumor pro-motion and tumor progression we propose is a quantitative extension of that described by Moses and Robinson (1982). In their model transformation frees a cell from a natural block in G(0) phase of the cell cycle, where it arrests due to deficiency in exogonous growth factor, by creating a source of endogonous growth factor. Our quantitative adaptation of this process (Meeker, Thompson and Herbst 1982; Meeker and Thompson, in prep.) is based on two as-sumptions: (a) *the activity of the endogonous growth factor*, GF, *is related to the number of oncogene related chemical interactions of the carcinogen with DNA of the cel-lular genome* and (b) *the level of GF activity determines the probability of neoplastic transformation of the ini-tiated cell and the rate of proliferation of its clone of daughter cells following transformation* and, thereby, the detection time of the induced mammary cancer. We cannot, at this stage, further identify these interactions. The hypothesized relationship between GF activity and number of interactions could result from any of the mechan-isms recently discussed in the literature (Land *et al* 1983; Cooper 1982; Astrin and Rothberg 1983; Sukumar *et al* 1983; Weiher, König and Grass 1983). The conclusions we draw from the model are independent of the particular causal mechanism underlying the assumed relationship.

While we view the process of neoplastic transformation as continuous, the model incorporates the three conceptual stages of initiation, promotion and progression. We assume that carcinogen exposure *initiates* a cell of the mammary epithelium with the potential for neoplasia through inter-action of the chemical with target sites in the cellular genome. The number of unrepaired lesions per cell of the target epithelium should follow the Poisson distribution with mean equal to agc/τ, where τ is the mean duration of the cell cycle (Russo and Russo 1980), c is the dose of carcinogen, g is the mean number of target sites per cell and a is a factor of proportionality. A cell undergoing precisely k such lesions (k = 1,2,...) is called a k-cell. N(k), the random variable denoting the number of k-cells per rat, is also approximated by a Poisson distribution and has mean

(1) $E(N(k)) = \lambda(k) = n_p (agc/\tau)^k \exp(-agc/\tau)$,

where n_p is the mean number of proliferating cells in the tissue.

We suppose that an initiated k-cell is *promoted* to the neoplastic state if the endogonous GF activity exceeds a threshold value. We suppose that GF activity is distributed about a mean which increases with k and let $\delta(k)$ denote the probability that the activity exceeds the threshold value and stimulates the biochemical mechanism(s) leading to transformation. While the m-hit model implies a single mode of transformation and a homogeneous population of induced cancers, the MP-model implies a heterogeneous cancer population composed of promoted 1-cells, 2-cells, etc., occuring with expected numbers $\lambda(1)\delta(1)$, $\lambda(2)\delta(2)$, etc. .

We assume that a promoted k-cell gives rise to a k-clone of transformed daughter cells which *progresses* through cell proliferation at a rate proportional to its GF activity to reach palpable size. Let $F(k,t) = P\{T \leq t\}$ be the cumulative distribution function (CDF) of the detection time, T, of a k-clone. Then the probability that a cell from the N(k) initiated k-cells is promoted and progresses to form a tumor detected in the time interval $[0,t]$ is $\delta(k)F(k,t)$. The number of such k-clones, J(k,t), is Poisson with mean $E(J(k,t)) = \delta(k)\lambda(k)F(k,t) \equiv \mu(k,t)$. If we assume that all promoted cells eventually reach a palpable size and are detected, $F(k,\infty) = 1$ and $\mu(k,\infty) \equiv \delta(k)\lambda(k)$ is the mean number of promoted k-cells.

The total number of cancers detected in $[0,t]$ is $J(t) = J(0,t) + J(1,t) +...$ where J(0,t), with mean $\mu(0,t)$, represents the number of spontaneous tumors induced in the tissue (these are rare and slow to develop (McCormick *et al* 1981)). J(t) has mean $\mu F(t)$ where $\mu = \mu(0,\infty) + \mu(1,\infty) + ...$ and $F(t) = [\mu(0,t)) + \mu(1,t) + \mu(2,t) + ...]/\mu$ is the unconditional CDF of the detection times of all induced tumors.

EXPERIMENTAL SUPPORT FOR MULTI-PATH THEORY

Dose Response

The proportionality expressed in Eq. (1) implies

(2) $\mu(k,t) = c^k \beta(k) F(k,t)$,

where $\beta(k)$ is a factor of proportionality. This has important implications. If, as we have assumed, the k-clones
progress significantly faster than the (k-1)-clones, then
most k-clones will be detected before (k-1)-clones begin to
appear. If this difference is sufficiently pronounced we
should expect to find times ... , $s'(k+1) < s(k+1) < s'(k) <
s(k) < s'(k-1)$... such that (a) most k-clones are detected
in the interval $s'(k) \le t \le s(k)$ and (b) $F(k,t) = 0$ for
$t < s'(k)$ while $F(k,t) = 1$ and $\mu(k,t) = \mu(k,\infty)$ for $t > s(k)$.
Under these conditions the number of tumors detected in
$(s'(k), s(k)]$, $J(s(k)) - J(s'(k))$, has mean

(3) $\mu[F(s(k)) - F(s'(k))] \cong \mu(k,\infty)$

$$= c^k \beta(k), \quad k = 1,2,\ldots .$$

Thus, while the m-hit model of carcinogenesis implies
a constant dose response proportional to c^m, the MP-model
suggests that the dose response of the number of detected
tumors may vary from time-interval to time-interval.

Figure 1(a) displays, as a function of dose of MNU,
the number of tumors/rat detected in the intervals 30 - 70
days, 71 - 125 days and 126 - 400 days estimated from Chart
4 of McCormick *et al* (1981). The response predicted by Eq.
(3) is strongly evident. It suggests that (a) the early
appearing tumors result from at least three oncogene
related MNU-genomic interactions; (b) the late appearing
tumors are due to a single interaction and (c) the tumors
appearing in the middle interval exhibit a transitional
response. Thus, there is evidence for at least two, and
possibly three, tumor subpopulations arising from different
patterns of interaction. This observation is incompatible
with a uniform m-hit origin of the detected cancers and
supports the assumptions underlying the MP-model.

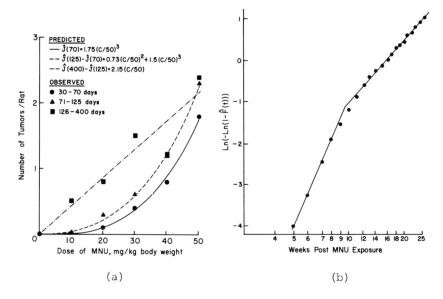

Fig. 1: (a) Dose response over three intervals. (Significance levels: 30-70 days, $\beta(1) = \beta(2) = 0$, $p > 0.90$; 71-125 days, $\beta(1) = 0$, $p > 0.90$; 125-400 days, $\beta(2) = \beta(3) = 0$, $p > 0.90$)

(b) Weibull plot of detection times of 443 tumors from 76 female Sprague-Dawley rats injected with 50 mg MNU/kg Body Weight at 50 days of age.

Figure 1(b) provides further support for the existance of at least two subpopulations, having distinct detection-time distribution parameters, among the induced cancers. It displays a Weibull plot of the time-to-detection distribution obtained by pooling the control group results from three recent experiments in our laboratory. In such a plot a random variable from a Weibull distribution would plot as a straight line. Note that the "break point", between the two lines suggestive of Weibull distributions, occurs near the 10 week (70 days) value consistent with Figure 1(a).

This analysis suggests that a single interaction can lead to transformation. However, since cancer yields can be increased by feeding promoting substances such as high

fat (Chan *et al* 1977; Dao and Chan 1983), we conclude that
it need not always do so. The observations are consistent
with the presence in the genome of a primary transforming
gene *c-onc-1* having the highest probability of activation
by MNU. Additional oncogene activation, of the same or
different types, then confers other properties on the
transformed cell leading to earlier detection and, we suspect, other distinguishable characteristics.

Detection Time vs. Number of Cancers

　　Table 1 describes the percentage decomposition of the
cancer population induced by a single dose of MNU in terms
of the total number of cancers detected on the animal and
cancer detection time. The distribution of detection times
shows a strong relationship ($p < 0.01$) with the number of
cancers. Clearly cancers on the rats bearing more cancers
tend to develop faster.

　　Neither the "m-hit" nor the MP-theory, as described,
can account for this phenomenon. However, if the MP-model
is modified to include the influence of estrous state at
time of exposure upon the animal's susceptibility to the
carcinogen, an explanation appears.

Detection	Number Detected Cancers			No. of
Time (days)	1 - 5	6 - 10	> 10	Cancers
30- 70	17	22	38	114
71-125	45	49	48	212
126-180	38	29	14	117
	100	100	100	443

Table 1: Classification of cancers induced in 76 female
Sprague-Dawley rats by s.c. injection of 50 mg MNU/kg bw at
50 days of age, by percent. Categories defined by number
of cancers detected on rat and time of detection.

　　Buffalo rats in diestrus at time of carcinogen exposure have been reported to be less than one-half as susceptible to tumor induction by MNU as those in proestrus or
estrus (Lindsy, Das Gupta and Beattie 1981). This is
believed to result from changes in those cell kinetic
parameters we have identified in Eq. 1: the size of the

proliferative pool and the mean cell cycle duration.
Changes in the size of the proliferative pool introduce
linear effects which cannot account for the pattern we
observe. However, small increases in cell cycle time,
which primarily extends the G(1) phase (Russo and Russo
1980), can greatly increase the time available for DNA
repair and, thereby, protect the animal from the short-
lived effects of MNU exposure. In contrast to changes in
proliferative pool, changes in cell cycle times introduce
non-linear effects into the detection-time distribution (in
the MP-model but not in the m-hit model) which imply that
the more susceptible animals (larger n_p and smaller τ, see
Eq. (1)) will have an increased proportion of early tumors
(2- and 3-clones) relative to those in diestrus at time of
MNU exposure (Meeker and Thompson in prep.). Thus, the MP-
model predicts that the more tumors an animal develops the
more likely it is to have been in the susceptible state
when exposed to MNU and, therefore, the more likely it is
to have an increased proportion of early "3-hit" tumors as
our experiments indicate.

Oncogene Identification

The recent report of malignant activation of H-*ras*-1
by a single point mutation in MNU-induced tumors (Sukumar
et al 1983) is also compatible with the MP-model. That
study, involving Buf/N rats, used an MNU dose (30mg/kg bw)
which, in Sprague Dawley rats, would induce a tumor population consisting of approximately 57% 1-clones, 26% 2-
clones and 17% 3-clones. Thus, of the 9 tumors examined,
the MP-model predicts that most (5/9) would be 1-clones.
It is possible that H-*ras*-1 possesses the properties we
have assigned to *c-onc-1* and that those tumors (one third
of those tested) exhibiting additional amplified, but non-
transforming, H-*ras* sequences are, in fact, among the 4
tumors predicted to be 2- or 3-clones by the model.

THE MP-MODEL AND THE M-HIT MODEL

The MP-model contains the multi-hit model as a special
case. For example, the successful two-hit model (Moolgavkar and Venzon 1979; Maskens 1981) corresponds to a low
probability of 1-cell promotion ($\delta(1) \cong 0$) and a relatively
large probability of 2-cell promotion ($\delta(2) \cong 1$). Under

continuous exposure to a carcinogen the rare DNA interaction creating a 1-cell would give it a proliferative advantage and create a clone of cells susceptible to an additional "hit" and ultimate promotion. This is, precisely, the role of the "intermediate cells" of Moolgavkar and Venzon. Thus the model of carcinogenesis presented here can be considered an extension of the multi-hit theory. An extension which incorporates, in a natural fashion, the recent contributions of molecular biology to our growing understanding of the neoplastic process.

References

Astrin SM, Rothberg PG (1983). Oncogenes and cancer. Cancer Investigation 1(4):355.
Brown CC, Koziol JA (1983). Statistical aspects of the estimation of human risk from suspected environmental carcinogens. SIAM REVIEW 25:151.
Cooper GM (1982). Cellular transforming genes. Science 218: 801.
Crump KS, Hoel DG, Langley CH, Peto R (1976). Fundamental carcinogenic processes and their implications for low dose risk assessment. Cancer Research 36:2973.
Chan C, Head JS, Cohen SA, Wynder EL (1977). Influence of dietary fat on induction of mammary tumors by N-nitroso methyl urea: Associated hormone changes and differences between Sprague Dawley and F344 rats. J. Natl. Canc. Inst. 59:1279.
Dao TL, Chan P. (1983). Effect of duration of high fat intake on enhancement of mammary carcinogenesis in rats. J. Natl. Canc. Inst. 71:201.
Gullino PM, Pettigrew HM, Grantham FH (1975). N-nitrosol-methylurea as mammary gland carcinogen in rats. J. Natl. Cancer Inst. 54:401.
Land H, Parada LF, Weinberg RA (1983). Cellular oncogenes and multistep carcinogenesis. Science 222:771.
Lindsey WWF, Das Gupta TK, Beattie CW (1981). Influence of estrous cycle during carcinogen exposure on nitrosomethyl-urea-induced rat mammary carcinoma. Cancer Research 41:3857.
Maskens A (1981). Confirmation of the 2-step nature of chemical carcinogenesis in the rat colon adenocarcinoma model. Cancer Research 41:1240.
McCormick, DL, Adamowski CB, Fiks A, Moon RC (1981). Lifetime dose-response relationship for mammary tumor in-

duction by a single administration of N-methyl-N-nitro-sourea. Cancer Research 41:1690.

Meeker LD, Thompson HJ, Herbst EJ (1982). A multi-stage model of mammary carcinogenesis and chemoprevention. Abstract, Biometrics 38:1115.

Meeker LD, Thompson HJ, in preparation.

Moolgavkar SH, Venzon DJ (1979). Two-event models for car-cinogenesis: Incidence curves for childhood and adult tumors. Math. Biosc. 47:55.

Moses HL, Robinson RA (1982). Growth factors, growth factor receptors, and cell cycle control mechanisms in chemical-ly transformed cells. Fed. Proceedings 41:3008.

Russo J, Russo IH (1980). Influence of differentiation and cell kinetics on the susceptibility of the rat mammary gland to carcinogenesis. Cancer Research 40:2677.

Sukumar, S, Notario V, Martin-Zanca D, Barbacid M (1983). Induction of mammary carcinomas in rats by nitroso-methylurea involves malignant activation of H-ras-1 locus by single point mutations. Nature 306:658.

Swan PF, Magee PN (1968). Nitrosomine-induced carcinogene-sis: the alkylation of nuclear acids of the rat by N-methyl-N-nitrosourea, dimethylnitrosomine, dimethyl sulfate, and methyl metanesulfate.

Thompson HJ, Meeker LD (1983). Induction of mammary gland carcinomas by the subcutaneous injection of 1-methyl-1-nitrosourea. Cancer Res. 43:1628.

Weiher H, Konig M, Gruss P (1983). Multiple point mutations affecting the simian virus 40 enhancer. Science 219:626.

Whittemore A, Keller JB (1978). Quantitative theories of carcinogenesis. SIAM REVIEW 20:1.

Acknowledgement

The authors would like to acknowledge the support of the National Cancer Institute in the form of USPHS Grants CA28109 and CA32465 and from the University of New Hamp-shire Research Office.

Molecular Basis of Cancer, Part A: Macromolecular Structure, Carcinogens, and Oncogenes, pages 389–399
© **1985 Alan R. Liss, Inc.**

CARCINOGEN-INDUCED INSERTION MUTATIONS IN E. COLI

Takeshita, Masaru, Van der Keyl, Harjeet,
and
Grollman, Arthur P.

Department of Pharmacological Sciences
State University of New York at Stony Brook
Stony Brook, New York 11794

Chemical carcinogens create lesions in DNA which activate cellular repair mechanisms and lead to base mutations. Point mutations and transposition of genetic elements are associated with the activation of cellular oncogenes (cf Bishop 1983); these processes represent essential events in carcinogenesis (Cairns 1981; Weinstein 1981).

We examined the mutagenic effects of carcinogen - DNA adducts located in the promoter-structural region of the plasmid gene which confers resistance to tetracycline in E. coli. N-acetoxy-N-acetyl-2-aminofluorene (AAAF) (McCann 1975) serves as a model for the ultimate carcinogen in these experiments. Plasmids with mutations in the tetracycline gene were isolated; several were found to carry the IS5 insertion element (Timmons 1983) and one had a single GC base pair addition. In contrast to the report of Fuchs et al (1981), no deletion mutants were detected.

MATERIALS AND METHODS

Bacterial strains and media - E. Coli Kl2 strains 803, HB101 and C600 were used as recipients for transformation experiments. Luria broth was used for cultivation of bacteria; ampicillin, 25 µg/ml; chloramphenicol, 100 µg/ml; and tetracycline, 15 µg/ml) were added to the media or agar plates.

Plasmid DNA –E. coli strains harboring plasmids were grown to logarithmic phase and amplified by cultivation in the presence of spectinomycin (Bolivar 1978). DNA was extracted by the cleared lysate method (Clewell and Helinski 1970) and purified by centrifugation in cesium chloride. The procedure of Holmes and Quigley (1981) was used for routine examination of plasmid DNA.

Gel electrophoresis and DNA sequence analysis – Agarose gel electrophoresis was performed in horizontal slab gels in a buffer composed of 40 mM Tris-acetate, pH 8.3, and 2 mM EDTA. DNA was identified by staining the gel with ethidium bromide. Appropriate fragments were excised from the gel and extracted by electroelution.

DNA sequences were determined by methods developed by Maxam and Gilbert (1980) and by Sanger (cf Messing 1981). For dideoxynucleotide sequencing, DNA fragments were excised, ligated into M13mp9 or M13mp8 and transfected directly into JM103 cells. Single strand DNA was isolated from the clones, annealed to a 15-mer primer (Messing 1983) and the sequence determined (Messing et al 1981).

Materials – Restriction endonucleases and pBR325 (Bolivar 1978) were purchased from BRL and T4 DNA ligase from P.L. Biochemicals. AAAF was obtained from the National Cancer Institute.

Nick translation and hybridization analysis. – Nick translation of pBR 325 DNA was carried out by a modification of the procedure by Rigby et al (1977). DNA hybridization was performed by the method of Southern as modified by Maniatis et al (1982).

Modification with AAF and bacterial transformation – The 346 bp Hind III–Bam Hl restriction fragment was excised from pBR325 and purified by agarose gel electrophoresis. This DNA (14 pmole) was incubated in the dark for 60 min at 37° in a 150 ul reaction mixture containing 50 mM Tris HCl, pH 7.2, 30% ethanol and varying concentrations of AAAF. Excess AAAF was removed by repeated extraction with ether and the modified DNA recovered by ethanol precipitation. The larger of the two fragments obtained by digestion of pBR325 with Hind III and Bam Hl was treated with alkaline phosphatase (Bolivar and Backman 1979) and used as vector. Ligations were conducted at 12° in the presence of a tenfold excess of the AAF-treated fragment (Weiss et al 1968). The ligation mixture was used directly to transform competent recipient cells (Dagert and Ehrlich 1979). $Ap^R Cm^R Tc^S$ colonies were identified by replica plating. In the following text, this phenotype is denoted as Tc^S and $Ap^R Cm^R Tc^R$ as Tc^R.

RESULTS

Effects of AAF - Effects of AAF-modification on efficiency of transformation and frequency of mutation in the Tc^R gene are shown in Fig 1. Transformation efficiency decreased by 85% when the DNA fragment was treated with 1 mM AAF. In the control experiment, the excised fragment was subjected to identical manipulations but AAF was omitted from the reaction. The mutation frequency (Tc^S/Ap^R) was 9.9% for AAF-treated DNA and 1.9% for the unmodified control. In experiments using other bacterial strains, the mutation frequency in the controls varied from 0.01% to 2%.

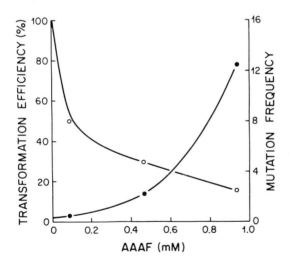

Fig 1. Effect of AAF on transformation efficiency and mutation frequency. The Hind III-Bam H1 region of pBR325 was modified with AAF and used to transform E.coli 803 as described under Materials and Methods. Transformation efficiency is shown relative to the number of Ap^R colonies. Mutation frequency is presented as the increase in the number of Tc^S colonies over control values following cyclo-serine enrichment (Bolivar and Backman 1979).

Isolation of transformants – Results of experiments in which the transforming plasmid DNA was modified with AAF are shown in Table 1. Seven transformants, isolated from 102 Tc^S colonies of strain 803, retained both restriction sites. Of these, six were found to contain inserted sequences. Single transformants with plasmids containing insertions were identified among 32 Tc^S colonies of C600 and 13 Tc^S colonies of HB101.

Table 1. Transformation with AAAF-modified plasmid DNA.

E. coli Strains	Ap^R	Tc^S	Transformants[a]	Plasmid size (kb)
803	1370	102	AT23	6.0
			AT33,AT34,BPT9,BPT11	7.2
			AT47,AT52	11.0
C600	396	32	BP12	7.2
HB101	337	13	BB17	7.2

[a] Yielding plasmid DNA with intact _Bam_ H1 and _Hind_ III sites.

All Tc^S colonies isolated from control experiments in which the transforming DNA was unmodified yielded plasmid DNA that lacked either _Hind_ III or _Bam_ H1 sites or both. Twenty-eight such colonies were isolated from 1296 Ap^R colonies of strain 803 of which seven were indistinguishable in size from pBR325. Three appear to be dimers and the remainder were less than 6.0 kb. In similar control experiments, six Tc^S transformants were isolated from 285 Ap^R colonies of strain C600 and 36 from 1705 Ap^R colonies of HB101.

Restriction enzyme mapping – Plasmid DNA isolated from AT23 produced a single linear fragment when digested with _Eco_ R1. (Fig 2). Double restriction digests with _Hind_ III and _Bam_ H1 produced fragments of 0.346 and 5.7 kb. Similar digests of pBB17 (Fig 2), pAT33, pAT34, pBPT9, pBPT11 and pBP12 (not shown) produced 1.54 and 5.7 kb fragments. These plasmids contained an additional _Eco_ R1 site (shown for pBB17, pAT33 and pBP12) and new _Bgl_ II and _Bst_ EII restriction sites (shown for pBB17 only).

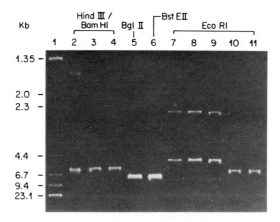

Fig. 2. *Restriction enzyme analysis of mutant plasmids. Plasmid DNA was purified and digested with the enzymes shown in the Figure. DNA fragments were separated by electrophoresis in 1.5% agarose and stained with ethidium bromide. Size markers are shown in Lane 1; Lanes 2, 5, 6 and 7 contained pBB17; Lane 3 and 10, pAT23; Lane 4 and 11, pBR325; Lane 8, pAT33; and Lane 9, pBP12.*

Plasmid DNA prepared from the remaining two transformants, AT47 and AT57, yielded fragments of 0.346 and 10.7 kb when digested with Bam Hl and Hind III. The inserted sequences in these mutants did not hybridize with a pBR325 probe and were located outside the region of AAF modification. The large (5 kb) insert in these plasmids was not analyzed further.

Restriction enzyme analysis of the six 7.2 kb mutants indicated that a 1.2 kb sequence had been inserted in the Tc gene. These mutants appeared to share a common structure. We determined the sequence of approximately 200 bases starting from the Hind III site and 500 bases between the Bam Hl and Eco Rl sites.

An autoradiogram, showing part of the sequence of mutant pBB17, is shown in Figure 3. The sequence, read from the Hind III to Bam Hl site and including the CTAA sequence located at positions 93-96, is identical to that of pBR325 (Prentki et al 1981). CTAA is one of several reported target sequences of IS5 (Engler and van Bree 1981). A 16 bp inverted repeat and full duplication of the CTAA target sequence appear at the end of the inserted sequence, 279 bp from the <u>Bam</u> Hl site. No mutations were found between the <u>Bam</u> Hl site and the end of the target sequence. As reported for IS5 (Schoner and Kahn 1981), there was one mismatch between the inverted repeat sequences.

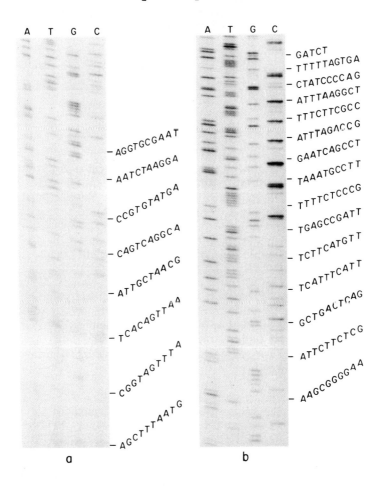

Fig. 3. *Sequence analysis of the Hind III-Bam H1 regions of pBB17. The Hind III-Bam H1 fragment of pBB17 was cloned into M13mp8 and analyzed by dideoxysequencing as described in Materials and Methods. Electrophoresis (6% polyacrylamide gel) was developed at 1500 V for 1.5 hrs (a) and 3 hrs (b). The four bases represent dideoxy ATP, dideoxy TTP, dideoxy GTP and dideoxy CTP reactions in the chain extension step.*

Although the complete sequence of the insert in pBB17 was not determined, its size, the location of Bgl II and Bst EII sites and the presence of an identical 354 base sequence clearly identify the inserted sequence as IS5. The remaining five 7.2 kb mutant plasmids also contain IS5. The target site for insertion was common to all mutants sequenced.

The 6.0 kb mutant plasmid (pAT23), was found to have a single additional GC base pair immediately adjacent to the Bam H1 site as shown below:

$$5' \quad T \; G \; G \; G \; A \; T$$
$$3' \quad A \; C \; C \; C \; T \; A$$

DISCUSSION

In these experiments, six plasmids acquired IS5 by transformation of E.coli with plasmids regionally modified with AAF. No insertion elements were identified in plasmids recovered from control experiments. The frequency of IS5 transposition observed in these experiments (0.25%) is much higher than the reported spontaneous transposition frequencies for IS5 of 10^{-6} (Schoner and Kahn 1981, Starlinger and Saedler 1976) and 10^{-9} (Nakamura and Inouye 1981).

There is no evidence to indicate that the host cell gains a selective advantage by acquiring IS5 under the conditions of our experiments. Furthermore, the observed frequency of transposition is too high to be accounted for by the possible instability of the plasmid. A number of Tc^S mutants were isolated in which one or both ligation sites were lost. These mutants appear to be artifacts of the ligation procedure and did not acquire IS5 elements.

The consensus target sequence for IS5 ($C \cdot T/A \cdot A \cdot G/A$) is present at 56 sites in pBR325. The presence of AAF-DNA adducts may increase the frequency of IS5 insertion at a preferred target site or serve to redirect the element to another target sequence. Due to the infrequency of IS5 insertions in unmodified pBR325, we cannot distinguish between these possibilities although there appears to be a preference for insertion at the CTAA sequence located at position 93-96. In either case, AAF modification promotes IS5 insertion through a recA independent process.

Since IS5 resides as multiple copies in the E. coli chromosome, the presence of AAF-DNA adducts in the plasmid must somehow provide a signal that increases the frequency of IS5 insertions. Several cellular mechanisms, including "stress" of various types, have been reported to promote transposition. Distortion of helical DNA by AAF (cf Grunberger and Santella 1983) could be a signal for this event. Repair processes involved in removal and repair of the AAF-DNA adduct could introduce nicks on opposite strands of the target sequence, thereby promoting insertion of IS5 (cf Kleckner 1981).

Our data differ somewhat from those reported by Fuchs et al (1981). These investigators, employing different strains of competent cells, treated pBR322 with AAAF, removed the Bam Hl-Sal I fragment, and ligated the carcinogen-modified sequence into an untreated vector. In our experiments, the Hind III-Bam Hl fragment was excised before treating the plasmid with AAF. It seems unlikely that the order of chemical modification and reconstruction would affect the outcome of these experiments; however, there is evidence that foreign sequences cloned in the Bam Hl site of the gene can increase the frequency of transposition (Amster et al 1982). It is therefore possible that the frequency of IS5 insertion could be higher in the Hind III-Bam Hl region of the Tc^R gene than in the Bam Hl-Sal I region.

In contrast to our results, Fuchs et al (1981) isolated several mutant plasmids bearing deletions. These investigators also reported a single GC "base addition" involving position 526-529 in pBR322. However, Peden (1983) recently reported that four GC base pairs normally appear in that region of the pBR322 sequence.

SUMMARY AND CONCLUSIONS

Mutagenic effects of AAF have been examined by transforming competent E. coli cells with plasmid DNA which were regionally-modified with this carcinogen. Transposition of IS5 from chromosomal DNA to target sequences in the AAF-modified region was detected in six plasmids obtained from wild type and recA strains. A single GC addition was identified in an additional plasmid; no deletions were detected. The observed frequency of IS5 insertion, 2.5 x 10^{-3}, exceeds that reported for naturally-occurring IS5 transposition in E.coli. These results suggest that the frequency of recombinational events in E.coli can be increased by the presence of a DNA-carcinogen adduct.

ACKNOWLEDGEMENT

We thank Dr. Keith Peden for helpful suggestions during the course of this work and Dr. Eriko Takeuchi for assistance with the M13 cloning experiments. These studies were supported by Grant CA 17395 from the National Institutes of Health.

REFERENCES

Amster O, Salomon D, Zamir A (1982). A cloned immuno-globulin cDNA fragment enhances transposition of IS elements into recombinant plasmids. Nucl Acids Res 10:4525.

Berg DE (1983). Structural requirement for IS50-mediated gene transposition. Proc Natl Acad Sci 80:792.

Bishop JM (1983). Cellular oncogenes and retroviruses. Ann Rev Biochem 52:301.

Bolivar F (1978). Construction and characterization of new cloning vehicles. III. Derivatives of plasmid pBR322 carrying unique EcoRl sites for selection of EcoRl generated recombinant DNA molecules. Gene 4:121.

Bolivar F, Backman K (1979). Plasmids of Escherichia coli as cloning vectors. In Wu R (ed): "Methods in Enzymology, Recombinant DNA", 68, Academic Press, p 245.

Cairns J, (1981). The origin of human cancers. Nature 289:353.

Calos MP, Miller JH (1980). Transposable elements. Cell 20:579.

Clewell DB, Helinski DR (1970). Properties of super-coiled DNA-protein relaxation complex and strand-specificity of the relaxation event. Biochemistry 9:4428.

Dagert M, Ehrlich SD (1979). Prolonged incubation in calcium chloride improves the competence of Escherichia coli cells. Gene 6:23.

Engler JA, van Bree MP (1981). The nucleotide sequence and protein-coding capability of the transposable element IS5. Gene 14:155.

Fuchs RPP, Schwartz N, Daune MP (1981). Hot spots of frameshift mutations induced by the ultimate carcinogen N-acetoxy-N-2-acetylaminofluorene. Nature 294:657.

Grunberger D, Santella R (1983). Conformational changes in DNA induced by chemical carcinogens. In Weinstein B and Vogel HJ (eds) "Genes and Proteins in Oncogenesis", Academic Press: New York p 13.

Holmes DS, Quigley M (1981). A rapid boiling method for the preparation of bacterial plasmids. Anal Biochem 114:193.

Kleckner N (1981). Transposable elements in prokaryotes. Ann Rev Genet 15:341.

McCann J, Choe E, Yamasaki E, Ames BN (1975). Detection of carcinogens as mutagens in the Salmonella/ microsome test assay of 300 chemicals. Proc Natl Acad Sci USA 72:5135.

Maniatis T, Fritsch EF, Sambrook J (1982). Molecular Cloning. Cold Spring Harbor Lab, p 382.

Maxam AM, Gilbert W (1980). Sequencing end-labeled DNA with base-specific chemical cleavages. In Grossman L and Moldave K (eds): "Methods in Enzymology", Nucleic Acids, Part 1, 65, Academic Press: p 499.

Messing J (1983). New M13 vectors for cloning. In Wu R and Grossman L (eds): "Methods in Enzymology, Recombinant DNA", Part C, 101, Academic Press: p 20.

Messing M, Crea R, and Seeburg PH (1981). A system for shotgun DNA sequencing. Nuc Acids Res 9:309.

Nakamura K, Inouye M (1981). Inactivation of the Serratia marcescens gene for the lipoprotein in Escherichia coli by insertion sequences, 1S1 and 1S5; sequence analysis of junction points. Mol Gen Genet 183:107.

Peden KWC (1983). Revised sequence of the tetracycline-resistance gene of pBR322. Gene 22:277.

Prentki P, Karch F, Lida S, Meyer J (1981). The plasmid cloning vector pBR325 contains a 482 base-pair-long inverted duplication. Gene 14:289.

Rechavi G, Givol D, Canaani E (1982). Activation of a cellular oncogene by DNA rearrangement: possible involvement of an IS-like element. Nature 300:607.

Rigby PWJ, Kieckmann M, Rhodes C, Berg P (1977).
Labeling deoxyribonucleic acid to high specific
activity in vitro by nick translation with DNA poly-
merase I. J Mol Biol 113:237.
Schoner B, Kahn M (1981). The nucleotide sequence of
IS5 from Escherichia coli. Gene 14:165.
Starlinger P, Saedler H (1976). IS-Elements in micro-
organisms. In Basle WA et al (eds): "Current Topics in
Microbiology and Immunology", 75. Springer-Verlag:
Berlin, Heidelberg, New York, p111.
Timmons MS, Bogardus AM, Deonier RC (1983). Mapping of
chromosomal IS5 elements that mediate type II F-prime
plasmid excision in Escherichia coli K-12. J Bact 153:395.
Weinstein IB (1981). Current Concepts and Controversies in
Chemical Carcinogenesis. J Supramol Struc Cellular Biochem
17:99.
Weiss B, Jacquemin-Sablon A, Live TR, Fareed GC,
Richardson CC (1968). Enzymatic breakage and joining
of deoxyribonucleic acid. J Biol Chem 243:4543.

**Molecular Basis of Cancer, Part A: Macromolecular
Structure, Carcinogens, and Oncogenes, pages 401–408
© 1985 Alan R. Liss, Inc.**

ULTRAVIOLET RADIATION-INDUCED DEREPRESSION OF THE LACTOSE
OPERON OF *E. COLI* : *IN VITRO* STUDIES

Spodheim-Maurizot, M., Culard, F., Charlier, M.,
and Maurizot, J.C.
Centre de Biophysique Moléculaire, C.N.R.S.,
1A, avenue de la Recherche Scientifique
45045 Orléans cedex, France

Disorganization is a general phenomenon occurring in
cancerous cells. Activation of normally silent cellular genes
C-onc, similar to transforming genes of oncoviruses is, in
several cases, at the origin of this phenomenon. This activation may occur, for instance, by transposition of genes (for
review see Dulbecco, 1983). In the case of chemical carcinogenesis (considered as a two steps process : initiation followed by promotion (Miller, 1978)) the presence of such genes
could be considered as corresponding to initiation, and their
activation by an exterior factor-to promotion step. It is
known that expression of genes is under the control of an
elaborate regulatory system involving proteins-nucleic acids
interactions in eukaryotic cells as well as in prokaryotes
(Jacob and Monod, 1961). Activation of otherwise silent genes
may, thus, result from a modification of such interaction by
a promotion factor. The protomer may induce this modification
in acting on the protein. For instance, the induction of phosphorylation of a protein by a well known promoter, TPA, was
recently reported (Gilmore and Martin, 1983).

To investigate the mechanism of action of a promoter on
a regulatory system we have chosen to study the effect of U.V.
radiation on the regulatory system of lactose metabolism of
E. coli. The promotional effect of U.V. radiation recently
observed in carcinoma cells (Rundel, 1983) suggested the use
of this agent as modifying factor. This *lac* repressor-*lac*
operator system is a good model of protein-nucleic acid interaction, since it has been extensively described from genetic, biochemical and biophysical point of view for several
years (e.g. Müller-Hill, 1975 ; Charlier *et al.*, 1980 ;

Barbier *et al.*, 1982). The lactose metabolism in *E. coli* is
under the negative control of the *lac* repressor. The *lac* repressor, a tetrameric protein, interacts specifically with a
sequence of about 20 base pairs of DNA, the *lac* operator,
preventing the expression of the structural genes of the *lac*
operon. The presence of a natural (allolactose) or synthetic
isopropyl-β-D-thiogalactoside (IPTG) inducer which binds to
repressor prevents operator binding and, thus, induces the
system.

A photochemical study of the *lac* repressor and the implications of its U.V. irradiation on the binding of the inducer has been previously published (Charlier *et al.*, 1977).

The questions to which we try to answer using this system are : a) Under the conditions in which the expression of
lac genes are repressed, does the genes become derepressed
when the repressor is U.V. irradiated ? b) If there is no derepression, is the system still sensitive to the effect of
inducer (IPTG) ? Or, in more general terms, can the modification of a protein by a promotion factor induce the misfunctioning of the regulatory system which it controls and, thus,
trigger the expression of the otherwise repressed genes ?

The repressor solution was irradiated in the wavelength
range 250-400 nm, at a fluence rate of 560 watts/m^2 for several time intervals.

The photochemical damage of the irradiated protein was
followed by the modification of fluorescence spectrum. A rapid decrease of fluorescence intensity without any change of
shape of the spectrum was observed upon irradiation (Fig. 1).
As it was previously shown (Charlier *et al.*, 1977) the decrease of fluorescence of *lac* repressor upon U.V. irradiation
is due to tryptophan photooxidation. Only one of the two
tryptophyl residues of the protomer is destroyed. Correlati-
vely, the IPTG binding activity of that protomer vanishes.
On the contrary, circular dichroism spectra remained unchanged upon irradiation for the same time intervals (until a decrease of fluorescence of 75 % from the initial intensity)
(results not shown) indicating that no serious conformational
change of the protein occurs in these conditions.

In a first set of experiments, the interaction of the
irradiated protein with DNA was compared to that of the non-
irradiated one by polyacrylamide gel electrophoresis. The DNA

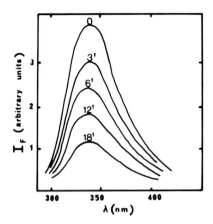

Fig. 1. Fluorescence spectra of irradiated *lac* repressor.
Irradiation times (in minutes) are given on the curves. Concentration : 10^{-6} M tetramer.

was a 203 base pairs restriction fragment bearing *lac* operator and pseudo-operator, prepared from pOP_{203_1} (derived from
pMB9) plasmid, and the repressor was a wild type one, isolated from BMH 493 strain of *E. coli* (Culard and Maurizot,
1982). Operator and pseudo-operator are partially homologous
and the affinity of repressor for pseudo-operator is 10 to
1000 times lower than that of the operator.

    DNA and repressor solution were mixed in the ratio 1:1
between DNA fragment and tetrameric protein concentrations
for the non-irradiated, as well as for the irradiated samples,
and electrophoresis was performed. Figure 2A shows the results
of microdensitometric scanning of a negative photograph of an
electrophoresis gel.

    Three bands are observed corresponding to free DNA (D),
to a first DNA-repressor complex (C_1),corresponding as previously proposed (Fried and Crothers, 1981 ; Winters and Von
Hippel, 1981) to a stoechiometry of 1 repressor for 1 DNA
fragment, and to a second complex (C_2), corresponding to a
stoechiometry of 2 repressors for 1 DNA fragment. We can attribute these bands to a specific repressor-operator complex
for C_1 and respectively, to both repressor-operator plus re-
pressor-pseudo-operator complex for C_2. Taking into account
the linearity of the peaks areas as a function of DNA quanti-

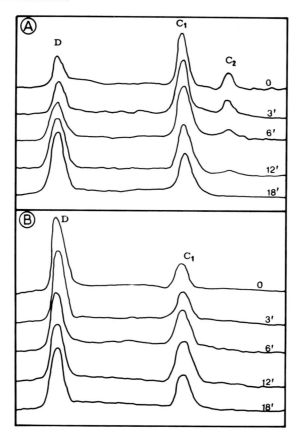

Fig. 2. Densitograms of photographs of electrophoresis gels. A : electrophoresis of the irradiated *lac* repressor and 203 base pairs DNA fragment in the ratio 1 tetramer for 1 fragment. Irradiation times (in minutes) are given on the curves. B : Same as A, but in presence of IPTG. Gel : 4.94 % acrylamide, 0.06 % bisacrylamide. Buffer : 10 mM Tris, 10 mM KCl, 0.1 mM EDTA, pH 7.25. Staining : ethidium bromide (BET).

ty, we determined the proportions of free DNA, DNA involved in the first complex and in the second one, for the two experiments, as shown in Fig. 3 A and B. The quantities of DNA are plotted as a function of decrease of fluorescence intensity as calculated from Fig. 1.

One observes that when the repressor is native, most of

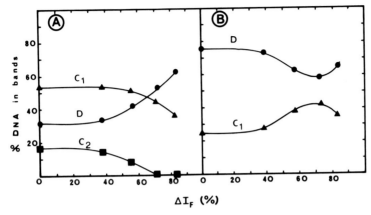

Fig. 3. Effect of irradiation on the relative amount of free DNA (D) and in the two complexes (C_1 and C_2). Data are plotted as a function of the relative irradiation-induced decrease of the fluorescence of repressor in the absence (A) and in the presence of IPTG (B).

DNA is complexed to it in the two types of complexes. Repressor binding is not affected by irradiation as long as the photochemical damage does not correspond to a fluorescence decrease of more than 40 %. Beyond this value, binding decreases as shown by the diminution of C_1 and C_2 bands.

Another set of experiments was performed in the presence of IPTG. The results of scannings of gel photographs are presented in Fig. 2B. One observes that in this case only one complex (C_1) is formed and only to a low extent for the native repressor. Upon irradiation the quantity of free DNA decreases, and that of the complex increases.

In fact, three regions are observed in the binding curve in the presence of IPTG. Until 40 % decrease of fluorescence intensity of the repressor, IPTG reduces strongly the extent of repressor binding to DNA as in the well known case of a native repressor (75 % from total DNA is free in the presence of IPTG as compared to only 30 % in the absence of the inducer). For a photodamage corresponding to a decrease of fluorescence intensity between 40 % and 70 %, binding of irradiated repressor to DNA increases as compared to that of native repressor. It is important to notice that in the ab-

sence of IPTG the same irradiated repressor binds less DNA
than does a native one.

For a decrease of fluorescence of more than 70 %, irradiated repressor binding to DNA is exactly the same in the
absence or in the presence of IPTG, and it decreases with
irradiation. We suggest the following explanation of this behaviour. Until a photodamage corresponding to a ΔI_F of 40 %,
an irradiated repressor behaves as a native one, and therefore IPTG reduces its binding to DNA. For a ΔI_F of 40 %, the
number of photodamaged protein becoming important, repressor
binding to DNA is modified (decreased in the absence of IPTG,
increased in the presence of this inducer). It was shown that
a photodamaged protomer does not bind IPTG any more since
the site of IPTG binding involves the photooxidized tryptophan (Charlier, 1977). A repressor containing such a protomer,
will thus bind DNA, even in the presence of IPTG. Or, in other
words irradiation "locks" this repressor on DNA, since the
inducer cannot dissociate anymore the DNA-protein complex.
The population of such repressor increases in the region
$\Delta I_F \in (40-70 \%)$. At a ΔI_F of 70 %, almost all repressors contain damaged protomers and thus IPTG becomes entirely inef-
fective.

Therefore binding of the strongly irradiated repressor
to DNA in the presence of IPTG is exactly the same as in the
absence of IPTG.

Another set of experiment was performed using the nitrocellulose filter binding method (Riggs *et al.*, 1970). In this
case, the operator was carried by a λ phage DNA (strain
λC_{I857} p*lac* S am 7) labelled with $\left[{}^3H\right]$ thymidine. The results
presented in Fig. 4 show that the amount of complexed DNA-
retained on the filter- decreases only when the protein is
irradiated so that the decrease of its fluorescence is larger than 40 %. In the presence of an inducer (IPTG), the native repressor binds a smaller amount of DNA than in the absence of the inducer. This amount is almost the same as the
background level. When the repressor is irradiated so that it
looses more than 40 % of its fluorescence, the binding is increased. Thus, the results of nitrocellulose filtration are
in perfect agreement with those of gel electrophoresis.

In view of these experiments we can conclude that :

- In conditions in which a native repressor is complexed

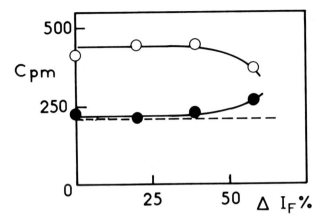

Fig. 4. Binding of repressor to *lac* operator, using λp*lac* phage DNA. The ratio repressor/operator is equal to 1 tetramer for 1 operator. DNA was labelled with $[^3H]$ thymidine, and complexes retained on the filter were assayed by liquid scintillation counting. Abscissa : see Fig. 3. o experiments in the absence of inducer. ● experiments in the presence of 5.10^{-3} M inducer (IPTG). Concentration of operator : 10^{-12} M. ---- Background level for DNA filtration alone.

to the operator (repressed gene), a low dose irradiated repressor still binds to the operator. On the contrary, a high dose irradiated repressor (ΔI_F higher than 40 %) binds to a lower extent to operator (derepression).

In condition in which no derepression occurs (low dose irradiated repressor), IPTG still induces the system. For irradiations corresponding to a decrease of fluorescence intensity between 40 and 70 % repressor gets "locked" on operator in a non-inducible way. This behaviour is similar to that observed for i[S] mutations (Müller-Hill, 1975).

It is obvious that one cannot extrapolate from such a simple prokaryotic system to the very complex system of regulation of gene expression in eukaryotes. However, the present study reports an example of misfunctioning of a simple genetic system induced just by the action of a carcinogenic (promoter) factor on a regulatory protein.

REFERENCES

Barbier B, Charlier M, Culard F, Durand M, Maurizot JC, Schnarr M (1982). The *lac* repressor, structure and interactions. In Helene C (ed) : "Structure, dynamics, interactions and evolution of biological macromolecules", Reidel D Publ Comp, Dordrecht, Holland, p 141.
Charlier M, Maurizot JC, Zaccaï G (1980). Neutron scattering of *lac* repressor. Nature 286:423.
Charlier M, Culard F, Maurizot JC, Hélène C (1977). Photochemical reactions of *lac* repressor. Effects on inducer binding. Biochem Biophys Res Comm 74:690.
Culard F, Maurizot JC (1982). Binding of *lac* repressor induces different conformational changes on operator and non-operator DNAs. FEBS Lett 146:153.
Dubelcco R (1983). La nature du cancer. La Recherche 13:1436.
Fried M and Crothers DM (1981). Equilibria and kinetics of *lac* repressor-operator interactions by polyacrylamide gel electrophoresis. Nucl Acids Res 9:6505.
Gilmore T, Martin GS (1983). Phorbol ester and diacyl-glycerol induce protein phosphorylation at tyrosine. Nature 306:487.
Jacob F, Monod J (1961). Genetic regulatory mechanisms in the synthesis of proteins. J Mol Biol 3:318.
Miller EC (1978). Some current perspectives on chemical carcinogenesis in human and experimental animals. Cancer Res 38:1479.
Müller-Hill B (1975). *Lac* repressor and *lac* operator. Prog Biophys Mol Biol 30:227.
Riggs A, Suzuki H, Bourgeois S (1970). *Lac* repressor-operator interactions. I. Equilibrium study. J Mol Biol 48:67.
Rundel RD (1983). Promotional effects of ultraviolet radiation on human basal and squamous cell carcinoma. Photochem Photobiol 38:569.
Winter RD, Von Hippel PH (1981). Diffusion-driven mechanisms of protein translocation on nucleic acids. The *Escherichia coli* repressor-operator interactions. Equilibrium measurements. Biochemistry 20:6948.

Molecular Basis of Cancer, Part A: Macromolecular Structure, Carcinogens, and Oncogenes, pages 409–416
© 1985 Alan R. Liss, Inc.

ATAXIA-TELANGIECTASIA: A HUMAN GENETIC DISORDER WITH
PREDISPOSITION TO CANCER

Martin Lavin, Jane Houldsworth, Rahmah Mohamed,
Paul Bates and Sharad Kumar
Department of Biochemistry, University of
Queensland, Brisbane, 4067 Australia

A number of human genetic disorders have been
described that exhibit sensitivity to one or more agents
(Setlow 1978; Lehmann 1981). In some cases this sensitivity can be attributed to a deficiency in DNA repair whereas
in others the evidence is indirect. The autosomal reces-
sive disorder ataxia telangiectasia (A-T) falls into both
camps. Paterson et al. (1979) demonstrated that levels of
repair replication, induced by exposure to γ-rays under
anoxic conditions, were significantly lower in three A-T
cell strains than in control cells. Subsequent to that
report studies in a number of different laboratories have
demonstrated that most A-T cells examined are not repair
deficient (Smith, Paterson 1979; Shiloh et al. 1980; Ford
et al. 1981), as determined by repair replication.

Epidemiological evidence suggests that >75% of all
cancers are due to environmental exposure. Cleaver (1968)
was the first to describe a human genetic disease where
hypersensitivity to an environmental agent and a defect in
DNA repair were linked to increased incidence of skin
cancer. Treatment of patients with ataxia telangiectastia
for lymphoma, using radiotherapy, gave rise to a hypersensitive response resulting in death (Gotoff et al. 1967;
Cunliffe et al. 1975). A large number of studies have
demonstrated this radiosensitivity in cells in culture.
The incidence of cancer in A-T patients has been reported
as high as 10% from a number of studies (Spector et al.
1982). The overall incidence of cancer in A-T patients is
approximately 1200 times that for the general population.
The pattern of malignancy in A-T patients in childhood

reflects that seen in a number of other immunodeficiency syndromes, lymphomas and acute lymphocytic leukaemia (ALL) being the major forms. This would suggest that these tumours, which are not the major malignancies seen after exposure to radiation, are due to the immunodeficiency in the syndrome and not due to the radiosensitivity. However, the appearance of other forms of cancer in adulthood in A-T as well as an increased frequency of a number of different tumours in close relative of A-T patients cannot be explained by abnormalities of immune function. Data collected by the Immunodeficiency Cancer Registry showed that one-fifth of 108 A-T patients with malignant disease had a carcinoma, and this was primarily evident in female adult A-T patients (Spector et al. 1982). Carcinoma development was excessive compared with age and sex matched controls. This is in contrast to results with other immunodeficiency disorders of childhood where few non-lymphoid cancers are ever observed. The occurrence of carcinomas was confined largely to the liver, stomach and ovaries. While A-T heterozygotes show none of the major clinical features of the disease, intermediate sensitivity to radiation between controls and A-T homozygotes as well as increased chromosome aberrations, have been demonstrated in cells from some A-T heterozygotes (Chen et al. 1978; Paterson et al. 1979b). A-T family studies also demonstrate that the incidence of cancer in close relatives of A-T homozygotes significantly exceeds the expected number (Swift et al. 1976). Higher incidence of cancer was most evident in individuals under the age of 45. One study has determined that the incidence of A-T homozygotes is 1 in 40,000, which would indicate that the frequency of heterozygotes is 1 in 100. Using an estimate of relative risk and this frequency of A-T heterozygotes it has been suggested that heterozygotes account for 6-10% of individuals dying from certain cancers (Swift et al. 1976).

Biochemical Defect in A-T

Taylor et al. (1975) were the first to describe an enhanced killing of A-T fibroblasts compared to control cells after exposure to γ-radiation. This hypersensitivity has also been observed after treatment with radiomimetic chemicals and in other A-T cell types. Nevertheless the increased sensitivity to radiation observed in this syndrome is not reflected in increased frequency of the

types of tumour observed after radiation exposure. As
pointed out previously, an obvious defect in DNA repair
synthesis in only some A-T cell lines has been established.
Increased levels of spontaneous chromosome aberrations
support a defect in some form of DNA repair or DNA processing in these cells. Further support comes from the very
high levels of radiation-induced aberrations seen in A-T
cells.

A more recent description of radioresistant DNA synthesis in A-T cells points to possible differences in chromatin structure or the recognition of chromatin structure
in these cells after exposure to γ-radiation (Houldsworth,
Lavin 1980; Painter, Young 1980; Edwards, Taylor 1980).
This radioresistant DNA synthesis is also observed after
exposure of A-T cells to high energy neutrons (Figure 1).

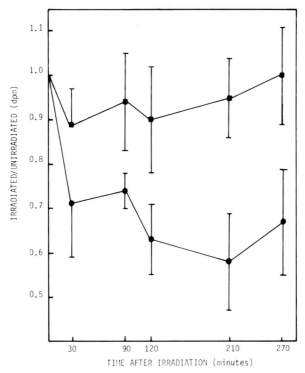

Fig. 1. Inhibition and recovery of DNA synthesis in
control (●) and A-T (■) lymphoblastoid cells after
exposure to 10 Gy of neutrons, mean energy 1.74 MeV.

Since ionizing radiation at low to moderate doses inhibits primarily initiation of DNA replication in sets of replicons it was possible that A-T cells had an altered form of chromatin structure that did not undergo conformational change leading to such an inhibition. We have used micrococcal nuclease in isolated nuclei as a probe for chromatin structure in control and A-T cells. The results in Figure 2 demonstrate that the kinetics of digestion of bulk-labelled chromatin from irradiated and unirradiated control cells are similar. Figure 3 describes similar kinetics in A-T cells indicating that bulk chromatin in A-T cells is not markedly different to that in controls and that irradiation does not alter appreciably the kinetics in either case.

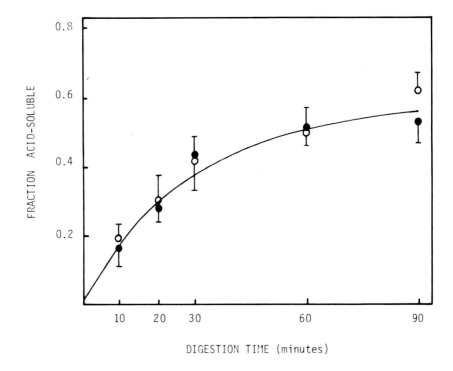

Fig. 2. Micrococcal nuclease digestion of bulk chromatin from unirradiated (○) and irradiated (●) control cells.

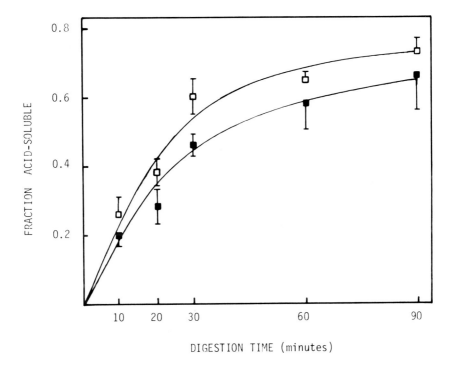

Fig. 3. Micrococcal nuclease digestion of bulk chromatin from unirradiated (□) and irradiated (■) A-T cells.

Failure to find gross differences at the level of chromatin or in newly-synthesized and chased DNA (results not shown), led us to investigate the possibility that some factor was produced in A-T cells which in binding to chromatin structure made it immune to the inhibitory effects of radiation damage. In these experiments control or A-T cells were temporarily made permeable with lysolecithin and extract from the different cell types was introduced into the cells prior to rendering the cells intact again in complete medium. The results obtained with two cell lines AT1ABR and C3ABR appear in Table 1.

EXTRACT	RECIPIENT CELL (DNA Synthesis-Irradiated/Unirradiated)	
	AT1ABR	C3ABR
No addition	0.98 + 0.05	0.60 + 0.02
AT1ABR	1.00 + 0.04	1.00 + 0.04
No addition	1.10 + 0.06	0.65 + 0.05
C3ABR	1.12 + 0.04	0.70 + 0.03

Table 1. Effect of addition of cell extract to control and A-T cells after exposure to ionizing radiation.

The most obvious effect is the ability of A-T cell extract to remove the inhibitory effect of radiation on DNA synthesis in control cells. Control extract on the other hand had no effect on DNA synthesis in either cell type.

The results presented in this paper together with recent observations on major perturbations to the cell cycle in A-T cells (Ford et al. 1984) are compatible with a mutation in a protein involved in organizing chromatin structure or in a regulatory gene. Isolation of the factor (with characteristics of a protein) may provide a means of isolating and cloning the defective gene in A-T. Identification of the product of this gene will help in explaining the sensitivity of A-T cells to radiation and may also provide further information on the predisposition to malignancy in this syndrome.

Chen PC, Lavin MF, Kidson C, Moss D (1978). Identification of ataxia telangiectasia heterozygotes, a cancer prone population. Nature 274:484-486.
Cleaver JE (1968). Defective repair replication of DNA in xeroderma pigmentosum. Nature 218:652-656.

Cunliffe PN, Mann JR, Cameron AH, Roberts KD, Ward HWC (1975). Radiosensitivity in ataxia telangiectasia. Br J Radiol 48:374-376.

Edwards MJ, Taylor AMR (1980). Unusual levels of (ADP-ribose) and DNA synthesis in ataxia telangiectasia cells following γ-ray irradiation. Nature 287:745-747.

Ford MD, Houldsworth J, Lavin MF (1981). DNA-repair synthesis in ataxia telangiectasia lymphoblastoid cells. Mutat Res 84:419-427.

Ford MD, Martin L, Lavin MF (1984). The effects of ionizing radiation on cell cycle progression; in ataxia telangiectasia. Mutat Res 125:115-122.

Gotoff SP, Amirmorki E, Liebner EJ (1967). Ataxia telangiectasia. Neoplasia, untoward response to x-irradiation, and tuberous sclerosis. Am J Dis Child 114:617-625.

Houldsworth J, Lavin MF (1980). Effect of ionizing radiation on DNA synthesis in ataxia telangiectasia cells. Nucleic Acids Res 8:3709-3720.

Lehmann AR (1981). Cancer-associated human genetic diseases with defects in DNA repair. J Cancer Res Clin Oncol 100:117-124.

Painter RB, Young BR (1980). Radiosensitivity in ataxia-telangiectasia: A new explanation. Proc Natl Acad Sci USA 77:7315-7317.

Paterson MC, Anderson AK, Smith BP, Smith PJ (1979b). Enhanced radiosensitivity of cultured fibroblasts from ataxia telangiectasia heterozygotes manifested by defective colony-forming ability and reduced DNA repair replication after hypoxic γ-irradiation. Cancer Res 39:3725-3734.

Paterson MC, Smith PJ (1979). Ataxia telangiectasia: an inherited disorder involving hypersensitivity to ionizing radiation and related DNA-damaging chemicals. Ann Rev Genet 13:291-318.

Paterson MC, Smith PJ, Bech-Hansen NT, Smith BP, Sell BM (1979). γ-Ray hypersensitivity and faulty DNA repair in cultured cells from humans exhibiting familial cancer proneness. In Okada S, Imamura M, Terashima T, Yamaguchi H (eds): "Radiation Research: Proceedings of the Sixth International Congress of Radiation Research", Tokyo: Toppan Printing, pp 484-495.

Setlow RB (1978). Repair deficient human disorders and cancer. Nature 271:713-717.

Shiloh Y, Cohen MM, Becker Y (1980). Ataxia-telangiectasia: studies on DNA repair synthesis in fibroblast strains. In Seeberg E, Kleppe K (eds): "Chromosome Damage and Repair", Plenum Press.

Spector BD, Filipovich AH, Perry III GS, Kersey JH (1982). Epidemiology of cancer in ataxia-telangiectasia. In Bridges BA, Harnden DG (eds): "A Cellular and Molecular Link between Cancer, Neuropathology and Immune Deficiency", John Wiley and Sons Ltd, pp 103-138.

Swift M, Sholman L, Perry M, Chase C (1976). Malignant neoplasms in the families of patients with ataxia-telangiectasia. Cancer Res 36:209-215.

Taylor AMR, Harnden DG, Arlett CF, Harcourt SA, Lehmann AR, Stevens S, Bridges BA (1975). Ataxia telangiectasia: a human mutation with abnormal radiation sensitivity. Nature 258:427-429.

III. ONCOGENES
B. STRUCTURE OF ONCOGENE
PROTEINS

Molecular Basis of Cancer, Part A: Macromolecular
Structure, Carcinogens, and Oncogenes, pages 419–430
© 1985 Alan R. Liss, Inc.

PROTEIN STRUCTURE AND ONCOGENESIS

Matthew R. Pincus, M.D., Ph.D.

Department of Pathology
Columbia College of Physicians & Surgeons
New York, New York 10032

It has recently been found(Tabin et al 1982;
Reddy et al 1982) that a specific tumor-causing
gene of the ras family can be cloned from a human
(EJ) bladder carcinoma cell line. This gene, if
transfected into normal NIH 3T3 cells in culture,
transforms them with high efficiency into malignant cells. This oncogene has been shown to be
virtually identical to a normal gene contained in
normal human bladder cells, the proto-oncogene,
except that it contains a different coding triplet
at position 12 in the first exon, i.e.,GTC in
place of the usual GGC (Tabin et al 1982; Reddy et
al 1982). Each gene codes for a single protein of
a molecular weight of approximately 21,000 daltons,
the so-called P21 protein product. The mutation
results in the substitution of Val for Gly at position 12 in the P21 protein. A number of studies
on this protein and on related protein products
indicate that it is involved in the regulation of
cell division (Wigler 1984).

The level of expression of both oncogene and
proto-oncogene is essentially the same (Tabin et
al 1982; Reddy et al 1982), indicating that the
protein product itself, rather than an abnormality
at the gene level, causes the malignant change in
the previously normal cells. The question naturally arises as to whether a single substitution
can cause a critical change in the structure of
the P21 protein that is responsible for its

causing the malignant changes observed.

Over the past several years, we have developed a theoretical approach employing conformational energy calculations that enables us to calculate the preferred structures for given sequences of polypeptides and proteins (Nemethy and Scheraga 1977; Pincus, Klausner 1982; Pincus, Klausner, Scheraga 1982) and thus that allows us to answer such a question.

METHODS

The basic method employed has been described at length elsewhere (Nemethy, Scheraga 1977). The method is based on the principle that the observed structure of a protein (or any molecule) will be the one of lowest free energy. Practically, by generating the allowed structures for a molecule like a protein and computing and minimizing the conformational energy of each, the observed structure (s) should be the one (s) of lowest conformational energy (energies). Briefly, the conformational energy for a given conformation of a peptide is computed as the sum of electrostatic, dispension, van der Waals repulsive and torsional energies (Nemethy, Scheraga 1977; Momany et al 1975; Pincus, Scheraga 1981). The allowed conformational states for a given starting dipeptide are generated as all possible combinations of the known single residue minima for each amino acid residue in the dipeptide (Zimmerman et al 1977; Vasquez et al 1983). The energies of these conformations are then selected. Succeeding amino acids are then added in all of their single residue minima to these resulting structures, and the process is repeated until all residues have been added. This directed search method has been modified so that fewer structures have to be considered at each stage of this "build-up" procedure (Pincus, Klausner 1982; Pincus, Klausner and Scheraga 1982) and can now be used to compute the preferred conformations for long polypeptide chains. This method has been used to compute the allowed conformations for all twenty blocked amino acid residues (Zimmerman et al 1977; Vasquez et al 1983), short peptides and longer peptides (Nemethy, Scheraga 1977) and enzyme-substrate complexes (Pincus, Scheraga 1981). New methods for proteins are now available (Pincus, Klausner 1982;Pincus et al 1982).

For example, in the case of the simplest membrane or membrane-active protein, melittin, which has 26 amino acids, we have computed the allowed structures for this protein and obtained, of many starting conformations considered in the build-up procedure, only two lowest energy structures that were quite similar to each other and to the x-ray crystallographic structure determined for this molecule (Terwiliger et al 1982;Pincus et al 1982).

In our computed melittin structure there are two long alpha helical segments that contain mostly hydrophobic residues. The axes of these two helical segments form an obtuse angle where the helix is broken by a Thr-Gly-Leu sequence. The Gly residue adopts either an alpha-helical (A) conformation or a D* conformation (PHI=-120°, PSI=60°, approximately; see Zimmerman et al 1977 for definitions of states of amino acid residues). The latter conformation is a left-handed twist structure and becomes a bend in combination with a C conformation at the preceding Thr residue (Pincus et al 1982). Gly is the only amino acid residue of all of the naturally occurring amino acids that can adopt the D* conformation. In the crystallographic structure of melittin the same features were observed, a bend occurring at the Thr-Gly sequence, between 2 long helical segments (Terwiliger et al 1982; Pincus et al 1982). We are therefore able to compute the three-dimensional structure from sequence for polypeptides in which intramolecular interactions predominate.

RESULTS ON THE P21 PROTEIN AND DISCUSSION

The problem of analyzing whether or not the substitution of single amino acid residues for Gly at position 12 in the P21 protein, whose sequence is known but whose structure is unknown, cause major structural changes readily lends itself to

the above approach, all the more so because the
critical position occurs in the middle of a long
stretch of hydrophobic residues in which intramolecular interactions may be expected to predominate.
The sequence for the first 20 amino acid residues
in this protein is Met-Thr-Glu-Tyr-Lys-Leu-Val-Val-
Val-Gly-Ala-Gly-Gly-Val-Gly-Lys-Ser-Ala-Leu-Thr-
(Tabin et al 1982;Reddy et al 1982).The nydropho-
bic sequence begins at Leu 6 and extends through
Gly 15. It is known that the P21 protein is very
likely membrane-bound (Shih et al 1982), and this
hydrophobic sequence may interact with the membrane.

        In applying the above-described methods to the
hydrophobic decapeptide, we first determined all
of the low energy conformations for N-Acetyl-Leu-
$(Val)_3$-Gly-Ala-$NHCH_3$. Here, as expected, the lowest energy form was an alpha-helix, but in other
conformations whose energies lie quite close to
that of the global minimum, the helix is broken
(Pincus et al 1983).

        The remaining amino acids in the hydrophobic
decapeptide were then added individually in all
of their sigle residue minima to each of the allowed conformations for the hexapeptide, with the
methods described above. Each peptide differs from
the others only at position 12. Tables I and II
summarize the results obtained for the "normal"
(Gly 12-containing) and oncogenic (Val 12-contain-
ing) peptides, respectively.

        It may at once be noted from a comparison of
the lowest energy structures in Tables I and II that
the global minimum for the "normal" protein (conformer 1, Table I) is a unique conformation in which
the alpha helix is broken at Ala 11 and Gly 12.
The latter residue adopts a unique conformation,
the D* state, one not available to L-amino acids
as noted above in the case of melittin. With Val
at position 12, the lowest energy structure (conformer 1, Table II) is different from that of the
Gly 12-containing peptide. In this case, the alpha
helix continues through Ala 11 and then breaks at
a chain reversal at Val 12 and Gly 13 (Pincus et al
1983). The two lowest energy structures from Tab-

Table I. Low Energy Conformations for the Hydrophobic Decapeptide in the Normal P21 Protein

	Conformational State[1]									
No.	Leu	Val	Val	Val	Gly	Ala	Gly	Gly	Val	Gly	E^2
1	A	A	A	A	A	C	D*	A	A	A	0.0
2	A	A	A	A	A	A	C	D*	A	A	0.8
3	A	A	A	C	D*	D	D*	A	C	F*	0.9
4	A	A	A	A	A	D	D	D*	A	A*	1.2
5	A	A	A	A	A	A	C	D*	A	A*	1.2
6	A	A	A	A	A	C	D*	A	A	A*	1.6
7	A	A	A	E	D*	D	D*	A	C	D*	1.7
8	A	A	A	A	A	C	D*	A	A	D*	1.7
9	A	A	A	A	A	C	D*	A	A	A	1.9
10	A	A	A	A	A	A	C	D*	A	D	1.9
11	A	A	A	E	D*	D	D*	A	C	E*	2.0
12	A	A	A	A	A	A	A	A	A	A	2.0

1. For detailed definition of states see Zimmerman et al 1977 and Pincus et al 1983.

2. Relative energy (relative to that of conformer 1) kcal/mole.

Table II. Low Energy Conformations for the Hydrophobic Decapeptide in an Abnormal P21 Protein (Val at Position 12)

	Conformational State									
No.	Leu	Val	Val	Val	Gly	Ala	Val	Gly	Val	Gly	E
1	A	A	A	A	A	A	C	D*	A	A	0.0
2	A	A	A	A	A	A	C	D*	A	A*	1.0
3	A	A	A	A	A	A	C	D*	A	D*	1.9
4	A	A	A	C	D*	A	A	A	A	A	2.0

See footnotes to Table I.

les I and II are superimposed and shown in stereo
view in Fig. 1. In this figure, the two chains are
virtually superimposable up to the region around
residue 12(arrows) where the chain direction proceeds in a left-handed twist for the Gly 12-con-
taining peptide (stippled) and in a right-handed
twist for the Val 12-containing peptide (unstippled). The fact that only the peptide with Gly at
position 12 can adopt this conformation suggests
that any L-amino acid that substitutes for Gly 12
may cause malignant changes in normal cells. This
prediction has been verified. Random substitutions
of amino acids such as Lys, Ser, Arg, and Asp,in
addition to Val, for Gly at position 12 in the P21
protein all cause malignant changes (Tabin et al
1982; Reddy et al 1982; Santos et al 1983; Pincus
et al 1983).

Comparison of conformer 2 in Table I with conformer 1 in Table II demonstrates that with a small
increase in energy, the Gly 12-containing protein
can adopt a conformation identical to that of the
lowest energy Val 12-containing protein. This result suggests that if the normal (proto-oncogene-
encoded) protein is present at significantly increased concentrations intracellularly,i.e., the
level of expression of the proto-oncogene is increased, the cells containing it should be transformed. Elevated concentrations of the normal protein would allow the alternate form of the Gly 12-
containing protein to be present in significant
concentrations. This conclusion is supported by the
results of experiments in which the proto-oncogene
has been spliced onto a viral LTR (long terminal
repeat) gene that is known to allow full expression of neighboring genes (Chang et al 1982). When
this newly synthesized proto-oncogene was used to
transfect NIH 3T3 cells with resulting increase in
intracellular P21 protein levels, malignant transformation resulted with an efficiency comparable
to that obtained with the EJ bladder oncogene
(Chang et al 1982).

It thus appears that the conformation of the
amino acid residue at position 12 is critical in
determining the local structure of the protein in

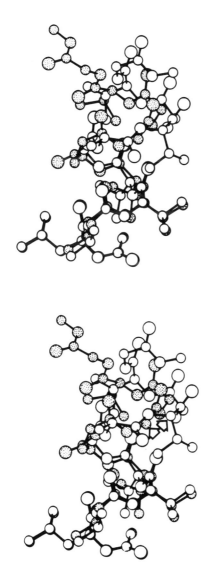

Fig. 1. Stereoview of superposition of the hydrophobic deca-peptides of the P21 Proteins containing Gly 12 (stippled) & Val 12 (unstippled). The chains progress from left to right amino to carboxyl terminus.

the region of the hydrophobic decapeptide. In order further to examine the conformational effects
of substituting different amino acids at position
12, we have recently studied the conformational
preferences for the hydrophobic decapeptides containing other known malignancy-producing substitutions at position 12 such as Ser, Lys, and Pro
(Pincus, Brandt-Rauf 1984; Pincus, Brandt-Rauf,
manuscript in preparation). Remarkably we find that
not only can these peptides (as expected) <u>not</u> adopt
the lowest energy conformation for the Gly 12-con-
taining protein (conformer 1, Table I) but <u>both</u>
Ser 12- and Lys 12-containing peptides adopt the
same lowest energy structure as that for the Val
12-containing peptide (confomer 1, Table II). This
result suggests that a "malignancy-causing" conformation may exist. Our preliminary results with Pro
at position 12 indicate that only Pro at this position gives distinctly different results in that it
induces a break in the alpha helix at positions 11
and 12. This result is expected because any amino
acid residue that immediately precedes Pro on its
amino terminal end, cannot adopt the alpha helical conformation (Pincus et al 1982; Zimmerman,
Scheraga 1977).

In the protein containing Pro at position 12,
the helix terminates in a chain reversal at the
same positions (11 and 12) as it does in the case
of the lowest energy minimum for the Gly 12-con-
taining protein (conformer 1, Table I). The conformation of the Pro 12-containing protein is different, however, because Pro cannot adopt the D*
conformation. The fact that only the Pro 12-con-
taining peptide does not adopt a conformation like
conformer 1 of Table II but rather adopts a conformation more like that of conformer 1 of Table I
may be indicative of a lower transformation potential for the Pro 12-containing protein. This conclusion is supported by the finding that transfection of NIH 3T3 cells with an oncogene coding for
Pro at position 12 of the P21 protein results in
a greatly lowered rate of cell transformation compared with that obtained with the other oncogenes
(Wigler 1984).

Table III. Comparison of Results
for Computed Preferred Structures
for the P21 Protein Sequence Leu
6-Gly 15 with Experimental Results

Theoretical

Experimental

1. In the "normal" pro-
tein, alpha helix ends
in CD* conformation at
Ala 11-Gly 12,unique in
Gly 12-containing pro-
tein. L-amino acids at
position 12 cause sig-
nificant structural al-
terations.

1. Random substitutions
at position 12 of L-amino
acids for Gly in P21 pro-
teins cause malignant
transformation.

2. L-amino acids such
as Lys&Ser but not Pro
substituting for Gly
12 all have the same
lowest energy confor-
mation. Pro promotes
break in helix at Ala
11-Pro 12, same as for
"normal" protein.

2. All L-amino acids that
substitute for Gly 12, except for Pro cause mali-
gnant transformation of
cells with high effiency.

3. Because Gly 12-cont-
aining P21 protein can
adopt "malignancy-cau-
sing" conformation with
higher energy, high con-
centrations of "normal"
P21 protein should cause
transformation.

3. Synthetic gene with
viral LTR spliced to pro-
to-oncogene causes high
intracellular levels of
P21 and malignant trans-
formation.

It appears, therefore, from the above correlations between structure and transforming activity that P21 proteins with amino acids at position 12 that cause a break in the helix at positions 11 and 12 and that can adopt the D* conformation (imparting a left-handed sense to the chain reversal at these positions) do not cause cell transformation unless malignancy-producing forms can also exist as discussed above. This finding raises the possibility that placing a helix-breaking D-amino acid residue at position 12 where now left-handed twist conformations such as D* are energetically favored may also result in a non-transforming product.

In Table III we summarize the results we have obtained in our calculations and compare them with genetic experimental findings. It appears that position 12 in the P21 protein is critical because simple substitutions for Gly at this position cause major changes in structure in the local vicinity of this position. These changes seem to correlate well with the transforming potential of the protein.

REFERENCES

Chang EH, Furth MA, Scolnick EM, Lowy DR (1982). Tumorigenic transformation of mammalian cells induced by a normal human gene homologous to the oncogene of Harvey murine sarcoma virus. Nature 297:479

Momany FA, McGuire RF, Burgess AW, Scheraga HA(1975). Energy parameters in polypeptides VII. Geometric parameters,partial atomic charges,non-bonded interactions and intrinsic torsional potentials for the naturally occurring amino acids. J Phys Chem 79:2361.

Nemethy G, Scheraga HA (1977). Protein Folding. Q Rev Biophys 10:239.

Pincus MR, Brandt-Rauf (1984). The Relationship of Structure to activity of the oncogene-encoded proteins. Eighteenth Middle Atlantic Regional Meeting of the American Chemical Society: 40.

Pincus MR, Klausner RD (1982). Prediction of the three dimensional structure of the leader sequence of pre-kappa light chain, a hexadecapeptide. Proc Natl Acad Sci USA 79:3413.

Pincus, MR, Klausner RD, Scheraga HA (1982). Calculation of the three-dimensional structure of the membrane-bound portionof melittin from its amino acid sequence. Proc Natl Acad Sci USA 79: 5107.

Pincus MR, Scheraga HA (1981). Theoretical calculations on enzyme-substrate complexes: The basis of molecular recognition and catalysis. Acc Chem Res 14:299.

Pincus MR, van Renswoude J, Harford JB, Chang EH, Carty RP, Klausner RD (1983). Prediction of the three dimensional structure of the transforming region of the EJ/T24 human bladder oncogene product and its normal cellular homologue. Proc Natl Acad Sci USA 80:5253.

Reddy EP, Reynolds RK, Santos E, Barbacid M (1982). A point mutation is responsible for the acquisition of transforming properties by the T24 human bladder carcinoma oncogene. Nature 300:149.

Santos E, Reddy EP, Pulciani S, Feldmann RJ, Barbacid M (1983). Spontaneous activation of a human proto-oncogene. Proc Natl Acad Sci USA 80:4679.

Shih TY, Weeks MO, Gruss P, Dhar, R, Oroszlan S, Scolnick EM (1982). Identification of a precursor in the biosynthesis of the P21 transforming protein of Harvey murine sarcoma virus. J Virol 42:253.

Tabin CJ, Bradley SM, Bargmann CI, Weinberg RA, Papgeorge AG, Scolnick EM, Dhar R, Lowy DR, Chang EH (1982). Mechanism of activation of a human oncogene. Nature 300:143.

Terwiliger TC, Weissman L, Eisenberg D (1982). The structure of melittin in the form I crystals and its implication for melittin's lytic & surface activity. Biophys J 37:353.

Vasquez M, Nemethy G, Scheraga HA (1983). Computed conformational states of the 20 naturally occurring amino acid residues and of the prototype residue alpha-aminobutyric acid. Macromolecules 16:1043.

Wigler M (1984). Oncogenes in eukaryotes from yeast to humans. In "Oncogenes and Oncogenic Polypep-

tides: Biological, Biophysical, and Theoretical,"
National Foundation for Cancer Research, New York,
to be published.

Zimmerman SS, Pottle MS, Nemethy G, Scheraga HA
(1977). Conformational analysis of the twenty
naturally occurring amino acid residues using
ECEPP. Macromolecules 10:1.

**Molecular Basis of Cancer, Part A: Macromolecular
Structure, Carcinogens, and Oncogenes, pages 431–441**
© **1985 Alan R. Liss, Inc.**

SOME COMMENTS ON PROTEIN TAXONOMY:
PROCEDURES FOR FUNCTIONAL AND STRUCTURAL CLASSIFICATION

Charles DeLisi, Petr Klein and Minoru Kanehisa

Laboratory of Mathematical Biology,
National Cancer Institute, Bldg. 10, Rm. 4B56
Bethesda, Maryland 20205

Introduction

    For the majority of proteins encoded by the more than 3
million nucleotides that have now been sequenced, neither
structure, function nor cellular location is known. On the
other hand, many of these proteins, such as those encoded by
oncogenes, are believed to bear on processes that are of
considerable fundamental, as well as practical, importance.
Consequently, an urgent need exists for methods that can
provide functional and positional information. A central
theoretical question is the extent to which function and
location can be predicted from sequence properties. The
coupled question related to structure has long eluded a
general solution, but it forms an integral part of the
complex of problems related to function and location of
deduced sequences. The approaches that we have begun to
take to attack these problems will be briefly reviewed in
this paper, and illustrated in the accompanying paper by
Minoru Kanehisa, with preliminary results from work in
progress on oncogenes.

The Database

The first step in any predictive endeavor is organizing the data upon which methods will be developed, and against which they will be tested. All available protein and nucleic acid structural data including sequences and atomic coordinates, have been assembled on the Laboratory's VAX 11/780 computer within a relational database management system (Fig. 1).

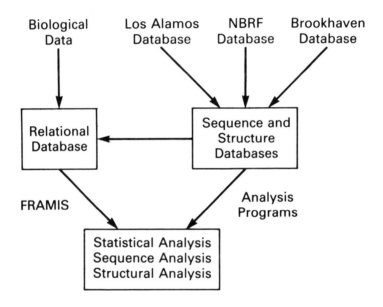

Fig. 1 Sequence attributes and sequence identification codes are organized within Framis, a relational database management system. A variety of specialized software has been developed for rapid retrieval of actual sequences with attributes specified by the user.

For any given application, usually only a small subset of sequences having specified properties--e.g. all mammalian immunoglobulins; all proteins with alpha helical content exceeding a certain value, etc-- will be required for analysis. A variety of software has therefore been developed to facilitate rapid retrieval and manipulation of specified subsets of these millions of bits of information. The files thus created can then be analyzed for particular structural or functional properties using software developed by ourselves and others (Kanehisa et al., 1984 and Fig. 2). We will briefly report on progress in the development and applications of two of these analytical methods, one relating to functional classification, and the other to structural prediction.

INTEGRATED STRUCTURAL ANALYSIS SYSTEM

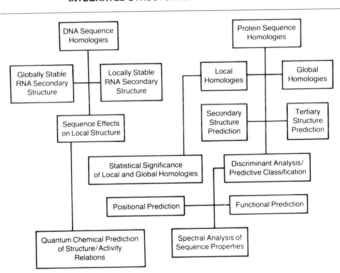

Fig. 2 Some of the analytical software currently available for molecular structure analysis.

Functional Classification (Klein, Kanehisa and DeLisi, 1984)

The objective is to segment the collection of proteins into functional categories that can be identified on the basis of sequence properties. For example the intensity of 3.6 residue per turn periodicity in hydrophobic residues tends to be much more pronounced in globins than in most other proteins. This property alone is sufficient to discriminate globins from all other proteins with nearly 95% reliability. At the current time, we have divided the protein data base into 27 functional categories, and usually only three or four variables are required to filter out one category from the rest by discriminant analysis with greater than 97% reliability (Table 1).

Table 1.

Examples of functional categories into which the protein database is currently segmented.

CATEGORY	NUMBER OF CCURRENCES	EXAMPLE OF IMPORTANT ATTRIBUTE	PROBABILITY OF CORRECT CLASSIFICATION*
cytochrome c'	16	frequency of alanine (3**)	1.00
phospholipase	24	frequency of cysteine (3)	1.00
plastocyanin	13	oligopeptide signature sequence, Asp-Glu-Asp-Glu (1)	1.00
ferrodoxin	48	net charge (4)	0.99
globins	69	average intensity of 3.6 hydrophobic periodicity (4)	0.99
histones	46	maximum local charge (3)	0.98

*
 Although in filtering out any single category the probability of correct classification is greater than 0.97, the overall probability of classifying a protein into the correct category is 0.87.
**
 Number of attributes required to achieve probability of correct classification indicated in last column.

It seems likely that many of the variables that allow generic classification on the basis of function will play an important role, either directly or indirectly, in determining general structural properties. Because at present the data base is coarsely divided; i.e. we have defined only 27 functional categories, the discriminant variables can be at best only general measures of structure.

In particular we cannot expect a relation between these variables and detailed geometric arrangements, but we might expect correspondence with general topological features of the folded molecule.

We are just beginning to pursue this aspect of the problem, but the idea can be understood by again considering globins. These molecules have a high alpha helical content; i.e. they are arranged in an ordered structure which twists in such a way that a residue occurs approximately every $100°$. Moreover, because of the globular nature of the molecules, much of its outer surface is defined by alpha helical regions. In an aqueous environment, one face of a surface helix contacts a predominantly polar environment, whereas the opposite face on the interior portion of the surface necessarily contacts a much less polar environment. Evidently, an energetically favorable structure would be highly amphipathic, having polar residues facing outward into the aqueous environment, and non polar residues facing inward. Amphipathicity is maximized when the occurrence of hydrophobic residues varies with a period of 3.6 per turn.

Sequence Properties and Molecular Topology

The relation between sequence properties and topological features of a folded globin is an example of what might be a more general principle. Eisenberg and his colleagues (1984) have suggested, based on a sample of some thirty odd proteins, that sequences tend to adopt ordered structures that maximize their amphipathicity. For example a sequence in which hydrophobicity tended to alternate between high and low values on every other residue would favor a beta strand structure. Let h_j be the hydrophobicity of the jth residue, assigned for example according to the values in Eisenberg et al. (1982), and let $\bar{h}_k$ be the average hydrophobicity of the kth segment. Then a quantitative measure of the contribution I, from a given period p, to the magnitude of hydrophobicity in a sequence segment of length ℓ is given by (Moore and Stroud, 1984; Eisenberg, Weiss and Terwilliger, 1984; Klein, Kanehisa and DeLisi, 1984)

$$I_k(p) = \left| \sum_{j=k}^{k+\ell-1} (h_j - \bar{h}_k) \exp(\omega j) \right| \qquad (1)$$

where

$$\omega = 2\pi i/p.$$

Equation 1 assigns values to the kth segment of length ℓ in the sequence, according to the period used. I is thus a function of two variables, and is visualized either as a surface in three dimensions, or as a series of contours in two dimensions. Much of the most important information, however, can be summarized by plotting position of the block against the period at which the intensity is maximum. Typically, such plots for beta rich structures show relatively frequent occurrence of stretches with highest intensity at periods close to 2 (Fig. 3).

SPECTRAL ANALYSIS OF HYDROPHOBICITY
OF HUMAN FC FRAGMENT

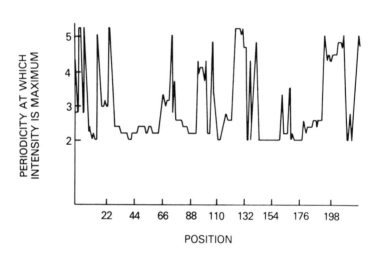

Fig. 3 Periodicity at which hydrophobic intensity of a sequence is maximum plotted against position of the segment. The immunoglobulin fragment used in this example is known to be beta rich.

It is important to notice that the result for a particular block number cannot be unambiguously ascribed to the corresponding residue number in the chain because of end effects. There is no rigorous way to take account of such effects, though reflecting the terminal portion of the sequence about the end residues might help place these residues on an equal footing with the more central residues in the sequence. For the results in Figs. 3 and 4, however, attempts at precise association between block number and corresponding residue number should be avoided, nor will the features of interest to us here depend on such an association.

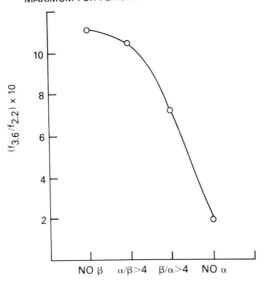

f_x = FRACTION OF RESIDUES AT WHICH INTENSITY IS MAXIMUM FOR PERIODICITY BETWEEN x AND x±Δx

Fig. 4 f_x is the fraction of sequence segments having maximum hydrophobic intensity for a period between x and x+Δx. The figure indicates a strong correlation between the value of periodicity in hydrophobicity and the type of ordered structure that is formed.

More generally, if we define a ratio

$$R = f_{3.6}/f_{2.2}$$

where f_x is the fraction of residues having maximum intensity at a periodicity between x and x +Δx, we are interested in the relation between R and the ratio of alpha to beta structure in proteins. A preliminary result using a rapid search of the Brookhaven database (Fig. 4) shows a strong correlation between periodicity and structure for the following proteins. (1) no alpha, high beta :con A, Ig bence Jones REI dimer, Ig Fc fragment (human(Hu) IGG1), neurotoxin B (laticauda semifasciata) (2) high beta, low alpha (ratios ranging from 12:1 to 4:1): alpha chymotrypsin A, Con A (3CHA); elastase (porcine,tosyl); hu lambda heavy chain; plastocyanin (poplar); prealbumin (hu); proteinase B (streptomyces criseus); Cu, Zn superoxide dismutase (bovine) (3) High alpha, low beta: adenylate kinase (porcine muscle), lysozyme (bacteriophage T4), phospholipase A2 (bovine) IBP2 and 2Bp2. (4) All alpha, no beta: erythrocruorin, hemoglobin (horse aquo met) alpha chain, hemoglobin beta chain (horse aquo leg hemoglobin), mellitin.

If the relation shown in Fig.4 holds more generally, it would be important not only in the development of discriminant variables for functional classification, but it might also be useful in conjunction with structural prediction algorithms. For example, current algorithms such as those based on the Chou and Fasman (1974) and Delphi (Garnier, Osguthorpe and Robson, 1978) methods distinguish poorly between alpha and beta structures. A preliminary Fourier analysis of the sequence prior to an energy minimization calculation would provide additional information that could be used in weighting the probabilities that a particular residue adopted a configuration compatible with one or another ordered structure. A more precise development of ideas concerning the role of hydrophobic periodicity and structure would be aided by systematic structural studies of selected sequences in different solvents. Spectral analyses such as Eq.1, and generalized versions of it for the analysis of higher order structural features, are being used to categorize and identify structurally and functionally related families of proteins.

Sequence Properties and Structure.

Although analysis of physical properties of linearly ordered residues might provide some insight into principles governing folding for certain classes of molecules, their implementation and integration into free energy minimization algorithms such as those of Scheraga (1975) and Jernigan (1979) and their colleagues, is essential for developing a detailed understanding of the relation between structure and function. One of our approaches to this problem proceeds from an attempt to answer the following question: given a class of functionally related molecules, to what extent and under what conditions can detailed structural information about some of its members aid us in calculating structural detail about other members for which information is more limited? In this section we will summarize one of the approaches we are taking to answer this question for immunoglobulin (Ig) related molecules.

Molecules of the immunoglobulin family, whether they be antibodies or products of the major histocompatibility complex (MHC), must be capable of recognizing a wide range of antigens. It is not surprising, therefore, that when antibodies of a subclass are aligned, a few regions stand out dramatically, showing large numbers of amino acid substitutions. As predicted by Wu and Kabat (1970), these regions of hypervariability form the antigen combining site. An important consequence of associating sequentially spaced, localized regions of hypervariability, with a single combining site, is the constraint it places on the way a chain folds; viz, folding must bring the hypervariable regions into spatial proximity.

Two other constraints are important, both having their basis in sequence homologies. First, all available evidence indicates that each of the compact, disulfide bonded domains comprising the Ig molecule have a common characteristic fold; viz. a four stranded beta sheet stacked on top of a three stranded beta sheet (Amzel and Poljak, 1979). Whether such a fold is also present in MHC proteins is not known with certainty, but theoretical considerations as well as experimental evidence suggests its likelihood. In particular both class 1 and class 2 MHC products are compatible with a discrete domain structure showing sequence homologies to the Ig domains, and stabilized by disulfide bonds. In addition all circular dichroism data of which we are aware indicate only beta structure. The assumption of a characteristic beta sandwich fold for all Ig like molecules therefore seems reasonable.

It is worth noting at this point that the environment of the interior of a beta sandwich is likely to be somewhat less polar than the exterior environment. One might therefore expect either that a sequence with maximum hydrophobic periodicity of two residues per turn would show some bias toward adopting such a structure, or alternatively, if such a structure is functionally necessary, some evolutionary pressure to evolve toward a period 2 sequence could be anticipated. In either case, the tendency illustrated in Fig. 3 is understandable in terms of a beta sandwich.

If a domain adopts the characteristic fold, and we impose the requirement, at least for the variable domains, that locations of high variability or polymorphism must be spatially proximate in the folded structure, the ability to correctly assign ordered regions; i.e. to predict correct secondary structure, becomes the central part of the problem of predicting the tertiary structure of the molecule. The standard secondary structural prediction methods, unfortunately, tend not to be successful for beta sheet structures, typically predicting from 50-60% correct structure.

There are a number of possible approaches one might try to improve on these methods. The simplest would be to search for homologies with other Ig related molecules whose structures are known, and to use the known structural information to bias the weights for choosing a beta state at a known position. The emphasis in the last sentence is important; one cannot be sure that a homologous, or even an identical, short sequence (e.g. seven residues) in one molecule, will adopt the same structure in another. A number of examples can be found in which identical sequences have entirely different structures in different molecules (Kabsch and Sander, 1984). The important question here is whether we can define conditions or indicators that will tell us when similar sequences will have similar structures. The problem can be approached by an extensive geometric homology search of the crystallographic data base. At present this project is not complete, but we speculate based on evidence obtained to date, that the relation between local sequence and local geometric homology is strong for functionally related molecules. Moreover we expect the variables used in our functional classification scheme to be useful in making the distinction.

References

Amzel LM, Poljak RJ (1979). Three dimensional structure of immunoglobulins. Ann Rev Biochem 48:961-997.

Chou PY, Fasman GD (1974). Conformational parameters for amino acids in helical β sheet and random coil regions calculated from proteins. Biochem 13:211.

Dygert M, Go N, Scheraga HA (1975). Use of symmetry condition to compute the conformation of gramicidin Sl. Macromolecules 8:750-761.

Eisenberg D, Weiss P, Terwilliger T, Wilcox W (1982). Faraday Symp Chem Soc 17:109-120.

Eisenberg D, Weiss RM, Terwilliger T (1984). The hydrophobic moment detects periodicity in protein hydrophobicity. Proc Nat Acad Sci USA 81:140-144.

Finer-Moore J, Stroud RM (1984). Amphipathic analysis and possible formation of the ion channel in an acetylcholine receptor. Proc Nat Acad Sci USA 81:155-159.

Garier J, Osguthorpe DJ, Robson B (1978). Analysis of the accuracy and implications of simple methods for predicting secondary structure of globular proteins. J Mol Biol 120:97-120.

Jernigan RJ, Szu SC (1979). Conformational energy minimization in the approximation of limited range interactions. Macromoleucles 12:1156-1159.

Kabsch W, Sander C (1984). On the use of sequence homologies to predict protein structure: identical pentapeptides can have completely different conformations. Proc Natl Acad Sci USA 81:1075-1078.

Kanehisa M, Klein P, Greif P, DeLisi C (1984). Computer analysis and structure prediction of nucleic acids and proteins. Nucl Acids Res 12:417-428.

Klein P, Kanehisa M, DeLisi C (1984). Prediction of protein function from sequence properties: discriminant analysis of a database. Biochim Biophys Acta, in press.

Wu TT, Kabat E (1970). An analysis of the sequences of the variable regions of Bence Jones Proteins and myeloma light chains and their implications for antibody complementarity. J Exp Med 132:211-250.

**Molecular Basis of Cancer, Part A: Macromolecular
Structure, Carcinogens, and Oncogenes, pages 443–452
© 1985 Alan R. Liss, Inc.**

SEQUENCE HOMOLOGIES OF ONCOGENE PROTEINS: A CRITICAL REVIEW

Minoru Kanehisa and Charles DeLisi

Laboratory of Mathematical Biology, National
Cancer Institute, National Institutes of Health,
Bethesda, Maryland 20205

1. INTRODUCTION

There is a growing belief that malfunction of
proto-oncogene encoded proteins, which by themselves appear
to be important in normal cellular activity, is somehow
involved in a step toward malignant transformation.
Oncogene products may be produced in excess quantities, in
wrong places, or at wrong times, or they may have locally
altered structure due to amino acid changes in the sequence.
Thus, functional identification of those proteins should
provide a clue to our understanding of cancer. Insight into
the general function of a protein sequence is sometimes
obtained through a homology search. The procedure is to try
to find a protein of known function whose sequence
properties resemble, to within some specified degree of
tolerance, those of the protein in question. Thus the
protein encoded by the simian sarcoma virus oncogene sis
shows roughly 80% homology with platlet-derived growth
factor (Doolittle et al. 1983; Waterfield et al. 1983),
suggesting the very reasonable possibility that this
oncogene product plays a role in cell growth. Similarly the
erb-B transforming protein of avian erythroblastosis virus
is strongly homologous to the epidermal growth factor
receptor (Downward et al. 1984). In this latter instance,
however, the portion of the receptor to which erb-B is
homologous shows kinase activity, whereas apparently the
erb-B protein does not.

Dayhoff, Barker, and colleagues (1978) have compiled a
superfamily classification of all published protein
sequences in their protein sequence database, Protein

Identification Resource (PIR). When two sequences are identical at over 50% of the amino acid positions, they are classified in the same family. When two sequences are less than 50% identical, but the probability of sequence similarity by chance is less than 10^{-6}, they are assumed to belong to the same superfamily of similar function. The similarity of two sequences is calculated, not by the number of identical amino acids, but by the weighted number of similar amino acids based on the observed frequency of amino acid mutations in related proteins.

According to their criteria, sis and PDGF, or erb-B and the EGF receptor should belong to the same family, or possibly to the same subfamily (more than 80% identical). Barker and Dayhoff (1982) also reported the sequence homology of src protein and bovine cAMP-dependent protein kinase. Although it contains only 20-30% identities, the two sequences belong to the same superfamily. The homology of ras protein and mitochondrial ATPase (Gay and Walker 1983) is based on the same criteria, but it extends only a portion of the sequneces. There are additional reports of sequence homologies which appear to depend on different criteria of similarity; including myc and adenovirus E1a (Ralston and Bishop 1983), Blym and transferrin (Goublin et al. 1983), and polyoma middle T and gastrin (Baldwin, 1982). We could not confirm any of these findings when Dayhoff's criteria were used. As reported elsewhere (DeLisi and Kanehisa 1984) different criteria of similarity and different penalties for insertions and deletions can produce different homology alignments.

Here we report another oncogene homology--between Blym and immunoglobulin related molecules. We have carried out a homology search of the Blym oncogene protein against the PIR protein sequence database. Different portions of the oncogene product were found to have local homologies to the second framework (FR2) regions of immunoglobulin (Ig) light and heavy chains and to a segment in the variable domain of class I major histocompatibility complex (MHC) antigens. These homologies are stronger than the previously observed homology with transferrin and the functional implications are somewhat different.

2. METHODS

Homology was searched by the protein version of the Goad-Kanehisa algorithm (1982) for identifying all homologous subsequences in two longer sequences. For the criteria of amino acid similarity, we use the amino acid mutation data compiled by Dayhoff (1978). Amino acid matches and favorable replacements among chemically similar amino acids take positive values and unfavorable replacements take negative values (see Fig. 84 in Dayhoff 1984). Given a set of weights for each amino acid match, mismatch, and deletion, the algorithm finds essentially all local segments where the sum of weights exceeds zero. One unknown quantitiy is the weight for an amino acid deletion, which we take equal to the highest penalty for an amino acid replacement. Note that the length of the aligned segment is not predefined in our search algorithm. It is determined by the optimization procedure; each alignment is extended as long as the criteria of similarity are met.

The significance of each alignment found was checked by a Monte Carlo calculation in the following way. Suppose that the optimum value of the homology score (i.e., the sum of weights) is D in the actual alignment of two local segments. We want to know the probability that two random sequences having the same respective compositions will have a score of D or higher. A standard procedure is to randomize the two segments many times and calculate the mean sample score μ and the sample standard deviation σ for the randomized pairs. Then, the quantity $(D - \mu)/\sigma$ represents, in standard deviation units, the difference between D and the mean value of the sample. For example, the probability that D is more than three standard deviation units from the sample mean is less than 0.00135 for the normal distribution. In practice we repeated the randomization procedure 1,000 times.

3. RESULTS AND DISCUSSION

Goubin et al. (1983) found that B lymphocytes infected with avian leukosis virus contain, in addition to an activated myc gene which has a viral homologue, another transforming gene, Blym, which has no viral homologue. They also reported that the portion of the polypeptide encoded by the second exon of the transforming gene is homologous to the amino terminus of transferrin. As shown in Table 1 this homology does not place the two sequences in the same superfamily. Table 1 also shows homology scores and their significance for the two best alignments, human Ig heavy chain Jon and HLA-A2 antigen, and for some additional good alignments found in our database search of over 360,000

```
                                      10        20        30        40        50        60
Blym                 MKARRSWTDATIPSKTLNYHRWRNQSIHEKTKFTQYLSMNSALQMIIMGKLQHKEGKRCPRKQES
                                      :       :::  ::::::
Ig kappa chain       SCRASKSVSTSGYSYMHWYQQKPGQPPKLLIYLASN
(mouse)

                                      10        20        30        40        50        60
Blym                 MKARRSWTDATIPSKTLNYHRWRNQSIHEKTKFTQYLSMNSALQMIIMGKLQHKEGKRCPRKQES
                       : :::: :  ::  : ::
Ig heavy chain       TAWMKWVRQA PGKGLEWVWRVEQVVEKA FANSVN
(human)

                                      10        20        30        40        50        60
Blym                 MKAR RSWTDATIPSKTLNYHRWRNQSIHEKTKFTQYLSMNSALQMIIMGKLQHKEGKRCPRKQES
                       : ::::: :  :::   :
HLA antigen          LKEDLRSWTAADMAAQITK HKWEAARVAEQRR A YLEGTCVE
(human)

                                      10        20        30        40        50        60
Blym                 MKARRSWTDATIPSKTLNYHRWRNQSIHEKTKFTQYLSMNSALQMIIMGKLQHKEGKRCPRKQES
                         :::
H2 antigen           KTWTAADMAALITK HKW EQA GEAERLRAYLE
(mouse)

                                      10        20        30        40        50        60
Blym                 MKARRSWTDATIPSKTLNYHRWRNQSIHEKTKFTQYLS MNSALQMIIMGKLQHKEGKRCPRKQES
                           :: ::  :::  ::
Transferrin          RWCAVSEHEATKCQSFRDHMKSVIP
(chicken)

                                      10        20        30        40        50        60
Blym                 MKARRSWTDATIPSKTLNYHRWRNQSIHEKTKFTQYLSMNSALQMIIMGKLQHKEGKRCPRKQES
                                               ::::::
Trypsin inhibitor                             QKIVPCTRETKPN?QCPRKQ
(nematode)

Mouse kappa chain (upper) and human heavy chain (lower)
           10        20        30          40        50          60        70        80          90
DIVLTQSPASLAVSLGQRATISCRASKSVSTSGYSYMHWYQQKPGQPPK LL I  YLASNLESGVPARFS GSGSGTD FTLNIHPVEEDAATYYCQH
 ::  :  :  ::   :   :::  ::              :  :         :
DVQLVESGGGL VKPGGSLRLSC AASGFTFST AWMKWVRQAPGKGLEWVWRVEQVVEKAFANSVNGRFTISRNDSKNTLYLQMISVTPZBTAVVYCAR
           10        20        30          40        50          60        70        80          90
```

Figure 1. Local homologies of Blym oncogene protein found by the search of the protein sequence database. The alignments with human Ig heavy chain and HLA antigen scored best among 2,145 proteins according to our weighting scheme (see text). The bottom entry is the alignment of mouse Ig κ chain (upper sequence) and human Ig heavy chain (lower sequence) variable regions with the same weighting scheme.

Table 1. Locally homologous segments of <u>Blym</u> protein

Sequence	Segment	Blym Segm	Homol Score	Significance S.D.	Prob.
Mouse kappa PC6684	22-57	5-40	54	5.7	6.0×10^{-9}
Mouse kappa PC2154	22-69	5-50	48	4.9	4.8×10^{-7}
Human heavy Was	36-65	7-38	51	4.3	8.5×10^{-6}
Human heavy Lay	34-65	5-38	56	5.2	1.0×10^{-7}
Human heavy Jon	31-65	2-38	65	6.2	2.8×10^{-10}
Human HLA-B7	131-161	5-38	50	4.2	1.3×10^{-5}
Human HLA-A2	126-161	1-38	62	5.7	6.0×10^{-9}
Mouse pH-2d-1(fragment)	1-29	7-38	49	4.6	2.1×10^{-6}
Mouse H-2Kb	131-161	5-38	55	5.4	3.3×10^{-8}
Chicken transferrin	7-31	21-44	35	3.7	1.1×10^{-4}
Ascaris trypsin inhibitor	23-42	44-63	43	5.1	1.7×10^{-7}

residues. The actual alignments corresponding to the results of Table 1 are shown in Fig. 1. Although the density of matched residues may not appear to be very large, it must be emphasized that rare, more conserved amino acids, e.g. Trp(W), Tyr(Y), and His(H), are aligned well. This is why many in Table 1 have the probability of less than 10^{-6} (or equivalently, larger than 4.75 standard deviation units). Note, however, that in Table 1 the probability values are assigned to segments, not to entire sequences.

A comparison of the mouse Ig kappa light chain sequence and human Ig heavy chain sequenece (bottom alignment of Fig. 1) indicates that the segments around position 40, <u>viz</u> WVRQAPG (human heavy chain) and WYQQKPG (mouse kappa chain) are homologous to one another. The two segments are also homologous to different portions of the oncogene protein as shown in the top two alignments of Fig. 1; namely, the oncogene sequence apparently contains a duplication. These segments are in fact both in the second framework (FR2) region of kappa and heavy chains (Kabat et al. 1983). FR2 is one of the four relatively conserved regions of the immunoglobulin variable domain (Kabat et al. 1979).

In order to obtain more information that might bear on this observation, all Ig kappa chain V regions and all Ig heavy chain V regions that were locally homologous to the <u>Blym</u> oncogene protein were collected and the amino acid positions found to be identical were tallied. The count was

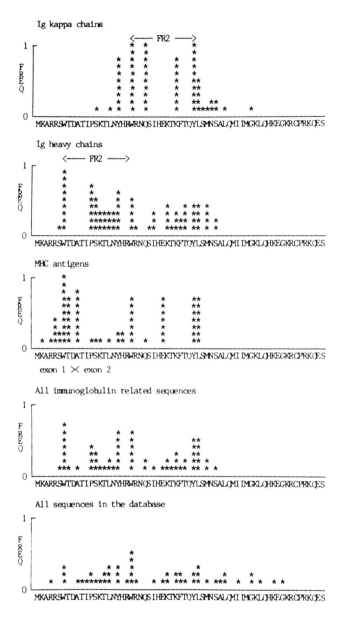

Figure 2. Fraction of amino acid matches at each position of Blym oncogene protein sequence when it is aligned with different groups of sequences in the database. The boundary of two exons in Blym sequence is noted in the third panel.

normalized to one by dividing by the total number of
homologous segments, and the fractional match plotted
against the oncogene sequence. The results (top two panels
of Fig. 2) are striking, clearly showing homologies to two
adjacent non-overlapping FR2 regions; one from heavy chains
and one from kappa light chains. These both appear largely
in the portion of the protein encoded by the second exon,
which starts at amino acid 10.

We have compared the location and degree of this
homology with the other sequence, Thy-1 glycoprotein, that
is known to be homologous to the immunoglobulin variable
domain (Williams and Gagnon 1982). Similar plots were made
(data not shown) by tallying locally homologous segments of
Thy-1 after the database search. The homology of the third
framework (FR3) region was the strongest in all groups of
immunoglobulin related sequences, including kappa, lambda,
and heavy chain variable domains, constant domains of both
light and heavy chains, and β_2 microglobulin. In addition,
the homology of the first framework (FR1) region was
observed in the light, especially kappa, chain variable
region. However, the homology of the FR2 region was not
significant in any group of sequences. It was this FR2
region that was found to be homologous in the Blym oncogene
encoded protein. The fourth framework (FR4) region, which
is encoded by a different exon, J segment, in immunoglobulin
genes, also lacked Thy-1 homologies.

The third panel of Fig. 2, a homology plot of the
oncogene protein against all histocompatibility antigens,
shows a dense homology pattern in exon 1 followed by diffuse
homology throughout the first half of the protein encoded by
the second exon. For class I histocompatibility antigens
there are now enough sequences accumulated to suggest
patterns of sequence variability along the chain (Coligan
and Kindt 1984). The homologous segments in Figs 1 and 2
were found to be located in the second variable domain, α_2
in mouse and C_1 in human; adjacent to, though not within,
what appear to be the regions of greatest variability. This
is therefore analogous to the finding above for FR2, which
is also in a variable region, though adjacent to rather than
within regions of highest variability. The remaining panels
are included for reference. As expected the panel showing
homologous segments of all proteins in the database is
rather featureless except that it exhibits the intrinsic
bias in the similarity weights used; Trp(W) has high values
reflecting the fact that the match with this residue

contributes most in the optimization procedure because it is
the most conserved amino acid in Dayhoff's compilation.

The picture that emerges from the above analysis is
that of an oncogene product with different portions
homologous to the evolutionary remnants of primordial
genetic segments coding for known protein regions; viz an
HLA variable region segment, followed sequentially by an Ig
heavy chain FR2 region and an Ig kappa chain FR2 region.
For example, starting with a single FR2 precursor, a second
FR2 could have arisen by gene duplication followed by gene
conversion, the latter mechanism being operative in highly
homologous sequences. A picture of this sort presupposes
the validity of ideas which regard FR2 as encoded by
minigenes (Kabat et al. 1979), i.e., nucleic acid sequences
that have segregational properties similar to those of
genes. The main difference is that here we are thinking of
genetic rearrangements that occur on the time scales of
evolutionary rather than developmental biology.

The striking gap in this picture of the oncogene as a
congeries of minigene encoded segments is the apparent
absence of proteins homologous to the terminal portion of
the protein. A homology search of this portion of the
sequnece, indicates a terminal segment homologous to Ascaris
lumbricoides trypsin inhibitor (Fig. 1), but its possible
biological significance is not clear. Unless this segment
has segregational properties, such as those of minigenes,
for example, the probability value in Table 1 should not be

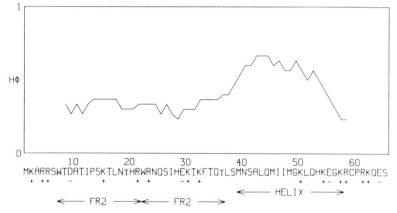

Figure 3. Relative hydrophobicity scale HΦ and charge
distribution in Blym protein. The predicted helical segment
and the FR2 homologies are also marked below the sequence.

taken too seriously. The sequence composition of the terminal portion is, however, noteworthy.

In Fig. 3 we have displayed the entire sequence in terms of a relative hydrophobicity scale, assigning 1 to Trp, Ile, Tyr, Phe, Leu Val, Met, Cys, Ala, and Gly, 0.5 to His, and 0 to the rest. The running average of these values for segments of 15 residues is plotted at the center of the segment. The stretch that falls roughly between amino acids 36 and 56 is unambiguously more hydrophobic than any other portion of the chain (Fig. 3). The stretch from 33 to 53 is uncharged except one lysine which is normally positively charged. Although an unambiguous prediction of secondary structure is not possible, estimates using the Jernigan et al. (1979) and Chou-Fasman (1978) methods and taking account of the tendency of polypeptides to form helices in nonpolar environments, indicate that a single helical core is favored at this hydrophobic stretch (Fig. 3). This probable helical segment can serve as a region of attachment to the membrane or as a hydrophobic core of a globular unit. Based on analogy with Igs and HLA, Blym protein could be involved in cell interactions. This, coupled with the small size of the molecule relative to HLA and Igs, suggests the possibility that it is a subunit, associated with other subunits either noncovalently or by a disulfide bond at amino acid 59.

We thank Dr. Robert Jernigan for performing secondary structure calculations, and Drs. Jay Berzofsky, Elvin Kabat, Rose Mage, Ronald Schwartz, and David Segal for valuable discussions.

REFERENCES

Baldwin GS (1982). Gastrin and the transforming protein of polyoma virus have evolved from a common ancestor. FEBS Lett 137:1.
Barker WC, Dayhoff MO (1982). Viral src gene products are related to the catalytic chain of mammalian cAMP-dependent protein kinase. Proc Natl Acad Sci USA 79:2836.
Chou PY, Fasman GD (1978). Prediction of the secondary structure of proteins from their amino acid sequence. Advan Enzymol 47:45.
Coligan JE, Kindt TJ (1984). In Weir DM, Herzenberg LA (eds): "Handbook of Experimental Immunology", Blackwell Scientific Publications.

Dayhoff MO (1978). "Atlas of Protein Seuquence and Structure", Volume 5, Supplement 3, National Biomedical Research Foundation, Washington, D.C.

DeLisi C, Kanehisa M (1984). Assessing the significance of local sequence homologies. Math Biosci 69:77.

Doolittle RF, Hunkapiller MW, Hood LE, Devare SG, Robbins KC, Aaronson SA, Antoniades HN (1983). Simian sarcoma virus onc gene, v-sis, is derived from the gene (or genes) encoding a platelet-derived growth factor. Science 221:275.

Downward J, Yarden Y, Mayes E, Scrace G, Totty N, Stockwell P, Ullrich A, Schlessinger J, Waterfield MD (1984). Close similarity of epidermal growth factor receptor and v-erb-B oncogene protein sequences. Nature 307:521.

Gay NJ, Walker JE (1983). Homology between human bladder carcinoma oncogene product and mitochondrial ATP-synthase. Nature 301:262.

Goad WB, Kanehisa MI (1982). Pattern recognition in nucleic acid sequences. I. A general method for findling local homologies and symmetries. Nucl Acids Res 10:247.

Goubin G, Goldman DS, Luce J, Neiman PE, Cooper GM (1983). Molecular cloning and nucleotide sequence of a transforming gene detected by transfection of chicken B-cell lymphoma DNA. Nature 302:114.

Jernigan RL, Szu SC (1979). Conformational energy minimization in the approximation of limited range interactions. Macromolecules 13:518.

Kabat EA, Wu TT, Bilofsky H (1979). Evidence supporting somatic assembly of the DNA segments (minigenes), coding for the framework, and complementarity-determining segments of immunoglobulin variable regions. J Exp Med 149:1299.

Kabat EA, Wu TT, Bilofsky H, Reid-Miller M, Perry H (1983). "Sequences of proteins of immunological interest", U.S. Department of Health and Human Services.

Ralston R, Bishop M (1983). The protein products of the myc and myb oncogenes and adenovirus E1a are structurally related. Nature 306:803.

Waterfield MD, Scrace GT, Whittle N, Stroobant P, Johnsson A, Wasteson A, Westermark B, Heldin CH, Huang JS, Deuel TF (1983). Platelet-derived growth factor is structurally related to the putative transforming protein p28sis of simian sarcoma virus. Nature 304:35.

Williams AF, Gagnon J (1982). Neuronal cell Thy-1 glycoprotein: Homology with immunoglobulin. Science 216:696.

Molecular Basis of Cancer, Part A: Macromolecular Structure, Carcinogens, and Oncogenes, pages 453–464
© **1985 Alan R. Liss, Inc.**

CONFORMATIONAL PROPERTIES OF ONCOGENE PRODUCTS

Thomas Kieber-Emmons, Joseph McDonald, Robert Rein

Unit of Theoretical Biology, Roswell Park
Memorial Institute, 666 Elm Street
Buffalo, New York 14263

Analysis of the oncogene sequences of EJ and T24 human
bladder carcinoma cell lines indicate that their activation
occurs via a localized genetic lesion in their normal cellular counterparts (Tabin et al. 1982; Reddy et al. 1982).
Sequence homologies with other ras p21 encoded sequences
suggest that mutations affecting the twelfth codon (the
loss of glycine in this position) may be sufficient to confer
transforming properties on the gene product to the respective human cell lines and retroviruses (Tabin et al. 1982;
Reddy et al. 1982; Santos et al. 1983). Transforming
properties can also be attributed to small changes in the
peptide sequence clustering around amino acids 59 to 63
(Yuasa et al. 1983). It appears that the transforming
properties of ras products represent abrupt changes in the
local stereochemistry in essential domains or a loss of
significant functional residues. The elucidation of the
structural characteristics of such domains is essential for
understanding oncogene product function.

In a broader context, one approach to the solution of
such problems has been to compare residue sequences of
unknown proteins with residue sequences of proteins whose
structures have been determined. Another aspect of such
comparisons is the superposition of crystal structures of
proteins to facilitate sequence alignments. The identification of structural homology by superposition of
proteins devoid of sequence homology is best represented
by dehydrogenases (Rossman 1975). Such studies have revealed conserved tertiary features representing particular
supersecondary folds. These features have been further

characterized in terms of residue sequence tracts. For example, comparisons of ATP binding proteins exhibit a conserved feature representing the $\beta\alpha\beta$ fold; notably the sequence tract G-X-X-X-X-G-K-(T)-X-X-X-X-X-X-I/V. This feature is observed in Bovine ATPase, E. coli ATPase (α,β forms), adenylate kinase (ADK), Rec A protein, and myosin (Walker et al. 1982).

Utilizing such an approach, a model for the domain encompassing the twelfth residue position in p21 has been suggested to involve the $\beta\alpha\beta$ fold (Gay, Walker 1983; Wierenga, Hol 1983). Here the salient features of such a model is discussed and compared with an alternative model involving the supersecondary fold $\alpha\alpha\beta$ which is observed in repressor proteins.

The superposition of dehydrogenases has revealed a common sequence feature within the $\beta\alpha\beta$ domain of these proteins. The sequence tract G-X-G-X-X-G (positions 10-15 in Table 1) which is a localized subset of ATP binding proteins, has been considered as a fingerprint for this domain (Wierenga, Hol 1983). In dehydrogenases, the fingerprint tract allows the polypeptide chain to make a sharp turn between the first β strand and the α helix. This sequence tract is identifiable in bovine protein kinase, ras p21, and other oncogene product families and allows a basis for sequence alignment (Wierenga, Hol 1983; Barker, Dayhoff 1982). This alignment is depicted in Table 1. The alignments are arranged with the intention of only emphasizing the fingerprint tract and are not intended to reflect any internal homology (i.e. insertions, deletions, or evolutionary relatedness). The sequence numbering is that of C-Ha-ras in which the second Gly in the fingerprint tract corresponds to position 12. By the same token, a sequence alignment of the $\beta\alpha\beta$ domain of adenylate kinase and ATPase with p21 exhibit the same degree of sequence homology as does the dehydrogenases with p21 (Gay, Walker 1983). These sequences are also shown in Table 1.

Since Harvey MuSV binds extensively to GTP and GDP as well as dGTP and dGDP (as opposed to the adenine forms), GTP binding proteins were examined for sequences which implied a $\beta\alpha\beta$ character. The tract G-X-X-X-X-G-K-(T)-X-X-X-X-X-I is present in EF-TU, corresponding to positions 10-23 in Table 1. In β-tubulin, the tract G-X-X-X-G-X-X-X-X-X-X-X-I corresponds to positions 11-25. A tract

TABLE 1
SEQUENCE ALIGNMENT OF FINGERPRINT TRACT

	5					10					15					20					25					30				STRUCTURE
C-Ha-ras	K	L	V	V	V	G	A	G	G	V	G	K	A	A	L	T	I	Q	L	I	Q	N	H	F	V	D				STRUCTURE
T24/EJ									V																					
Ha-MUSV									R																					
RaSV									R																					
rat H-ras-1									E																					
K1-MUSV									S																					
Balb									K																					
LDH	K	I	T	V	V	G	V	G	A	V	G	M	A	C	A	I	S	I	L	M	L	N	L	A	D	E				βαβ
ADH	T	C	A	V	F	G	L	G	G	V	G	L	S	V	I	M	G	C	K	A	A	G	A	A	R	I				βαβ
GPD	K	I	G	I	D	G	F	G	R	I	G	R	L	V	L	R	A	A	L	S	C	G	A	Q	V	V				βαβ
GR	D	Y	L	V	I	G	G	G	S	G	G	L	A	S	A	R	R	A	A	E	L	G	A	R	A	A				βαβ
PHBH	Q	V	A	I	I	G	A	G	P	S	G	L	L	L	G	Q	L	L	H	K	A	G	I	D	N	V				βαβ
MMSV	L	M	H	R	L	G	S	G	G	F	G	S	V	Y	K	A	T	Y	H	G	V	P	V	A	I	K				
RSV-PC	L	E	A	K	L	G	Q	G	C	F	G	E	V	W	M	G	T	W	N	D	T	T	R	V	A	I				
BOV-PK	R	I	K	T	L	G	T	G	S	F	G	R	V	M	L	V	K	H	M	E	T	G	M	H	Y	A				
A-MULV	N	K	H	K	L	G	G	G	Q	Y	G	V	Y	E	G	V	W	K	K	Y	S	L	T	V	A	A				
β-TUBULIN	L	T	H	S	L	G	G	G	T	G	S	G	M	G	T	L	L	I	S	K	I	R	E	E	Y	P				
α-TUBULIN	V	F	H	S	F	G	G	G	T	G	S	G	F	T	S	L	L	M	E	R	L	S	V	D	Y	G				
CI	V	A	D	K	M	G	M	G	Q	S	G	V	G	A	L	F	N	G	I	N	A	L	N	A	Y	N				αα β
CRO	T	A	K	D	L	G	V	Y	Q	S	A	I	N	K	A	I	H	A	G	R	K	I	F	L	T	I				ααβ
LAC	V	A	E	Y	A	G	V	S	Y	Q	T	V	S	R	V	V	N	Q	A	S	H	V	S	A	L	T				ααβ
CII	T	A	E	A	V	G	V	D	K	S	Q	I	S	R	W	K	R	D	W	I	T	K	F	S	M	L				
434 CRO	L	A	T	K	A	G	V	K	Q	Q	S	I	Q	L	I	E	A	G	V	T	K	R	P	R	F	L				
P22	L	G	K	M	V	G	V	S	N	V	A	I	S	Q	W	E	R	S	E	T	E	P	N	G	E	N				
A. KINASE	I	I	F	V	V	G	G	P	G	S	G	K	G	T	Q	S	E	K	I	V	Q	K	Y	G	Y	T				βαβ
BOV ATPase	K	I	G	L	F	G	G	A	G	V	G	K	T	V	F	I	M	E	L	I	N	N	V	A	K	A				
EF-TU	N	V	G	T	I	G	H	V	D	H	G	K	T	T	L	T	A	A	I	T	T	V	L	A	K	T				
EF-G	N	I	G	I	S	A	H	I	D	A	G	K	T	T	E	R	I	L	F	Y	T	G	V	N	H	K				
fes	L	G	E	Q	I	G	R	G	N	F	G	E	V	F	S	G	R	L	R	A	D	N	T	L	V	A				
fps	L	G	E	R	I	G	R	G	N	F	G	E	V	F	S	G	R	L	R	A	D	N	T	P	V	A				
ves	L	E	V	K	L	G	Q	G	C	F	G	E	V	W	M	G	T	W	N	G	T	T	K	V	A	Y				
fms	F	G	K	T	L	G	T	G	A	F	G	K	V	V	E	A	T	A	F	G	L	G	K	E	D	A				
erbB	K	V	K	V	L	G	S	G	A	F	G	T	I	Y	K	G	L	W	I	P	E	G	E	K	V	K				
REC-A	I	V	E	I	Y	G	P	E	S	S	G	K	T	T	L	T	L	Q	E	I	A									
mil	L	S	T	R	I	G	S	G	S	F	G	T	V	Y	K	G	K	W	H	G	D	V	A	V	K	I				
YP2	K	L	L	L	I	G	N	S	G	V	G	K	S	C	L	L	L	R	F	S	D	D	T	Y	T	N				

similar to that of the aforementioned ATP binding proteins
is observed in p21, namely, G-X-X-X-X-G-K-X-X-X-X-X-X-X-I,
corresponding to positions 10-24 in Table 1.

Contrary to the βαβ model, secondary prediction methods
and conformational energy calculations suggest that the

domain is more representative of an $\alpha\alpha\beta$ fold (Reddy et al. 1982; Pincus et al. 1983). Comparisons between repressor proteins, which are characterized by an $\alpha\alpha\beta$ supersecondary fold (Matthews et al. 1982) and p21 show that the CI repressor exhibits the subset sequence feature G-X-G-X-X-G. A superset of this tract, namely G-X-X-X-S-G-X-(G)-X-G-X-X-X-I is observed in the CI repressor (positions 10-23) and adenylate kinase (positions 10-23). For the CI repressor, the fingerprint is central to the recognition helix, with the region X-X-G (positions 13-15) beginning the N-terminus of the supersecondary fold's second helix.

The structurally aligned repressors (as determined by Matthews and co-workers) in Table 1 show that other residues are acceptable (positionally equivalent) within the $\alpha\alpha\beta$ domain corresponding to the subset sequence feature. The alignment of YP2, which has been suggested to be evolutionarily related to p21 (Gallwitz et al. 1983) exhibits a simulated substitution at position 12. Substituted residues for this position are also found in the $\beta\alpha\beta$ domain of Bovine ATPase (β subunit), adenylate kinase, and EF-TU (Table 1). This suggests that the structural integrity of the $\beta\alpha\beta$ fold may be maintained with positional substitutions, just as the $\alpha\alpha\beta$ motif has been observed in aligned repressors.

The alignment of adenylate kinase, ADH, and the repressors with human C-Has-ras provides for some geometrical perspectives on the effect of substitutions, since the structures in the fingerprint region are known for the two models. For the $\beta\alpha\beta$ model, Gly is at position 12 in ADH and therefore mimics the C-Ha-ras sequence. Adenylate kinases, with a proline at position 12 mimics a substitution at this position. For the $\alpha\alpha\beta$ model, Tyr is at position 12 and Ala at position 15. In Table 2, the $C\alpha$ distances (Å) between the residues at positions 10, 12, and 15 are presented and should be considered only for modelling purposes since each crystal structure has been refined to different degrees. The coordinates for ADH and adenylate kinase were obtained from the Brookhaven Protein Bank, while for cro, the coordinates were obtained through the courtesy of Brian Matthews.

For the G-X-G segment, it is observed that the distance between positions 10 and 12 is practically the same in the $\beta\alpha$ (ADK) model and the $\alpha\alpha$ (cro) model. Comparing ADH and cro for the G-X-X-G (12-15) portion of the fingerprint it appears that a substitution of Tyr in position 12 has

little effect on this region. On the other hand, considering the entire fingerprint, a progression to larger values
is clearly observed from the βαβ to ααβ model. It is
clear when considering ADH and ADK that the fingerprint
region is of wider radius in ADK. The result of the
wider radius is evident in comparing the topology of ADK
and ADH. Due to the similarity of some of the distances
between the two models, there is some implication that with
a substitution at position 12 a beta to alpha transition
may occur. Ser, Arg, and Lys substitutions in position 12
are found in several of the repressors (Table 1). Ser is
found in this position in YP2, with Val found in EF-TU.

TABLE 2

DISTANCES BETWEEN Cα ATOMS OF FINGERPRINT REGION

	DISTANCE	PROTEIN	DOMAIN
G-X-G	5.0	ADH	βαβ
G-X-P	7.3	ADK	βαβ
G-X-Y	7.1	CRO	ααβ
G-X-X-G	5.5	ADH	
P-X-X-G	8.8	ADK	
Y-X-X-A	5.7	CRO	
G-X-G-X-X-G	5.0	ADH	
G-X-P-X-X-G	8.4	ADK	
G-X-Y-X-X-A	10.2	CRO	

From another model building approach, the domain can
be built up from structural information derived from tripeptide sequences found in proteins whose crystal structures
are known. This technique provides for useful starting
points in conformational energy analysis and has shown
utility in describing detailed three-dimensional structure
of the backbones of small peptides and antibodies (Stanford, Wu 1980). The buildup of peptide fragments from these
starting conformations is akin to the method of combination
of nondegenerate minima (Pincus, Klausner 1983; Pincus et
al. 1982). Utilizing this approach, Table 3 lists the
occurrences of the middle residue G-X-G being in alpha,
beta, or other conformations as deduced from x-ray analysis
of 19 proteins (Wu et al. 1978). Second row values are
for cases in which the middle residue is in a stretch of
four or more residues lying in the appropriate conformation.

TABLE 3
TRIPEPTIDE OCCURRENCES FOR RESIDUE POSITIONS
5-14 FOR p21 AND ITS VARIANTS

	ALPHA	BETA	OTHER
G-X-G	3	4	14
	2	0	0
G-X-P	0	6	9
	0	0	0
G-X-Y	5	4	3
	1	2	0
G-X-V	5	5	5
	4	1	0
G-X-R	0	2	6
	0	1	0
G-X-K	3	3	5
	3	0	1
G-X-S	3	5	22
	7	3	6
G-X-D	3	1	0
	1	0	0
G-X-E	7	2	7
	6	0	0
A-X-G	9	3	16
	8	1	0
V-X-V	4	10	7
	4	8	0
V-X-G	7	5	17
	7	3	0
V-X-A	23	8	12
	20	6	1
K-X-V	7	2	4
	6	1	0
L-X-V	6	1	10
	6	1	0

It appears that the G-X-G tract is restricted to alpha
helical forms when contained in a stretch of four or more
residues which exhibit helical tendencies. The A-X-G tract
also shows this tendency. The conformational calculations
of Pincus et al., (1983) suggest that the residues preceding the G-X-G tract (i.e. residues 5-9) exhibit alpha
helical tendency and therefore the G-X-G would just continue this tendency. From a modelling perspective, the
tracts V-X-V, V-X-G, and V-X-A corresponding to position
7-9, 8-10, and 9-11 respectively, suggest an alpha helical

strating configuration for residues 8-11, while 7-9 suggests
a beta starting point. On the other hand, considering
K-X-V and L-X-V tracts corresponding to position 5-7, and
6-8 respectively, the results suggest starting configurations
of alpha helical form. It is clear that this approach
results in the same conformational conclusions as the
sequence alignments and provides some insight as to the
potential for conformational transitions. For example,
G-X-R in Table 3 exhibits no alpha helical tendencies,
while G-X-K does.

In considering the structural range of G-X-G and
the Val substituted G-X-V tracts, it appears that these
two tracts have the intrinsic ability to exhibit conformational properties which are similar. That is one may
anticipate that low energy forms of G-X-G and G-X-V are very
close and therefore G-X-G tracts may populate conformational
states which are shared by G-X-V. Since the frequency of
occurrences of a particular conformation is larger for the
G-X-G tract, one may anticipate that the G-X-V sequence
is more restricted in its conformational blends.   This has
been observed from calculations (Pincus et al. 1983) and
provides a rationale as to why over expression of normal
ras p21 may induce phenotypic transformation (Chang et al.
1982).

To obtain information on the general folding behavior
of oncogene products, studies have been initiated to
determine whether the calculation of antigenic determinants
of proteins with known structure, allows for correlates
to be established between epitopes and the tertiary
configuration of a protein. One interpretation of such
results is that the determinants define spatial constraints
in the tertiary structure which may be exploited in protein
reconstruction schemes utilizing other geometry constraints
and potential energy functions.

In Table 4, the antigenic determinants as evaluated by
the method of Hopp (1981), for adenylate kinase (ADK) and
ras p21, are presented. It is noteworthy that in three
cases the residue numbering for the determinants of the
two proteins is within 1 residue, while in another case
they are within four positions. Aligning p21 with ADK,
it is observed that 19 residue positions (including a Cys)
are preserved. The comparative size, general supersecondary structural characteristics, and positionally conserved

hydrophilic areas suggest that the two proteins may exhibit
a similar tertiary configuration.

TABLE 4
PROPOSED ANTIGENIC SITES

AK	(2.20)	(2.08)	(1.97)	(1.48)	(1.4)	(1.3)	(1.28)	(1.23)	(1.2)	(1.15)
	2	103	140	131	127	176	96	83	171	123
Ha-ras	(1.80)	(1.73)	(1.67)	(1.28)	(1.23)	(1.15)	(1.13)	(1.08)	(1.07)	(0.93)
	102	97	37	149	123	164	33	172	87	68

Sequence alignments of several oncogene products which
exhibit positive or negative protein kinase activity can be
partially aligned with Bovine-PK (Table 5) (Barker, Dayhoff
1982). The Lys at position 23 corresponding to position
32 in Table 1 has been reported to participate in binding
ATP.

TABLE 5
SEQUENCE ALIGNMENT WITH BOVINE-PK

```
A. G T G S F G R V M L V K H M E T G N H Y A M K
B. G S G G F G S V - - Y K A T Y H G V P V A I K
C. G Q G C F G E V - W M G T W N D T T R V A I K
D. G T G A F G K V V E A T A F G L G K E D A V L K
E. G S G A F G T I - - Y K G L W I P E G E K V K
F. G S G S F G T V - - Y K G K W H G D - V A V K
G. G G G Q Y G E V Y E G V W K K Y S L T V A V K
H. G R G N F G E V F S G R L R A D N T L V A V K
I. G R G N F G E V F S G R L R A D N T P V A V K
J. G Q G C F G E V - W M G T W N G T T K V A I K
```
A) BOV-PK, B) MMSV, C) RSV-PC, D) fms, E) erbB, F) mil,
G) abl, H) fes, I) fps, J) yes.

From a general binding perspective interaction calculations suggest that the βαβ supersecondary fold interacts with adenine moieties primarily through hydrophobic
interactions (Janin, Chothia 1978; Kieber-Emmons, Rein
1981). Examination of ribonuclease T shows that selective
binding of guanine is mediated by interactions with tyrosine.
A tyrosine is located at position 32 in ras p21 and YP2 and
position 31 in EF-TU (not shown in Table 1). Calculations
have shown that this position is adequate for adenine
interaction in models of GPD binding to ATP. Depending
upon the orientation of guanine, it is known that tyrosine
will selectively interact with guanine over adenine. This

point is presently under study. However, it is clear that
for this interaction to occur, some conformational changes
in this domain must be realized. It may be suggested that
the normal form of p21 can not adequately bind GTP. Only
after the conformational change with the substitution
can it do so. This would make some sense considering the
sequences for EF-TU and YP2.

Considering the $\alpha\alpha\beta$ model, the G-X-G tract in CI
repressor is located at the juncture of $\alpha2$ (defined by
residues 5-9) and the DNA recognition helix $\alpha3$ (defined by
residues 13-22). Both P22 and cro 434 repressors exhibit
simulated substitutions for Gly 12 in p21 products. In
addition, CII repressor has an Asp residue in the position
which mimics Glu. Helical wheel analysis displaying the
asymmetric charge distribution in the central recognition
helix of the repressors, have indicated that the central
helical segments orient with the grooves of DNA in a variety
of ways (Rein 1983). Substitution of the residues at
position 12 of lac and cro result in diminished nucleic
acid binding. With substitution of more functional residues,
perhaps binding to nucleic acids is fostered. Sequence
alignment of repressors show that either Val or Ile at
position 16 is conserved (see Table 1). It has been
suggested that Val or Ile participates in the search
procedure to find the repressor binding loci in DNA (Rein
1983). While Lys is observed in this position in the ras
products, Val is observed in A-MuLV.

Fluorescence assays have indicated a diffuse cytoplasmic
distribution of v-mil with v-mil possibly being associated
with RNA (Bunte et al. 1983). This is not to imply that
the model is solely responsible for the interaction of
oncogene products with nucleic acids. Helical wheel
analysis of heptapeptide fragments in ribosomal proteins
and alike suggest that basic charges at position 3, 6, and
7 of helical fragments provide for a general mode of
binding of helicies to a phosphate backbone (Argos 1981).
Cro is the only aligned repressor which exhibits such a
tract (positions 21, 24, 25) observed as part of the
recognition helix. Table 6 lists such tracts for the
oncogene products. Considering ribosomal proteins, there
appears to be some conservation of Ala in the fourth
position (Argos 1981). This is observed for cro as well
as for v-mil.

TABLE 6
ALIGNMENTS OF POSSIBLE RNA BINDING TRACTS

```
cro         K-A-I-H-A-G-K-K-I-F
fes         K-N-I-H-L-E-K-K-Y-V
EF-TU       V-L-L-R-G-I-K-R-E-E
            Y-F-G-K-I-T-R-R-G-S
Src         O-V-M-K-K-L-R-H-E-K
            S-L-Q-K-L-V-K-H-Y-R
gag-yes     Q-I-M-K-K-L-R-H-D-K
            A-V-M-K-E-I-K-H-P-N
abl         E-S-K-H-C-I-H-R-D-L
            E-E-R-R-L-V-H-R-D-L
erbB        R-R-R-H-I-V-R-K-R-T
                            I
mil         K-N-C-P-K-A- -K-R-L-V
                          M
v-has       I-R-W-H-K-L-R-K-L-N
```

In summary: One, structural interpretation of sequence
tracts involving the 12th position indicates two supersecondary models for this domain. Two, partial sequence
alignments of the supersecondary folds contain residues
other than Gly at the 12th position. This suggests that
the microdomain itself can participate in normal cellular
function. A single point mutation in ras may instill
competitive GTP binding or foster the misuse of GTP in a
particular pathway. Three, the identification of possible
supersecondary transitions in ras p21 is consistent with
observations that GTP binding proteins experience conformational transitions upon GTP binding. Four, the
identification of two possible supersecondary folds suggest
that oncogene products may actually have multifunctional
characteristics. This may include nucleic acid binding.

ACKNOWLEDGEMENTS

These studies were partially conducted pursuant to a
contract with the National Foundation for Cancer Research,
and partially by a grant from NASA #NSG-7305. The authors
would like to thank Deborah Raye and Karen Kennedy for
their assistance in the preparation of this manuscript.

REFERENCES

Argos P (1981). Protein structural models for nucleic acid
    interactions. J Theor Bio 93:609.
Barker WC, Dayhoff MO (1982). Viral src gene products are

related to the catalytic chain of mammalian AMP-dependent protein kinase. Proc Natl Acad Sci 79:2836.

Bunte T, Greiser-Wilke I, Moelling K (1983). The transforming protein of the MC29-related virus CM II is a nuclear DNA-binding protein whereas MH2 codes for a cytoplasmic RNA-DNA binding poly protein. Embo J 2:1087.

Chang EH, Furth MA, Scolnick EM, Lowy DR (1982). Tumorigenic transformation of mammalian cells induced by a normal gene homologues to the oncogene of harvey murine sarcoma virus. Nature 297:479.

Gallwitz D, Donath G, Sander C (1983). A yeast gene encoding a protein homologous to the human c-has/bas proto-oncogene product. Nature 306:704.

Gay NJ, Walker JE (1983). Homology between human bladder carcinoma oncogene product and mitochondrial ATP-synthase. Nature 301:262.

Hopp TP, Woods KR (1981). Prediction of protein antigenic determinants from amino acid sequences. Proc Natl Acad Sci 78:3824.

Janin J, Chothia C (1979). Structural aspects of protein interactions: Accessible surface area and the role of hydrophobicity. In Hofman E, Pfeil W, Aurich H (eds): "FEBS Federation of European Biochemical Societies 12th Meeting Dresden 1978. Protein: Structure, Function, and Industrial Applications", New York: Pergamon Press, p 227.

Kieber-Emmons T, Rein R (1981). Evolving nucleotide binding surfaces. In Wolman Y (ed): "Origin of Life", New York: D. Reidel Publ. Co., p 415.

Matthews BW, Ohlendorf DH, Anderson WF, Takeda Y (1982). Structure of the DNA-binding region of lac repressor inferred from its homology with cro repressor. Proc Natl Acad Sci 79:1428.

Pincus MR, Renswoude J, Harford JB, Chang EH, Carty RP, Klausner RD (1983). Prediction of three-dimensional structure of the transforming region of the EJ/T24 human bladder oncogene product and its normal cellular homologue. Proc Natl Acad Sci 80:5253.

Pincus MR, Klausner RD (1982). Prediction of the three-dimensional structure of the leader sequence of pre-K light chain, a hexapeptide. Proc Natl Acad Sci 79:343.

Pincus MR, Klausner RD, Scheraga HA (1982). Calculation of the three-dimensional structure of the membrane-bound portion of melittin from its amino acid sequence. Proc Natl Acad Sci 79:5107.

Reddy EP, Reynolds RK, Santos E, Barbacid M (1982). A point mutation is responsible for the acquisition of transforming properties by the T24 human bladder carcinoma oncogene. Nature 300:149.

Rein R, Kieber-Emmons T, Haydock K, Garduno-Juarez R, Shibata M (1983). Molecular modelling of protein-nucleic acid interactions. J Biomol Struc Dyn 1:1051.

Rossman MG (1974). A comparison of the binding and function of NAD with respect to lactate dehydrogenase and glyceraldehyde-3-phosphate dehydrogenase. In Sundaralingam M, Rao ST (eds): "Structure and Conformation of Nucleic Acids and Protein-Nucleic Acid Interactions", Baltimore: University Park Press, p 353.

Santos E, Reddy EP, Pulciani S, Feldmann RJ (1983). Spontaneous activation of a human proto-oncogene. Proc Natl Acad Sci 80:4679.

Stanford JM, Wu TT (1981). A predictive method for determining possible three-dimensional foldings of immunoglobin backbones around antibody combining sites. J Theor Bio 88:421.

Tabin CJ, Bradley SM, Bargmann CI, Weinberg RA, Papageorge AG, Scolnick EM, Dhar R, Lowy DR, Chang EH (1982). Mechanism of activation of a human oncogene. Nature 300: 143.

Wierenga RK, Hol WG (1983). Predicted nucleotide-binding properties of p21 protein and its cancer-associated variant. Nature 302:842.

Wu TT, Szu SC, Jernigan RL, Bilofsky H, Kabat EA (1978). Prediction of β-sheets in immunoglobin chains. Comparison of various methods and an expanded 20 x 20 table for evaluation of the effects of nearest-neighbors on the conformations of middle amino acids in proteins. Biopolymers 17:555.

Yuasa Y, Srivasta SK, Dunn CY, Rhim JS, Reddy EP, Aaronson SA (1983). Acquisition of transforming properties by alternative point mutations within c-bas/has human proto-oncogene. Nature 303:775.

III. ONCOGENES
C. FUNCTION OF ONCOGENE PROTEINS, MEMBRANE REACTIONS, AND CELL TRANSFORMATIONS

**Molecular Basis of Cancer, Part A: Macromolecular
Structure, Carcinogens, and Oncogenes, pages 467–487**
© **1985 Alan R. Liss, Inc.**

ONCOGENES: TARGETS FOR IMMUNODIAGNOSIS AND CHEMOTHERAPY?

Timothy E. O'Connor, PhD

Associate Institute Director for Scientific Affairs
Roswell Park Memorial Institute
666 Elm Street
Buffalo, New York 14263

SUMMARY

A hypothesis is presented that cellular proto-oncogenes
encode proteins that play a regulatory role in embryonic
development and in the terminal differentiations of cells in
various tissues and that alterations in these genes yield
oncogenes whose expression results in neoplasia. The
hypothesis suggests that study of the disturbance in cell
regulation introduced by oncogenes could permit the rational
design of inhibitors capable of restoring neoplastic cells
to normal differentiation lineages. Proteins encoded by
oncogenes may be immunogenic and thus provide diagnostic
markers in the tumor-bearing host.

Forty years have elapsed since Avery and his
associates provided the first experimental evidence that
DNA encodes genetic information (Avery et al, 1944). In
the interval, considerable information on the molecular
functioning of the cells has been gleaned in terms of DNA
replication and the transcription, processing and translation of its encoded information. Yet, information on the
molecular mechanisms by which cells become committed during
embryonic development and undergo terminal differentiations
into particular tissues is still sparse. Developments in
two areas now show promise of alleviating this deficiency.
First is observation that retroviruses, which can rapidly
transform cells in vitro and rapidly induce malignancies
in vivo, owe these capacities to the transduction of a
modified member of a limited class of cellular genes
(proto-oncogenes). (Reviewed by Bishop, 1981, 1983.) The
second development is the frequent observation that cells of

tumors of different pathological types (including breast carcinoma, neuroblastoma and a range of leukemias) can be induced by exposure to appropriate specific reagents in vitro to resume differentiation along their normal differentiation pathways with consequent loss of their malignant phenotypes. These observations have led to the postulate that neoplasia represents a lesion in tissue renewal processes arising from a blockage in the differentiation processes (Pierce, B., 1974). Consideration of these two sets of observations and viewpoints leads to a hypothesis which envisions proto-oncogenes (also designated c-oncs) as encoding regulatory proteins that are critical to development and differentiation processes. Such a hypothesis may prove useful in that it suggests that the study of particular proto-oncogene to oncogene conversions and the biochemistries of the changes in associated proteins may provide clues for the design of effective antagonists. The objective of such studies would be a chemotherapy which aims not at death of the malignant cell but rather at its reformation along normal differentiation pathways. Furthermore the realization that oncogene proteins may represent an aberrancy in normal differentiation processes raises the question of the immunogenicity of such proteins in the host and their usefulness as immunological markers of specific neoplasias. This paper is intended to provide a selective overview of the emerging information on the biology and biochemistry of oncogenes. Note will be made in passing of oncogene protein products that may provide candidates for immunodiagnosis of cancer.

Information on oncogenes as found in retrovirus isolates (v-oncs) is summarized in Table 1, together with information on the v-onc proteins. The list of v-oncs is divided into five groups based on nucleic acid homology patterns, and the sites and modes of action of their proteins. The sixth group is a miscellaneous one where insufficient evidence presently exists for assignments. The first group shows mutual nucleic acid homology to the catalytic site of the cAMP-dependent protein kinase (Baker, W.C. and Dayhoff, M.D., 1982). Their protein products are typified by the pp60^{src} protein product of v-src which, on the basis of nucleotide sequence, is postulated to contain a hydrophobic region for binding to the cell membrane and a hydrophilic region that contains a tyrosine-specific kinase (Czernilofsky, A.P. et al, 1980). The purified pp60^{src} protein has recently been shown to phosphorylate diacylglycerol and phosphatidyl inositol and may therefore operate at the cell membrane via the kinase c/inositol pathway (Sugimoto, Y. et al,

Table 1

PROPERTIES OF ONCOGENE PROTEINS

Oncogene	Location C-ONC and Human Chromosomes	Nature of Protein Product on Potential Biochemical Role
c-src	20q	Tyrosine-Specific Kinase Action on Membrane Kinase C/Phospholipid System through Phosphorylation of Phosphatidyl-inositol.
c-fes		
c-fgr		
c-ros		
c-yes		
c-abl	9q	
c-erb A	17	
c-ert B	7 pter→q22	Membrane Glycoprotein EGF Receptor Homology Apparently lack Tyrosine Kinase
c-sis	22q	Growth Factor (PDGF)
c-Ha ras 1	11p15	p21 GTP Binding Protein
c-Ha ras 2		p21 GTP Binding Protein
c-K_1 ras 1	6	p21 GTP Binding Protein
c-K_1 ras 2	12p12.1	p21 GTP Binding Protein
c-N ras		Competitors for membrane Cyclic AMP G Proteins?
c-myc	8q24	Nucleus
N-myc	2p23→pter	Cell Cycle Dependent Stimulated by PDGF
c-myb		
ets		Presently Unknown
rel		
ski		

1984) as well as through influence on cAMP-dependent protein
kinase. The c-erb B has recently been shown to encode the
membrane-attached glycopeptide epidermal growth factor (EGF)
receptor with tyrosine kinase activity (Lin, C.R. et al,
1984) while the v-erb B encodes a protein devoid of tyrosine-
kinase activity (Downard, J. et al, 1984). The c-sis
oncogene has been shown to encode platelet-derived growth
factor (PDGF). The c-ras oncogenes encompass the related
but distinct H-ras, K-ras and N-ras members that are detected
as both functional and pseudogenes. Each member of this
family encodes a 21 kilo-Dalton protein that has the capacity
to bind GTP at equivalent sites at amino acids 12 and 58
respectively. The ras proteins are located in the cell
membrane, lack tyrosine kinase activity but may operate
through competition with G proteins of the cyclic AMP system.
Finally, the c-myc, N-myc and c-myb oncogenes show mutual
nucleic acid homology and also homology to the DNA of adenovirus and of polyoma virus that encode the EIA and large T-
antigens respectively. The products of each of these genes
appear to act within the nucleus.

Oncogenes have also been characterized by transfection
of DNA of animal and human tumors into mouse NIH/3T3 cells
with concomitant transformation of these indicator cells
(for review see Cooper, G.M., 1982). These experiments have
identified modified members of c-ras as involved in human
bladder, colon and lung carcinomas (Tobin, C.J. et al, 1982;
Shimizu et al, 1983; Reddy, E.P. et al, 1982) but in some
instances have also identified other oncogenes not previously
identified in viral isolates. Nevertheless, the total number
of oncogenes identified to date is about two dozen. This
number should be viewed in the context of an expression of
$\sim 10^4$ genes in a typical cell from a probable repertoire of
approximately 10^5 available genes. This implies that neoplasia may arise only from mutation in a small set of genes
that regulate specific functions.

Studies on the expression of c-onc genes during embryonic
development (Table 2) as revealed by measurement of mRNA with
an appropriate labeled cloned DNA probe have revealed that
while c-ras is expressed at a low level in all stages of
embryonic development, other c-onc genes show predominant
expression in particular tissues at specific stages of development (Muller, R. et al, 1983). Particularly noteworthy is the
peak expression of c-abl at day 10 in the mouse embryo development and the tissue-specific high level of expression of c-abl
in the adult testis, spleen and thymus. The c-fms shows

Table 2

EXPRESSION OF C-ONC GENES AS m-RNA IN EMBRYONIC DEVELOPMENT AND ADULT TISSUES

cH-ras mRNA detected at low levels at all stages of embryonic development

c-abl mRNA peaks at day 10 in mouse embryonic development. Also detected in adult spleen, thymus and testes.

c-fos mRNA found at high levels in human amnion and chorion

c-fms mRNA found at high level in human term placenta

(Muller, R. et al 1982, 1983)

tissue-specific expression in the human term placenta. In other studies c-src has recently been shown to be expressed in developing retinal neurons at the onset of differentiation and persists in mature neurons (Sorge, L.K. et al, 1984).

While transduction of a c-onc gene by a retrovirus places the transduced gene under the control of the powerful viral promoters that are contained in the viral long terminal repeat (LTR), thus ensuring abnormally high levels of transcription, it is noteworthy that in every case examined the c-onc has undergone some molecular rearrangement in forming the v-onc that is transduced. Representative examples of these molecular alterations are presented in Table 3. Such changes in the oncogenic DNA can range from considerable rearrangements in converting c-src to v-src to a single point mutation in conversion of c-ras to v-ras.

A range of animal and human cancers and the lesions that have been identified in specific c-onc genes are presented in Table 4. Expression of an altered c-ras or c-myc appears to be associated with a range of tumors of different pathologies. While chromosomal alterations involving new homogenously staining regions (HRS), double minutes, and/or chromosomal translations have frequently characterized human tumors, it is of great significance that these lesions are now shown to

Table 3

GENOMIC CHANGES IN
CONVERTING *C-ONC* TO *V-ONC*

c-src versus *v-src* (Swanstrom, R et al 1983)

v-src arose from transduction of c-src by retrovirus.
In the process:

(a) An exon portion of c-src was lost.

(b) Recombination occurred at an intron and involved a
splice of the c-src with a repeat of the virus.

(c) Processes (a) and (b) ensure considerable differences
in the carboxyl terminal regions of the respective
proteins.

c-myc versus *v-myc*. For details see (Watson, D.K., 1983)

c-abl versus *v-abl*. For details see (Wang, J.Y.J., 1983)

involve chromosomal translocations and/or amplifications of
particular c-onc genes. Typical examples are the amplification
of c-myc in neuroblastoma; the translocation of c-myc in
Burkitt lymphoma; and the translocation of c-abl in chronic
myeloid leukemia. Such translations introduce lesions into
the transferred c-onc due to variability in the site of welding to the recipient chromosome. Such studies have revealed
a range of welding arrangements but have failed to pinpoint
a particular sequence of nucleotides in the transferred onc
and adjacent chromosomal regulator region that underlie the
oncogenicity of the transferred and altered c-myc gene. Particularly intriguing are observations by Croce and associates
on expression of myc in cell hybrids that suggest that expression of genes may be influenced by localized chromosomal
environments in a developmental pattern (Mishikura, K. et al,
1983). In contrast to these uncertainties the examination of
c-ras molecular lesions associated with neoplasia have all
been shown in plasmid reconstruction experiments to involve
point mutations at one of the two sites of GTP binding (Tobin,
C.J. et al, 1982; Shimizu et al, 1983; Reddy, E.P. et al,
1982).

Table 4

ANuMAL MORBIDITIES ASSOCIATED WITH ONCOGENES

Morbidity	Lesion Identified	References
ALV-induced B-cell avian lymphoma	Insertion of virus with LTR adjacent to *c-myc* gene	W.S. Hayward et al, 1981
Human Burkitt Lymphoma	Translocation segment chromosome 8 bearing *c-myc* to chromosome 14 with imperfect welding adjacent to promoter of Ig	R. Della-Favera et al, 1983 P.H. Hamlyn & Rabbitts, 1983 R. Taub et al, 1984
Mouse Plasmacytomas	Equivalent transfer of *c-myc*	J.M. Adams et al, 1983 R. Taub et al, 1982 M. Dean et al, 1983
Human small cell lung carcinoma	Amplification of *c-myc*	C.D. Little et al, 1983
Carcinogen-induced mouse thymoma Radiation-induced mouse thymoma	Amplification of *N-ras* Amplification of *K-ras*	I. Guerrero et al, 1984
Human chronic myelocytic leukemia	Translocation *c-abl* from human chromosome 9 to chromosome 22 in formation of Philadelphia chromosome	A. deKlein et al, 1982
Human neuroblastomas	Translocation and amplification of *c-myc*	N.E. Kohl, et al, 1983
Human bladder carcinoma Human colonic carcinoma Human lung carcinoma	Single nucleotide substitutions with single amino acid substitution at amino acid 12 of *c-ras*	L. Parada et al, 1982 E.P. Reddy et al, 1982 M.G. Goldfarb et al, 1982
Feline T-cell leukemia	Transduction of *c-myc* by FeLV	J.C. Neil et al, 1984 J.J. Mullins et al, 1984 L.S. Levy et al, 1984

Two recent experimental developments have enriched our understanding of the pathogenicity of oncogenes. One set of experimental data correlates the action of oncogenes with tumor growth factors (TGFs) while the second set of data illuminate a necessary complementary activity of oncogenes operating within the nucleus and oncogenes operating at the cell surface.

Tumor growth factors (TGFs) were originally observed as low molecular weight proteins that were shed by cells transformed by rapidly-transforming retroviruses (Todaro, G. 1982), or by human tumor cells (Marquardt, H. and Todaro, G., 1982), and that had the capacity to transiently induce a transformed phenotype when added to cultures of normal fibroblasts. The initial suggestion of an association between oncogenes and TGFs arose from the observation that transfection of DNA from an Abelson-like human leukemia (Lane, M.A. et al, 1982) or cells of a murine leukemia induced by AbLV resulted in transformation of mouse 3T3 cells with concomitant shedding of a TGF that was physiologically similar to the TGF shed by the parent leukemia. The recipient 3T3 cells were found not to contain the v-abl oncogene (Ozanne, B. et al, 1982). This data implied that the v-abl onc had activated a gene encoding the TGF and that this gene was recovered in the transfection experiment. More recently computer comparisons of amino acid sequences derived from nucleotide sequences have established that c-sis encodes platelet-derived growth factor PDGF (Robbins, K.C. et al, 1983; Doolittle, R.F. et al, 1983; Deul, T. et al, 1983; that c-erb B encodes the EGF receptor (Downward, J. et al, 1984; Lin, C.R. et al, 1984); and that B-lym (see below) encodes transferrin (Goubin, G. et al, 1983; Diamond, A. et al, 1983).

Early studies on transformation of cells with v-onc genes had employed transforming retroviruses. Since such transforming retroviruses usually contain a single v-onc the conclusion was widely drawn that such transformations solely involved the transduced v-onc. The roles of the then unknown promoter sequences and enhancing sequences (for review see Khoury, G. and Gruss, P., 1983; Parker, M., 1983) that are now known to be contained within the viral LTRs was unappreciated. Experiments with plasmids bearing only the v-onc sequences have now established that transformation of fibroblasts into cells that are tumorigenic in the nude mouse requires the complementary action of v-oncs that operate within the nucleus and at the cell membrane respectively. The nuclear-acting v-oncs include v-myc, v-abl and plasmids containing sequences encoding the EIA antigen of transforming adenoviruses or the polyoma large T antigen while the membrane-acting v-oncs include ras, src, abl, erb and plasmids containing sequences that encode the middle T antigen of polyoma virus (Land, H. et al, 1983; Ruley, H. E. et al, 1983).

In view of these developments it is instructive to review the pathogenesis of tumors where the oncogenic lesion is associated with the nucleus, the cell membrane, or is unknown. In this context the available data on lymphoid leukemias, erythroblastosis and mammary carcinoma will be examined.

Our examination of the pathogenesis of leukemias-lymphomas begins with the observation that normal fibroblasts stimulated with PDGF or normal lymphocytes stimulated with mitogen subsequently show a pulse of mRNA or c-myc at a specific stage (G_1/S) in the cell cycle. Note that a specific membrane, stimulus subsequently results in a specific nuclear event involving c-myc (Kelly, K. et al, 1983). In contrast to this behavior carcinogen-transformed 3T3 cells show constitutive production of the myc gene (Campisi, R. et al, 1984). Normal human cord lymphocytes can be immortalized by infection with EBV without evidence of malignancy, chromosomal translocations or recoverability of transforming DNA. In contrast Burkitt lymphoma cells show chromosomal rearrangements involving c-myc translocations and alterations and yield transforming DNA that transforms NIH/3T3 cells with a restriction enzyme digestion pattern characteristic of pre-B human or mouse lymphomas (Diamond, A. et al, 1982). Interestingly the transformed NIH/3T3 cell shows no nucleotide sequences characteristic of EBV. Other lymphoid leukemias, whether of spontaneous origin in man or arising from infection with slow leukosis virus in animals, can be classified in terms of B or T cell involvement and stage of maturation (as judged by cytology and antigenic markers) of the cell lineage at the point of leukemic arrest. Very significantly, cells arrested in leukemias of mouse or man show common stage-specific transforming DNAs as evaluated by DNA restriction patterns (Lane, M.A. et al, 1982). The gene which is recovered in transfection of DNA from pre-B leukemias has been designated B-lym I. It has been shown to be a member of a small family of genes and to encode a protein which is homologous both to the 5' segment of transferrin and to a surface antigen associated with human melanoma (Goubin, G. et al, 1983). These proteins differ from transferrin in showing homology at the 5' end, in being smaller and in lacking hydrophobic regions that appear necessary for anchorage in the cell membrane. The relationship of genes associated

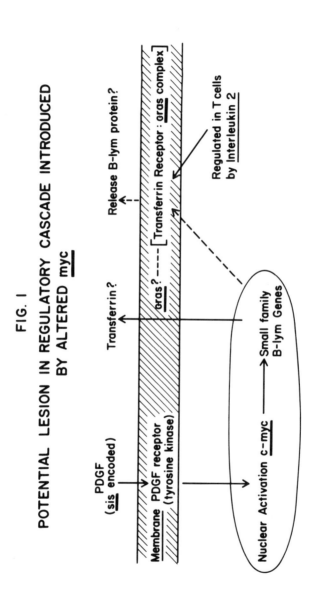

FIG. I

POTENTIAL LESION IN REGULATORY CASCADE INTRODUCED
BY ALTERED myc

with other stage leukemias to the other members of the family of lym genes awaits elucidation.

Transferrin is essential for cell growth and has recently been shown to be essential for differentiation of the metanephric mesenchyme following the inductive tissue interaction between the ureter bud and the mesenchyme (Ekblom, P. et al, 1983). The transferrin receptor has also been shown to be induced in the mitogen-stimulated T-lymphocyte by Interleukin-2 and to be essential for DNA synthesis (Neckers, L.M. and Cossman, J., 1983). Finally, the transferrin receptor has recently been shown to form a molecular complex with ras proteins in the cell membrance (Finkel, T. and Cooper, G.M., 1984).

These findings permit a tentative description of the molecular lesions in a biochemical cascade as shown in Figure 1. Normal cells are activated for cellular division through an appropriate initial stimulus of a membrane-associated event: binding of the sis-encoded PDGF to its receptor in fibroblasts or binding of mitogen to specific receptor on T lymphocytes. In each case the binding of the exogenous agent activates the the tyrosine kinase capacities of the specific receptors. In the normal cell this activation is followed by a pulse of transcription of the c-myc. In turn this probably results in transcription of one of the lym genes which encode a transferrin. In leukemic cells, however, signals arriving from the cellular membrane to the cell nucleus are interrupted by a lesion in c-myc. This lesion we can speculate results in a misreading of a lym gene, so that instead of transferrin, a shorter analog is produced. This analog possibly competes with transferrin for the transferrin receptor and results both in release of the c-ras protein with concomitant initiation of a different biochemical cascade and also in release of the transferrin receptor (at least in T-cell membranes) from control by Interleukin-2. Additionally, the modified B-lym protein, which lacks a hydrophobic region for membrane binding, may well be excreted and behave as a TGF through binding of transferrin receptors on adjacent cells. Note that the molecular lesion, while situated in an onc gene operative in the nucleus, ultimately produces its effect in the cell membrane through competition with a mediator of differentiation (transferrin).

The role of v-erb in neoplasia (Figure 2) is interesting in that the nucleotide sequence of v-erb B shows considerable homology to v-oncogenes such as src which encode proteins that

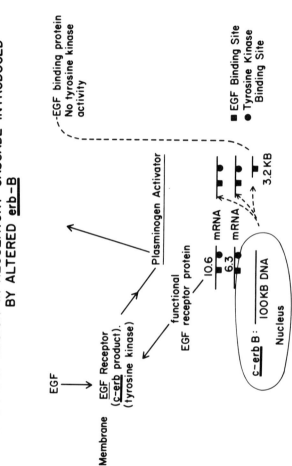

FIG. 2

POTENTIAL LESION IN REGULATORY CASCADE INTRODUCED
BY ALTERED erb-B

are membrane-associated and contain tyrosine-kinase activity. The v-erb B protein however does not show kinase activity. This anomaly has now been resolved by the finding that the nucleotide sequence of v-erb B protein represents a shortened version of the normal EGF receptor that lacks the tyrosine-kinase activity of this receptor (Lin, C.R. et al, 1984). Further light has recently been shed on this problem by the observation that A-431 carcinoma cells that show elevated levels of EGF receptor show an amplification of the EGF receptor gene. In addition this cell line shows a lesion in processing the RNA transcript of the 100 kilobase DNA region that encodes the full EGF receptor, so that a small 3.2 kilobase RNA that encodes a TGF binding site but not a tyrosine kinase site is produced in addition to the 6.3 and 10.6 kilobase RNA species that encode both the TGF binding and kinase sites. Significantly, the short fragment that carries only the TGF binding site is the predominant protein and is exported from the cell (Weber, W. et al, 1984). We may also note that down regulation of EGF receptors has recently been linked to pro-duction of plasminogen activator (Gross, J.L. et al, 1983), thus further extending the cascade.

Breast carcinoma has long been suspected of having a viral association but investigations of this relationship have been impeded by some of the technical difficulties associated with the MMTV that induces breast carcinoma in mice. Some recent advances deserve comment (Figure 3). First is the important observation that wild mice that do not transmit MMTV through the germ line may lack complete MMTV but harbor scattered nucle-otide sequences in their DNA that are homologous (albeit under relaxed hybridization conditions) to MMTV. Similar sequences homologous to MMTV are detectable in the human genome (Callaghan, R. et al, 1982). These findings can presently be interpreted as involving rearrangement of these elements in inbred mice in maturation of infectious MMTV or as fossil relics of an earlier MMTV-like infection. Second is the observation that a major fraction of MMTV-induced mammary carcinoma in C3H mice involve an insertion of MMTV adjacent to a gene designated Int I on mouse chromosome 15. Interestingly, the orientation of the MMTV inserts 5' or 3' to the Int I region is such as to preclude read out of the Int I gene under the influence of the viral promoter. In this dilemma the possible role of the enhancing elements in the MMTV-LTR has been invoked (Nusse, R. et al, 1984). In the BR6 strain mouse 17 of 40 tumors examined showed insertion of MMTV adjacent to a common gene designated Int 2 (Peters, G. et al, 1983). A third set of data from Cooper and

FIG. 3

POTENTIAL ROLE OF MTV IN MOUSE AND HUMAN BREAST CARCINOMA

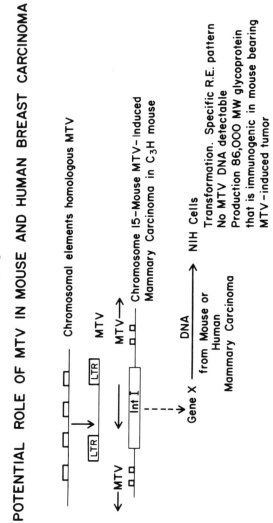

his associates involves observations or transformation of mouse NIH/3T3 cells on transfection with DNA either from mouse mammary carcinomas induced with MMTV or spontaneous human mammary carcinomas. The transfecting DNA in all cases gave a common enzyme restriction pattern, but no DNA homologous to MMTV-DNA was detectable in the transformed cells (Lane, M.A., Sainten, A. and Cooper, G.M., 1981). While the transforming gene (x) remains to be identified, its apparent product was precipitated with antisera from mice bearing tumors induced with MMTV (Becker, D. et al, 1982) as a glycopeptide (MW = 86,000). This strongly implies that the x gene product is associated with mammary carcinoma and its protein is immunogenic in the host. Further evaluation of the utility of this protein as a marker for breast cancer will be awaited with interest.

Potential biochemical mechanisms by which membrane-associated onc gene products mediate their effects can be tentatively postulated in light of recent developments in membrane biochemistry. The adenylate-cyclase mechanisms (Gilman, A., 1984; Figure 4) involves both stimulation and repression channels which are activated on binding of appropriate agonists to specific receptors. Activation of the receptors initiates a cascade of events including the key dissociation of either an activating $45K\alpha$ stimulating protein or a $41K\alpha$ inhibitory protein from binary or ternary complexes with simultaneous binding of GTP to the $45K\alpha s$ or $41K\alpha i$ proteins respectively. The GTP modified proteins then activate or repress the catalytic site of adenylate cyclase with consequent elevation or diminution of intracellular cyclic AMP. In turn the level of c-AMP regulates the activity of a c-AMP dependent kinase. In this scheme any of onc gene proteins with homology to the c-AMP dependent kinase site (src, fes, abl, erb B) could directly effect the c-AMP regulated pathway. The ras oncogene proteins can also be envisioned as providing competitive binding for GTP and thus deactivating the $45K\alpha s$ or $41K\alpha i$ proteins respectively. A second membrane-transduction system, which can be viewed as separate or coupled to the adenylate cyclase system and which involves the kinase C and phospholipids is shown in Figure 5. In this pathway phosphorylation of phosphatidyl insitol results in phosphatidyl-inositol-4,5 diphosphate (PI-4, 5P) Hydrolysis of PI-4,5P yields inositol triphosphate, which regulates elevation of Ca^{++}, and diacyl glycerol (DAG) which activates protein kinase C. The purified $pp60^{src}$ protein has recently been shown to successively convert PI to PI-4 and PI-4,5 (Y. Sugimoto el al, 1984).

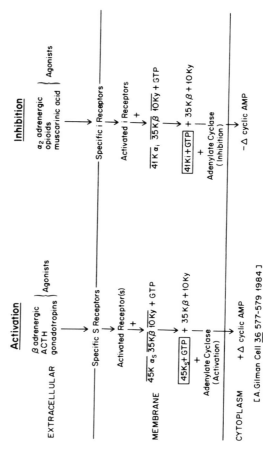

FIG. 4

Regulation of Cell via Adenylate Cyclase / G Proteins

FIG. 5

Role of SRC Oncogene on Kinase C / Phospholipid / Ca⁺⁺ Regulation

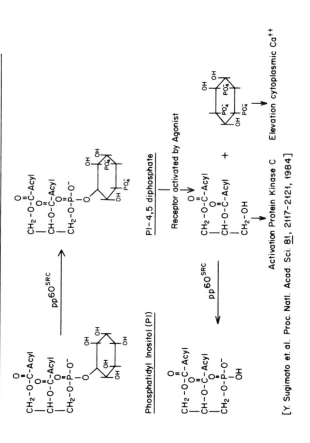

[Y. Sugimoto et. al. Proc. Natl. Acad. Sci. 81, 2117–2121, 1984]

Thus the src class of proto-oncogenes may also exert regulatory control through the protein kinase C/phospholipid pathway. It is of particular interest that phorbol diesters, which can act as tumor promoters, can also induce normal differentiation in myeloid leukemia cell lines. A direct action of the phorbol esters on kinase C, with subversion of the c-src regulatory element, is suggested by the recent finding of copurification of protein kinase C and the phorbol diester membrane receptor (Niedel, J. et al, 1983).

The rapidly expanding knowledge of the biochemical pathways that can be affected by oncogene proteins could well provide a rationale for the design of competitive inhibitors for restoration of normal differentiation to cells transformed by corresponding oncogenes. This knowledge might well rapidly expand the repertoire of reagents presently available as illustrated by differentiation agents currently available for reversion of the mouse myeloid leukemia cell line PU5-1.8 (Table 5) or human myeloid leukemia cell lines (Table 6). A delineation

Table 5

**INDUCED DIFFERENTIATION IN
MOUSE MONOCYTIC LEUKEMIA CELL LINE PU5-1.8**

Treatment	Products
Phorbol Myristate	MGF
Zymosan	Interleukin I
LPS	TNF
Lipid A	Plasminogen Activator
PPD	Elastase
	Collagenase
	Prostaglandins

[Ralph P. Broxmeyer HA, and Nakoinz I. J Expt Med 146,611; 1977]
[Mannel DN, Moore RN, and Mergenhagen SE. Infection and Immunity 523 1980]

Table 6

HUMAN MYELOID LEUKEMIA CELL LINES

Cell Line	Stage of Differentiation	Differentiation Inducer	Differentiated State	Reference
KG-1a	Early Myeloblast	None Known	—	Koeffler, H.P., et. al. Blood 56:265, 1980.
KG-1	Myeloblast	Phorbol Diesters. Teleocidin	Macrophage	Koeffler, H.P., Golde, D.W. Science. 200:1153, 1978.
ML-1*	Myelomonoblast	Phorbol Diesters. Teleocidin	Macrophage	Takeda, K., et. al. Cancer Res. 42:5152, 1981.
ML-2*	Myeloblast	?	?	— —
ML-3*	Myelomonoblast	Phorbol Diesters. Teleocidin	Macrophage	Takeda, K., et. al. Cancer Res. 42:5151, 1981.
U-937	Monocyte Like	Phorbol Diesters. Teleocidin	Macrophage	Sundstrom, C., Nillson, K. Int. J. Cancer. 17:565, 1976.
THP-1-(O)-(R)	Monoblast	Phorbol Diesters. Teleocidin	Macrophage	Tsuchiya, et. al. Int. J. Cancer. 26:171, 1980.
SU-DHL-1	Monocyte Precursor	?	?	Epstein, A.L., et. al. Cancer. 34: 1851, 1974.
HL-60	Promyelocyte	DMSO. DMF. Piperidone. HMBA Hypoxanthine Actinomycin 1,25 (OH)$_2$D$_3$ Retinoic Acid	Granulocyte + Macrophage	Collins, S.J., et. al. Nature. 270:347, 1977.

*Initiated at RPMI.

of the action of particular agents with specific onc gene
biochemical pathways could be informative. It also appears
pertinent to explore previously unsuspected links between
biochemical pathways that are known to regulate differentiation
processes and proto-oncogenes. In this context a possible
association between thyroxin receptors or steroid receptors
and oncogenes may merit examination in view of the roles of
thyroxin in metamorphosis of the frog, of ecdysone in moulting
of insects and of sex steriods in animal sexual differentiations
respectively. Clearly the rapidly evolving information on
proto-oncogenes and oncogenes is enlarging our biological
perspectives and providing promising new avenues for the
control of neoplasia.

REFERENCES

Adams, JM et al (1983). Proc Nat Acad Sci 80: 1982-1986.
Avery, OT, MacLeod, CM and McCary, M (1944). J Expt Med 79:
 137-158.
Barker, WC and Dayhoff, MO (1982). Proc Nat Acad Sci 79:
 2836-2839.
Becker, D, Lane, MA and Cooper, GM (1982). Proc Nat Acad
 Sci 79: 3315-3319.
Bishop, JM (1981). Cell 23: 5-6.
Callaghan, R, Drohan, W, Tronick, W and Schlom, J (1982).
 J Proc Nat Acad Sci
Callaghan, R et al (1982). Proc Nat Acad Sci 79: 4113-4117.
Campisi, J et al (1984). Cell 36: 241-247.
Cooper, GM (1982). Science 218: 801-806.
Czernilofsky, AP et al (1980). Nature 287: 198-203.
Dalla Favera et al (1983). Science 219: 963-967.
Dean, M et al (1983). Nature 305: 443.
deKlein, A et al (1982). Nature 300: 765-767.
Deul, TF et al (1983). Science 221: 1348-1350.
Diamond, A (1983). Nature 305: 112-116.
Doolittle, RF et al (1983). Science 221: 275-277.
Downward, J et al (1984). Nature 307: 521.
Gilman, AG (1984). Cell 36: 577-579.
Goldfarb, M et al (1982). Nature 296: 404.
Goubin, G et al (1983). Nature 302: 114-119.
Gross, JL et al (1983). Proc Nat Acad Sci 80: 2276-2280.
Guerrero, I et al (1984). Proc Nat Acad Sci 81: 202-205.
Hamlyn, PH and Rabbitts, TH (1983). Nature 304: 135-139.
Hayward, WS, Neel, BG and Astran, SM (1981). Nature 290: 475.
Housley, M (1983). Nature 303: 133.
Kelly, K et al (1983). Cell 35: 603-610.
Khoury, G and Gruss, P (1983). Cell 33: 313-314.

Kohl, NE et al (1983). Cell 35: 359-367.
Lane, MA, Sainten, A and Cooper, GM (1981). Proc Nat Acad Sci 78: 5185-5189.
Lane, MA, Neary, D and Cooper, GM (1982). Nature 300: 659-661.
Land, H et al (1983). Nature 305: 596.
Levy, LS, Gardner, MB and Casey, JW (1984). Nature 308: 853.
Lin, RC et al (1984). Science 224: 843-848.
Marquardt, H and Todaro, GJ (1982). J Biol Chem 257: 5220.
Mishikura, K et al (1983). Proc Nat Acad Sci 80: 4822-4826.
Muller, R et al (1982). Nature 229: 640.
Muller, R et al (1983). Nature 304: 454.
Mullins, JI et al (1984). Nature 308: 856.
Neil, JC et al (1984). Nature 308: 814-820.
Niedel, JE et al (1983). Proc Nat Acad Sci 80: 36-40.
Nusse, R et al (1984). Nature 307: 131-136.
Ozanne, R et al (1982). Nature 299: 744-747.
Parada, LF et al (1982). Nature 297: 474.
Parker, M (1983). Nature 304: 687-688.
Peters, G et al (1983). Cell 33: 369-377.
Pierce, GB (1974). Amer J Path 77: 103.
Reddy, EP et al (1982). Nature 300: 149-152.
Robbins, KC et al (1983). Nature 305: 605-608.
Ruley, HE et al (1983). Nature 304: 602.
Shimizu, K et al (1983). Proc Nat Acad Sci 80: 2112-2116.
Sorge, LK, Levy, BT and Maness, PF (1984). Cell 36: 249-257.
Swanstrom, R et al (1984). Proc Nat Acad Sci 81: 2117-2121.
Taub, R (1982). Proc Nat Acad Sci 79: 7837-7841.
Taub, R et al (1982). Nature 300: 143.
Tobin, CJ (1982). Nature 300: 143.
Todaro, G et al (1982). In: Tumor Cell Heterogeneity: Origins and Implications. A. Owens (ed). Academic Press, New York, Vol 4: 205-224.
Wang, JYJ et al (1984). Cell 36: 349-356.
Watson, DK et al (1983). Proc Nat Acad Sci 80: 2146.
Weber, W, Gill, GN and Spiess, J (1984). Science 224: 294.

**Molecular Basis of Cancer, Part A: Macromolecular
Structure, Carcinogens, and Oncogenes, pages 489–512**
© **1985 Alan R. Liss, Inc.**

CHEMICAL-VIRAL INTERACTIONS IN CELL TRANSFORMATION:
ENHANCEMENT OF HUMAN ADENOVIRUS TRANSFORMATION OF CLONED
RAT EMBRYO FIBROBLAST (CREF) CELLS BY ALKYLATING
CARCINOGENS

H. Hermo Jr., L.E. Babiss, W.S. Liaw, I.M.
Pinto,R.J. McDonald, P.B. Fisher[+]

Department of Microbiology, Cancer
Center/Institute of Cancer Research,
Columbia University,College of Physicians
and Surgeons, New York, NY 10032

INTRODUCTION

Although the majority of human cancers are believed to
be the consequence of exposure to chemical or physical
carcinogens (Hiatt et al, 1977; Weinstein et al, 1979),
there is now extensive evidence that chemicals and viruses
can interact synergistically in inducing specific cancers
in vivo and transformation in vitro (Fisher and Weinstein,
1980; Fisher, 1983a). The ability to study the
multifactor nature of carcinogenesis has been aided by the
development of well defined cell culture systems capable
of responding to the combined action of carcinogens and
viruses (For review see Fisher and Weinstein, 1981;
Fisher, 1983b). Analysis of the interactions between
chemical carcinogens and DNA tumor viruses, including
simian adenovirus 7, type 5 adenovirus (Ad5) and simian
virus 40, indicate that many carcinogens must be added to
cells either prior to or during viral infection for
enhancement of transformation (Casto, 1973; Casto et al,
1976; Fisher et al, 1978; Milo et al, 1978). This
temporal requirement suggests that the role of carcinogens
in modifying transformation by DNA viruses may involve
carcinogen-induced DNA damage and repair processes (Casto
et al, 1976). In contrast, carcinogen enhancement of cell
transformation induced by RNA viruses such as Rauscher
leukemia virus and mouse mammary tumor virus requires that
carcinogens be added to previously infected cells (Rhim et
al, 1971; Price et al, 1971; Howard et al, 1983). In
these systems enhancement of transformation may involve
the activation of cellular genes which interact

cooperatively with viral gene products in inducing stable transformation (Howard et al, 1983).

In addition to being multifactor in origin, the carcinogenic process also appears to involve multiple steps in its development. The most extensively studied animal model displaying the multistep nature of carcinogenesis is the two-stage mouse skin assay (For review see Boutwell, 1974; Hecker, 1975; Berenblum, 1975; Slaga et al, 1978). In this system, two qualitatively different stages, called initiation and promotion, have been identified. Initiating carcinogens are carcinogenic by themselves (solitary carcinogens), mutagenic and generate electrophiles which bind covalently to cell macromolecules, whereas tumor promoters are not solitary carcinogens or mutagenic and do not appear to require covalent binding to cell macromolecules as a prerequisite for biological activity (Weinstein et al, 1978a, 1978b; Slaga et al, 1978). A further complexity in attempting to define the stages of carcinogenesis has been the recent observation that even tumor promotion may involve several stages (Mufson et al, 1979; Slaga et al, 1980). A significant advance in studying the molecular basis of tumor promoter action has been the development of well characterized cell culture systems responsive to these agents. The most potent tumor promoting agents in cell culture as well as in vivo include TPA (12-0-tetradecanol-phorbol-13-acetate) and related diterpene esters and teleocidin and related indole alkaloids (For review see Fisher, 1983b). When added to cell cultures at concentrations as low as 10^{-8} to 10^{-11}M TPA and teleocidin induce numerous changes, including alterations in growth properties, programs of cell differentiation, cell membrane structure and function and enzymatic processes. The use of cell culture models for analyzing the process of initiation and promotion is further substantiated by the observation that TPA can enhance transformation of cells exposed to chemical carcinogens, UV-light, X-irradiation, and several DNA and RNA tumor viruses (For review see Fisher, 1983b).

ANALYSIS OF TYPE 5 ADENOVIRUS (Ad5) TRANSFORMATION USING THE CREF CELL LINE

The ability to analyze the molecular events involved

in adenovirus transformation of mammalian cells has been difficult because of the lack of a highly transformable cell culture system. Infection of heterogeneous rat embryo (RE) cells with group C adenoviruses, i.e. serotypes 1, 2 or 5, results in only a small fraction of cells integrating viral DNA and becoming stably transformed (usually $<10^{-5}$ transformants per infected cell) (Gallimore, 1974; Ginsberg et al, 1974). By systematically screening a series of cloned rat embryo cell cultures, a specific clone of Fischer rat embryo cells (CREF) was isolated which is transformed by Ad5 at a 100- to 200-fold higher frequency than primary or secondary RE cells (Fisher et al, 1982a). In addition, CREF cells remain contact inhibited at confluency, can be maintained at confluency for extended periods (>7 weeks at 37°C), do not form macroscopic colonies when seeded in agar, and do not induce tumors when injected into nude mice or syngeneic rats. Using the CREF system we have demonstrated that the potent tumor promoting agents TPA and teleocidin, epidermal growth factor and the bee venom polypeptide melittin enhance viral transformation when continually applied to cells previously infected with a temperature sensitive mutant of Ad5, H5ts125 (Fisher et al, 1980, 1981, 1982b). These observations indicate that the CREF-Ad transformation system should prove valuable in defining the molecular basis of tumor promoter action and the role of multiple factors in modulating viral transformation.

Infection of CREF cells with wild type Ad5 (H5wt) and growth at 39.5°C results in approximately a 3-fold higher transformation frequency than observed when infected cells are grown at 32 or 37°C (Fig. 1) (Fisher et al, 1982a). Infection of CREF cells with H5ts125 induces similar transformation efficiencies at 37 or 39.5°C, which are approximately 4-fold higher than found in H5ts125 infected cultures grown at 32°C (Fig. 1). When infected cells are grown at 32°C the frequency of H5wt and H5ts125 transformation is similar (Fisher et al, 1982a). Analysis of the pattern of DNA-integration by Southern blotting hybridization in H5wt-and H5ts125-transformed CREF clones isolated from 37 and 39.5°C cultures indicate that the complete Ad5 genome is present in the majority of transformants, whereas at 32°C the majority of H5wt transformed clones contain incomplete copies of the Ad5 genome while H5ts125 transformants contain complete copies

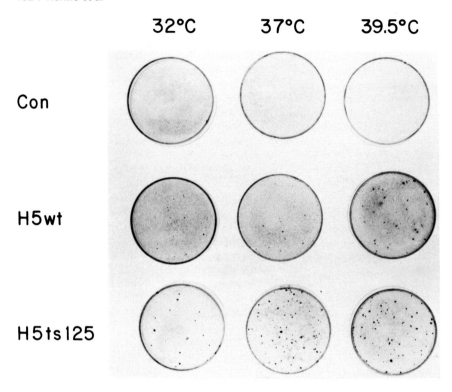

Figure 1. Effect of temperature on transformation of CREF cells by wild type 5 adenovirus (H5wt) and a temperature-sensitive mutant of Ad5 (H5ts125). CREF cells were mock-infected (control) or infected with 10 PFU/cell of H5wt or H5ts125, replated at 10^5 cells/5 cm dish and incubated at 32, 37 or 39.5°C. Four (39.5°C), five (37°C) or six (32°C) weeks post-infection plates were fixed with formaldehyde and stained with Giemsa. Further details can be found in Fisher et al (1981a, 1982a).

of the viral genome (Fisher et al, 1982a). Studies employing primary or secondary RE cells indicate that only part of the Ad5 genome (including the left end 15%, which contains the transforming genes of Ad5) is integrated in H5wt transformed clones isolated from infected cells grown at all three temperatures, whereas H5ts125 transformed RE clones isolated from cultures grown at 37 or 39.5°C contain the complete viral genome. In contrast, H5ts125 transformed RE clones isolated from 32°C cultures contain only the left end 15% of the viral genome. Since H5ts125 contains a mutation in the gene which encodes a 72,000-dalton (72-kd) DNA-binding protein, this viral gene product is functional at 32°C and is nonfunctional because of its temperature sensitivity at 37 or 39.5°C, a possible relationship may exist, therefore, between expression of this protein and viral DNA integration in RE cells (Ginsberg et al, 1974; Mayer and Ginsberg, 1977; Dorsch-Hasler et al, 1980). The observation that CREF cells can still integrate complete copies of the Ad5 genome at 32°C when infected with H5ts125 while at 32°C the transformation frequency is reduced to that found with H5wt indicates a dissociation between the effects of the 72-kd DNA-binding protein on viral DNA integration and transformation in CREF cells.

Studies utilizing host range (Graham et al, 1978; Solnick and Anderson, 1982) and host range deletion (Jones and Shenk, 1979) mutants of Ad5 suggest that the E1a (0 to 4.5 map units) and E1b (4.5 to 11.5 map units) transcriptional units are associated with the initiation and maintenance of transformation of rodent cells. A direct role of these Ad5 gene regions in transformation has come from studies in which the E1a or E1a + E1b region of Ad5 has been transferred into the appropriate target cells by Ca^{2+}-mediated DNA transfection (Graham et al, 1974; van der Eb et al, 1977; Houweling et al, 1980). Utilizing the CREF-transformation system we have demonstrated that the host range Ad5 mutant Hr1, which contains a single base pair deletion in E1a at position 1055 resulting in a 28,000 dalton instead of a 51,000 dalton protein, is cold sensitive for both establishment and maintenance of transformation (Babiss et al, 1983). When CREF cells are infected with Hr1 and grown at 37°C the frequency of transformation is approximately 5-fold higher than that observed in H5wt infected cells (Babiss et al, 1983; Montell et al, 1984). In contrast, growth of Hr1 infected CREF cells at 32°C for 6 weeks results in no or few discernible transformed foci depending on serum composition. Similarly, Hr1 transformed CREF clones display the transformed phenotype when grown at 37°C, but resemble the phenotype of untransformed CREF-cells when grown at 32°C. Temperature shift studies indicate that the defect in transformation is not at the level of DNA integration, transcription or mRNA production but most

likely is an effect resulting from the abnormal 28-kd
protein encoded by the defective E1a region of Hr1. To
directly determine whether the cold sensitive phenotype of
Hr1 was a consequence of the identified single-base
deletion in Hr1 or the result of a second missence
mutation a series of deletion and insertion mutations in
E1a were constructed (Babiss et al, 1984a). Analysis of a
series of mutant viruses containing engineered changes in
E1a and transfection analysis using the E1a and E1a + E1b
regions of Hr1 and the newly constructed viruses indicate
that cold sensitivity is a consequence of the defined
single-base change in E1a of Hr1. In addition, these
studies indicate that the cold sensitive transformation
phenotype is a consequence of E1a interacting with
cellular genes and does not require viral E1b gene
expression (Babiss et al, 1984a). These newly designed
viral mutants and their transforming E1a and E1b regions
(which have been cloned into plasmids, some of which carry
dominant selectable genes conferring neomycin or
mycophenolic acid resistance to transfected cells) should
prove valuable in defining the role of E1a and E1b gene
products in regulating initiation and maintenance of the
transformed phenotype (Babiss et al, 1983b, 1984a, 1984b).

EFFECT OF METHYLMETHANE SULFONATE (MMS) ON TRANSFORMATION
OF CREF CELLS BY WILD TYPE AND MUTANTS OF TYPE 5 ADENOVIRUS

In previous studies we have demonstrated that
pretreatment of secondary Sprague-Dawley RE cultures with
benzo(a)pyrene or 7,12-dimethylbenz(a)anthracene for 18 hr
prior to infection with H5ts125 results in a 2- to 4-fold
enhancement of transformation (Fisher et al, 1978). A
difficulty in attempting to use early passage cultures of
RE to investigate the mechanism(s) involved in
carcinogen-viral synergy is the heterogeneity of the
target cell population and the low efficiency of
transformation. The degree of carcinogen-induced
enhancement of viral transformation as well as the degree
of toxicity observed with specific carcinogens in
secondary RE cultures varies from experiment to experiment
and makes comparative studies difficult (Casto et al,
1976; Fisher et al, 1978). These problems may result
because RE cells are semipermissive for Ad2 and Ad5 and
contain at least two different cell populations: (a)
cells which can synthesize viral DNA, viral structural

Table 1

Effect of methylmethane sulfonate (MMS) on H5wt
and H5ts125 transformation of CREF cells

MMS (µg/ml)	Incubation Temperature (°C)[a]	Plating Efficiency (Fraction of Control)[b]	Transformed foci/10^5cells[c]	Transformation Frequency	Enhancement factor[d]
H5wt					
12	37	0.25	7.1	2.8×10^{-4}	3.4
	39.5	0.57	77.7	1.4×10^{-3}	0.9
25	37	0.07	3.2	4.6×10^{-4}	5.6
	39.5	0.38	65.4	1.7×10^{-3}	1.1
Solvent	37	1.00	8.2	8.2×10^{-5}	–
	39.5	1.00	145.0	1.5×10^{-3}	–
H5ts125					
12	37	0.12	81.0	6.8×10^{-3}	4.3
	39.5	0.42	262.0	6.2×10^{-3}	2.2
25	37	0.03	31.2	1.0×10^{-2}	6.3
	39.5	0.13	165.2	1.3×10^{-2}	4.6
Solvent	37	1.00	155.0	1.6×10^{-3}	–
	39.5	1.00	275.8	2.8×10^{-3}	–

[a]Following viral infection at 32°C CREF cells were replated at 10^5/50-mm
tissue culture plate and were grown at the indicated temperture for 6 weeks.
[b]Five 50-mm tissue culture plates were seeded with 250 or 500 cells each and
colonies were scored after 8 to 12 days at 37 or 39.5°C. The fraction of
cells surviving chemical treatment was obtained by dividing the total number
of colonies in treated cultures by the total number in solvent controls.
[c]Transformation assays were performed by plating 10^5 infected cells (10 PFU/cell
H5wt 37 and 39.5°C assays, 10 PFU/cell H5ts125 37°C assay or 20 PFU/cell
H5ts125 39.5°C assay) in each of ten 50-mm plates and feeding with reduced
calcium medium (0.1mM) twice per week. The mean number of transformed foci per
plate was determined after 6 weeks growth at 37°C. Transformation frequency is
expressed as the number of foci per 10^6 surviving cells. This calculation is
based on the assumption that, under these conditions, cell survival is not a
function of cell number.
[d]Enhancement factor is the transformation frequency in cells treated with MMS
relative to untreated controls.

proteins and infectious virus; and (b) cells which are
nonpermissive for viral replicative functions and can
integrate viral DNA and become stably transformed
(Gallimore, 1974; Fisher, 1983a). Different batches of RE
cultures may contain different proportions of the two cell
types which would explain the observed variations in
transformation frequencies between experiments employing
early passage RE cells.

Based on observations with RE cell cultures we
reasoned that a subset of RE cells should exist which were
resistant to Ad5 replication and consequently would
display an enhanced frequency of transformation. By
screening large numbers of cloned RE cultures from both
primary and established cell lines we have identified a
specific clone of the Fischer F2408 rat embryo cell line,

Table 2

Effect of MMS on H5hr1 transformation of CREF
cells grown at 39.5°C

MMS (μg/ml)	Plating Efficiency (Fraction of Control)[a]	Transformed foci/10⁵cells[b]	Transformation Frequency	Enhancement factor[c]
12	1.0	144	1.4×10^{-3}	1.4
18	1.0	143	1.4×10^{-3}	1.4
25	0.9	174	1.9×10^{-3}	1.9
37	0.6	197	3.3×10^{-3}	3.3
50	0.4	230	5.8×10^{-3}	5.8
Solvent	1.0	101	1.0×10^{-3}	–

[a]Plating efficiency was determined as described in Table 1.
[b]CREF cells were infected with 5 PFU/cell of Hr1. Assays were performed as described in Table 1 except assays were conducted for 5 weeks at 39.5°C.
[c]Determined as described in Table 1.

designated CREF, which is nonpermissive for Ad5 replication and is highly transformable by Ad5 (Fisher et al, 1980, 1981, 1982a). Pretreatment of CREF cells with MMS (6 to 25 μg/ml) results in enhanced H5ts125 transformation at both 37 and 39.5°C, but only enhances H5wt transformation at 37°C (Table 1). With both H5ts125 and H5wt, enhancement of transformation did not involve an increase in the absolute number of transformed foci above solvent treated controls but rather reflects an increase in transformation frequency when normalized for cell toxicity (Casto, 1973). In contrast, pretreatment of CREF cells with 25 to 100 μg/ml MMS prior to infection with Hr1 and growth at 32, 37 or 39.5°C results in an increase in the absolute number of transformed foci in comparison with solvent pretreated controls as well as an increase in transformation frequency when normalized for cell toxicity (Table 2 and Fig. 2). With all three viruses, transformed foci developed faster in carcinogen-pretreated cultures.

The mechanism underlying the difference in viral-chemical synergy between Hr1 and the other viral preparations (H5wt and H5ts125) is not known. Studies employing permissive human cell cultures, such as HeLa and KB, suggest that Hr1 is deficient in its ability to accumulate virus-specific early RNA (Berk et al, 1979; Jones and Shenk, 1979). Experiments using protein synthesis inhibitors, such as cycloheximide or anisomycin, suggest that one function of E1a is to inactivate a cellular gene product which functions as a negative

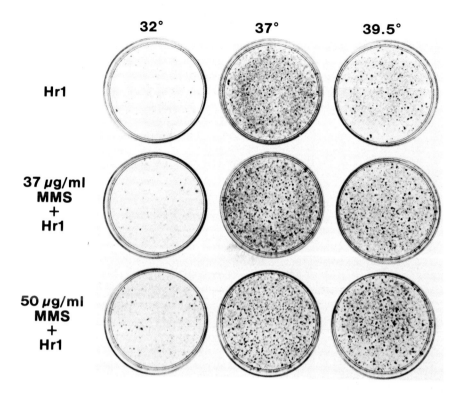

Figure 2. Effect of methylmethane sulfonate (MMS) on transformation of CREF cells at 32, 37 and 39.5°C by a host-range mutant of type 5 adenovirus (Hr1). CREF cells were pretreated for 2 hr with solvent or various levels (3 to 100 µg/ml) of MMS, infected with 5 PFU/cell of Hr1, replated at 10^5 cells/5 cm dish and incubated at 32, 37 or 39.5°C. Five weeks post-infection plates were fixed with formaldehyde and stained with Giemsa. Further details can be found in Fisher et al (1981a, 1982a) and Babiss et al (1983a).

regulator of viral gene expression (Nevins, 1981; Katze et al, 1982, 1983). We have recently shown that the tumor promoter TPA can suppress the transcription-delay phenotype of Hr1 without restoring its ability to replicate (Carter et al, 1984) and can induce transformation at 32°C in Hr1 infected CREF cells (Babiss, Carter, Milovanovic and Fisher, unpublished data). Based on these observations it is possible that MMS treatment of CREF cells results in the inactivation of a cellular repressor, thereby, permitting more efficient expression of early Ad5 genes and consequently a faster appearance of foci as well as an increase in the frequency of Hr1 transformation of CREF cells. By using viral mutants with specific transformation phenotypes and transfection analysis with the E1a and E1b regions of H5wt and recently engineered mutant viruses it should now be possible to directly test this hypothesis.

EFFECT OF MMS ON VIRAL DNA INTEGRATION IN Hr1-TRANSFORMED CREF CELLS

Carcinogen pretreatment could enhance viral transformation by: (a) increasing the number of copies, or specific regions, of viral DNA integrated on a per cell basis, thereby increasing the probability of individual cells becoming transformed; or (b) increasing the number of cells in an infected population that integrate viral DNA, thereby increasing the likelihood that more cells will become stably transformed (Fisher et al, 1980, 1981b). To test the hypothesis that carcinogens alter the pattern of viral DNA integration in transformed cells we have analyzed by liquid hybridization (C_0t analysis) and filter hybridization (Southern blotting) a series of H5ts125 transformed RE clones which were isolated from cultures pretreated with solvent or carcinogen (benzo(a) pyrene or dimethylbenz(a)anthracene) prior to viral infection (Fisher et al, 1980; Dorsch-Hasler et al, 1980). No specific differences were detected in either the location of viral DNA or in the number of copies of the transforming genes (E1a and E1b) in cells pretreated with solvent or carcinogen prior to infection with H5ts125 (Dorsch-Hasler et al, 1980). Possible explanations for the absence of differences in integration patterns between carcinogen- and solvent-pretreated cultures include: (a) Viral DNA integration does not involve a specific chromosomal site and carcinogens only randomly increase the number of potential integration sites; (b) Specific viral integration sites do exist in RE cells but these regions differ for different cell types within the heterogeneous RE population and a much larger analysis of transformed clones would be required to detect these differences; or (c) Carcinogen enhancement of transformation does not involve a specific alteration in the site of integration or the number of transforming genes which are integrated.

To determine what effect MMS pretreatment has on the pattern of viral DNA integration in Hr1-transformed CREF clones, chromosomal DNA was isolated from 6 solvent and 6 MMS pretreated clones and analyzed by filter hybridization (Fig. 3). Cellular DNA was cleaved with the restriction endonucleases BamH1 and Xba1, the fragments were separated by electrophoresis in 0.6% agarose, transferred to nitrocellulose sheets by blotting and hybridized to a 0 to 3.85 map unit Ad5 DNA fragment labeled with ^{32}P by nick-translation (Dorsch-Hasler et al, 1980; Fisher et al, 1982a). The pattern of integration of the E1a transforming gene was distinct for each cloned cell line and no consistent alteration was found in either the site of viral DNA integration or the number of integration sites following carcinogen pretreatment. These findings with the cloned CREF cell line support the observations with RE transformants indicating that carcinogens do not enhance viral transformation by specifically altering the pattern of viral DNA integration in transformed cells. Experiments now in progress suggest that the ability of carcinogens to enhance CREF transformation results because more CREF cells within the infected cell population originally contain and subsequently integrate viral DNA following carcinogen treatment.

EFFECT OF MMS PRETREATMENT ON THE PHENOTYPE OF Hr1-TRANSFORMED CREF CLONES

When compared to normal secondary Sprague-Dawley RE cells, most H5ts125-transformed clones display reduced population doubling times, reduced serum requirements, reduced calcium dependence, increased saturation densities, increased plasminogen activator production, reduced quantities of a large external transformation sensitive (LETS) protein, reduced [^{125}I]-epidermal growth factor binding, increased lectin agglutinability and decreased anchorage dependence (Fisher et al, 1979a, 1979b, 1980b; Goldstein and Fisher, 1980; Fisher and Weinstein, 1981b). Certain phenotypes, i.e. growth in

**Solvent
Pretreated** **Carcinogen (MMS)
Pretreated**

C C C C C   37 37 50 50 50
1 2 3 6 8 M   1 4 1 3 4

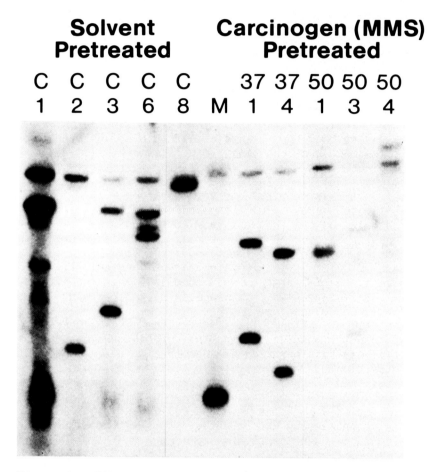

Figure 3. Filter hybridization (Southern blotting) analysis of type 5 adenovirus E1a sequences integrated into chromosomal DNA in solvent- and MMS-pretreated Hr1-transformed CREF clones. A 10µg quantity of cellular DNA isolated from the cloned cell lines indicated was cleaved with BamH1 and XbaI (which will generate a 0 to 3.85 map unit Ad5 fragment if the E1a gene is present). The fragments were separated by electrophoresis in 0.6% agarose, transferred to nitrocellulose sheets by blotting and hybridized to a 0 to 3.85 map unit Ad5 DNA fragment (isolated from pLB213, which contains the 0 to 4.5 map unit region of H5wt) labeled with ^{32}P by nick translation. Further details can be found in Fisher et al (1982a) and Babiss et al (1983a).

agar or reduced calcium and altered cell surface glycoproteins, were acquired earlier in transformed clones obtained from carcinogen-plus-virus treatment (Fisher et al, 1979a; Goldstein and Fisher, 1980; Fisher and Weinstein, 1981b). With repeated serial subculture or exposure to TPA certain phenotypes were either transiently or stably induced in early passage solvent-pretreated H5ts125-transformed RE clones (Fisher et al, 1979a, 1979b, 1979c; Fisher and Weinstein, 1981b).

In previous studies we have demonstrated that Hrl-transformed CREF cells are cold sensitive for maintenance of the transformed phenotype (Babiss et al, 1983a). When Hrl-transformed CREF clones are grown at 37°C they exhibit similar saturation densities, growth rates and agar cloning efficiencies as H5wt-transformed CREF cells. However, when grown at 32°C cells transformed by Hrl at 37°C display a similar saturation density as normal CREF cells and grow with a lower efficiency in agar than H5wt-transformed clones. To determine if carcinogen pretreatment alters the transformation phenotype of Hrl-transformed cells, a series of transformed foci were isolated from cells pretreated with solvent or MMS before infection with Hrl and pure single cell clones from each focus were generated (Fisher et al, 1978, 1982a). The agar cloning efficiency of solvent pretreated clones isolated from 39.5°C cultures varied between 6 and 37%, whereas the agar cloning efficiency of MMS-pretreated Hrl-transformed clones varied from 38 to 87% (Table 3). In addition, the average size of agar colonies from carcinogen-pretreated Hrl-transformed clones was larger than in solvent-pretreated Hrl-transformed clones. Carcinogen pretreatment did not alter cold sensitive expression of anchorage-independence in Hrl-transformed clones, i.e. growth at 32°C still resulted in a lower efficiency in agar growth and smaller colonies than observed when the same Hrl-transformed clone was grown in agar at 37 or 39.5°C (Table 3). The differential in agar growth between 32 and 39.5°C in solvent-pretreated and MMS-pretreated Hrl-transformed clones varied from only a 2-fold to a >2900-fold reduction at 32°C. With some clones, such as Hrl-39-C2, Hrl-39-C6 and Hrl-39-37-6, no colonies developed when 5×10^3 cells were seeded at 32°C, whereas with other clones, such as Hrl-39-C8, Hrl-39-50-3 and Hrl-39-50-4, agar cloning efficiencies of >13% were observed at 32°C. A direct relationship between relative

Table 3

Agar Cloning Efficiencies of Adenovirus (hrl) Transformed
CREF Clones Isolated from Cultures Pretreated with Solvent
or MMS Prior to Virus Infection

| Cell Type[a] | Agar Cloning Efficiency (%)[b] | | | |
	39.5°C	Colony Size	32°C	Colony Size
CREF	<0.001	–	<0.001	–
E11-NMT	38 ± 4	5	36 ± 3	5
wt-3A	37 ± 4	2+	40 ± 3	2+
A2-Agar	63 ± 5	4+	27 ± 2	2
Hrl-g8t	29 ± 2	2	<0.02	–
Solvent-Pretreated Hrl-Transformed				
Hrl-39-C1	14 ± 0.7	1	7 ± 0.3	1
Hrl-39-C2	20 ± 1.4	1	<0.02	–
Hrl-39-C3	10 + 0.2	1	1 ± 0.2	1+
Hrl-39-C6	11 ± 0.5	1	<0.02	–
Hrl-39-C7	6 ± 0.3	1	0.06 ± 0.02	1
Hrl-39-C8	37 ± 1.2	1	13.8 ± 0.3	1
MMS-Pretreated Hrl-Transformed				
Hrl-39-37-1	87 ± 3.0	2+	9.2 ± 0.3	1+
Hrl-39-37-4	38 ± 0.8	1+	8.7 ± 0.4	1
Hrl-39-37-6	58 ± 4.4	1+	<0.02	–
Hrl-39-50-1	42 ± 1.5	2	3.7 ± 0.2	1+
Hrl-39-50-3	73 ± 3.7	2	24.3 ± 0.5	1+
Hrl-39-50-4	42 ± 2.4	1+	14.0 ± 0.4	1

[a]E11-NMT: a nude mouse tumor-derived subclone of E11 cells (E11 is an H5ts125–
transformed Sprague-Dawley RE clone); wt-3A: an H5wt-transformed CREF clone;
A2-Agar: an H5hrl-transformed CREF clone selected from a colony growing in
0.4% agar; hrl-g8t: a CREF clone transformed by the 0 to 15.5 map unit region
of H5hrl; Solvent-pretreated Hrl-transformed clones: single cell clones isolated
from cultures originally preexposed to 0.01% solvent (95% ethanol) prior to
infection with hrl; MMS-pretreated hrl-transformed clones: single cell clones
isolated from cultures originally preexposed to MMS (37 or 50 μg/ml) prior to
infection with hrl.
[b]Agar assays were performed as previously described (Fisher et al, 1979a; 1983).
CREF cells were seeded at 10^5 cells/50–mm plate and all other cell types were
seeded at $5x10^3$ cells/50–mm plate. Base layers consisted of 0.8% agar and
overlay medium with cells was 0.4% agar prepared in Dulbecco's modified Eagle's
medium with 10% fetal bovine serum. Colony size is based on a 1 to 5 rating
with 5 being ≥2mm and 1 being ≤0.2mm.

cloning efficiency at 39.5°C and growth at 32°C in the
various Hrl-transformed clones was not apparent, i.e.
clones with high agar growth potential at 39.5°C did not
always display high growth potential at 32°C and clones
with low agar growth potential at 39.5°C did not always
display low growth potential at 32°C.

The complex biochemical changes involved in the
conversion of a normal cell into a transformed cell are
not known. Potentially important mediators of these
changes may be polypeptide growth factors which are

produced in large quantities by cells transformed by a diverse group of agents, including RNA tumor viruses, chemical carcinogens and DNA viruses (De Larco and Todaro, 1978, 1980; Ozanne et al, 1980; Moses et al, 1981; Kaplan et al, 1981; Kaplan and Ozanne, 1982; Twardzik et al, 1982; Fisher et al, 1983). In the case of murine sarcoma virus transformed rodent cells, De Larco and Todaro (1978, 1980) have identified polypeptides with molecular weights of 7 to 10,000 which can induce thymidine incorporation in serum-depleted untransformed normal rat kidney (NRK) cells, morphological changes in NRK cells which mimic those observed in transformed NRK cells and can also induce growth in agar of normally anchorage-dependent NRK cells. In addition, this transforming growth factor (TGF) was able to inhibit the binding of $[^{125}I]$-EGF to cell surface receptors presumably because it can occupy the EGF receptor, although there is evidence from immunoreactivity and molecular weight that this TGF is distinct from EGF (De Larco and Todaro, 1980) and specific receptors for TGFs which are distinct from EGF have been identified (Colburn and Gindhart, 1981). In contrast, although TGFs have been isolated from SV40- and polyoma virus-transformed rodent cells which induce growth in agar of normal cells, SV40- and polyoma virus-transformed cells do not display a reduction in $[^{125}I]$-EGF binding and presumably do not produce TGFs which can bind to the EGF receptor (Todaro et al, 1976). The importance of TGFs in the continued expression of the transformed phenotype is suggested by recent studies employing rat cells transformed by a temperature-sensitive (ts) mutant of Kirsten murine sarcoma virus (Ozanne et al, 1980; De Larco et al, 1981). In these cells, growth at the permissive viral temperature (32 or 33°C) was associated with a reduced $[^{125}I]$-EGF binding, a transformed morphology and TGF production, whereas at the nonpermissive viral temperature (39°C) the cells regained the ability to bind $[^{125}I]$-EGF, exhibited a more normal appearance and did not produce TGFs capable of inducing growth in agar of untransformed cells. Purification of TGFs from the ts mutants at 32°C indicated that it was not temperature-sensitive, suggesting that growth factor production was regulated by viral transforming genes and that the TGFs were probably of cellular origin (De Larco et al, 1981).

In previous studies, we have demonstrated that

Table 4

Epidermal Growth Factor (EGF) Binding in Hrl-Transformed CREF
Clones Isolated from Cultures Pretreated with Solvent or
MMS Prior to Virus Infection

Cell Type[a]	^{125}I-EGF Binding (cpm/10^6 cells)[b]					
	Specific Binding 32°C	% of Control 32°C	Specific Binding 37°C	% of Control 37°C	Specific Binding 39.5°C	% of Control 39.5°C
CREF	4277	100	4914	100	4674	100
E11-NMT	155	4	29	<1	166	4
A2-Agar	3984	93	1562	32	683	15
Solvent-Pretreated Hrl-Transformed						
Hrl-39-C1	4576	107	2243	46	2602	56
Hrl-39-C2	6185	145	3061	62	2554	55
Hrl-39-C3	6991	163	4037	82	3362	71
Hrl-39-C6	7479	175	2322	47	2179	47
Hrl-39-C7	7751	181	2828	58	2336	50
Hrl-39-C8	6235	146	2737	56	2488	53
MMS-Pretreated Hrl-Transformed						
Hrl-39-37-1	9214	215	2633	54	2021	43
Hrl-39-37-4	7294	171	2485	51	2075	44
Hrl-39-37-6	5081	119	2484	51	1338	29
Hrl-39-50-1	7872	184	4198	85	3464	74
Hrl-39-50-3	7306	171	2361	48	1969	42
Hrl-39-50-4	6276	147	2685	55	1999	43

[a] For designation of cell types refer to Table 3.
[b] ^{125}I-EGF binding assays were performed as previously described by Fisher
et al (1983). Specific binding is calculated by subtracting binding in the
presence of excess unlabelled EGF from binding in samples receiving ^{125}I-EGF.
Cells were grown at the indicated temperature for 1 week prior to performing
binding assay studies.

Ad5-transformed RE cells behave differently than SV40- or
polyoma virus-transformed cells in that they display a
dramatic (>97%) reduction in [^{125}I]-EGF binding to cell
surface receptors (Fisher et al, 1980b). In subsequent
studies, we have found that Ad5- (H5wt or H5ts125)
transformed CREF cells and Ad5-transformed Syrian hamster
embryo cells also bind lower levels of EGF than
untransformed cells, whereas Ad5-transformed human
embryonic kidney cells (cell line 293) and KB cells
containing and expressing the transforming genes of Ad5 do
not exhibit a reduction in EGF-binding (Fisher et al,
1983). Concentrated serum-free medium from
Ad5-transformed RE cells was able to stimulate growth in
agar of CREF cells and inhibit [^{125}I]-EGF binding in
CREF cells (Fisher et al, 1983). As can be seen in Table
4, when assayed at 39.5°C Hrl-transformed CREF clones
bound less EGF than untransformed CREF cells. In general,

the level of reduction of EGF binding in comparison with CREF cells was somewhat less for most transformed-clones when they were grown and subsequently assayed for EGF-binding at 37°C as opposed to 39.5°C. When binding assays were conducted at 32°C in cells which had been previously grown for 1 week at 32°, the level of EGF-binding in all of the solvent- and carcinogen-pretreated Hr1-transformed clones either exceeded or were similar to the level of EGF-binding observed in CREF cells (Table 4). Studies are presently in progress to determine: (a) if cold sensitive expression in [^{125}I]-EGF binding in Hr1-transformed clones results because production of TGFs are regulated in a cold sensitive manner or if the TGFs are themselves cold sensitive; and (b) if the type of TGFs produced by carcinogen-pretreated Hr1-transformed cells are the same or different than those produced by solvent-pretreated Hr1-transformed cells. In addition, by constructing cells (via Ca^{2+}-mediated DNA-transfection) which contain only the E1a (0 to 4.5 map units) or E1a + E1b (0 to 11.5 map units) region of H5wt and Hr1 it will also be possible to determine which transformation phenotypes are regulated by E1a (or E1a + E1b) gene products and what effect carcinogens have on the expression of these phenotypes in E1a and E1a + E1b transformed clones.

SUMMARY

A major advance in studying carcinogenesis has been the development of well defined cell culture systems which mimic in vitro carcinogenesis as it occurs in vivo. Utilizing these systems, stages analogous to initiation, promotion and progression have been identified and important insights into the molecular events involved in these processes should be forthcoming. In this review we describe some of our recent studies using the highly transformable CREF cell line to investigate the interactions between MMS and Ad5 in regulating the frequency of viral transformation and expression of the transformed phenotype. Our findings indicate that carcinogens enhance Ad5 transformation, but do not alter the pattern of viral DNA integration into cellular DNA or the qualitative expression of the transformed state. A likely hypothesis is that certain carcinogens exert their enhancing effect on DNA virus transformation by increasing the proportion of cells in an infected culture which can stably integrate viral DNA and thereby become transformed. In other cases, carcinogens may enhance DNA virus transformation by altering the expression of viral and/or cellular genes required for establishment of the transformed state.

Human T-cell leukemia virus, herpes viruses and Hepatitis B virus have been implicated in the development of specific human malignancies, but a direct link between viruses and the majority of human neoplasms has not been demonstrated. A possible reason for this apparent negative correlation may be that in most human malignancies putative viruses cause cancer via synergistic interactions with initiating chemical carcinogens, tumor promoters, hormones or other yet to be defined cofactors. Well characterized cell culture systems should prove instrumental in elucidating the role of multiple-factor interactions in the etiology of human cancer, as well as lead to an understanding of the basic principles underlying the processes of tumor promotion and progression.

ACKNOWLEDGEMENTS

We thank Barbara Hamilton for assistance in the preparation of this review article. This research was supported by a grant from the Council for Tobacco Research (CTR-1532 and CTR-1532/R1).

REFERENCES

Babiss LE, Fisher PB, Ginsberg HS (1984a). Deletion and insertion mutations in early region 1a of type 5 adenovirus that produce cold-sensitive or defective phenotypes for transformation. J Virol 49:731.
Babiss LE, Fisher PB, Ginsberg HS (1984b). Mutational analysis of the functional domains of the Ad5 E1a gene products effecting cell transformation. In Ginsberg HS, Vogel HJ (eds): "Transfer and Expression of Eukaryotic Genes," Arden House Conference: New York, in press.
Babiss LE, Ginsberg HS, Fisher PB (1983a). Cold sensitive expression of transformation by a host-range mutant of

type 5 adenovirus. Proc Natl Acad Sci USA 80:1352.

Babiss LE, Young CSH, Fisher PB, Ginsberg HS (1983b). Expression of adenovirus E1A and E1B gene products and the Escherichia coli XGPRT gene in KB cells. J Virol 46:454.

Berenblum I (1975). Origin of the concept of sequential stages of skin carcinogenesis. In Becker FF (ed): "Cancer, A Comprehensive Treatise," vol 1, New York: Plenum Pub Corp, p 323.

Berk AJ, Lee F, Harrison T, Williams J, Sharp PA (1979). Pre-early adenovirus 5 genome product regulates synthesis of early viral messenger RNAs. Cell 17:935.

Boutwell RK (1974). The function and mechanism of promoters of carcinogenesis. CRC Crit Rev Toxicol 2:419.

Carter TH, Milovanovic ZZ, Babiss LE, Fisher PB (1984). Accelerated onset of viral transcription in adenovirus-infected HeLa cells treated with the tumor promoter 12-0-tetradecanoyl-phorbol-13-acetate. Mol Cell Biol 4:563.

Casto BC (1973). Enhancement of adenovirus transformation by treatment of hamster cells with ultraviolet-irradiation, DNA base analogs and dibenz (a,h)-anthracene. Cancer Res 33:402.

Casto BC, Pieczynski WJ, Janosko N, DiPaolo JA (1976). Significance of treatment interval and DNA repair in the enhancement of viral transformation by chemical carcinogens and mutagens. Chem Biol Interact 13:105.

Colburn NH, Gindhart TD (1981). Specific binding of transforming growth factor correlates with promotion of anchorage independence in EGF receptorless mouse JB6 cells. Biochem Biophys Res Commun 102:799.

De Larco JE, Todaro GJ (1978). Growth factors from murine sarcoma virus-transformed cells. Proc Natl Acad Sci USA 75:4001.

De Larco JE, Todaro GJ (1980). Sarcoma growth factor (SGF): specific binding to epidermal growth factor (EGF) membrane receptors. J Cell Physiol 102:267.

De Larco JE, Peston, YA, Todaro GJ (1981). Properties of a sarcoma-growth-factor-like peptide from cells transformed by a temperature-sensitive sarcoma virus. J Cell Physiol 109:143.

Dorsch-Hasler K, Fisher PB, Weinstein IB, Ginsberg HS (1980). Patterns of viral DNA integration in cells transformed by wild type or DNA-binding protein mutants of type 5 adenovirus and the effect of chemical carcinogens on integration. J Virol 34:305.

Fisher PB, Weinstein IB, Eisenberg D, Ginsberg HS (1978). Interactions between adenovirus, a tumor promoter, and chemical carcinogens in the transformation of rat embryo cell cultures. Proc Natl Acad Sci USA 75:2311.

Fisher PB, Goldstein NI, Weinstein IB (1979a). Phenotypic properties and tumor promoter induced alterations in rat embryo cells transformed by adenovirus. Cancer Res 39:3051.

Fisher PB, Dorsch-Hasler K, Weinstein IB, Ginsberg HS (1979b). Tumor promoters enhance anchorage-independent growth of adenovirus-transformed cells without altering the integration pattern of viral sequences. Nature 281:591.

Fisher PB, Bozzone JH, Weinstein IB (1979c). Tumor promoters and epidermal growth factor stimulate anchorage-independent growth of adenovirus transformed rat embryo cells. Cell 18:695.

Fisher PB, Weinstein IB (1980). Chemical-viral interactions and multistep aspects of cell transformation. In Montesano R, Bartsch H, Tomatis L (eds): "Molecular and Cellular Aspects of Carcinogen Screening Tests," Intl Agency Res Cancer, IARC Sci Pub No 27, p 113.

Fisher PB, Dorsch-Hasler K, Weinstein IB, Ginsberg HS (1980a). Interactions between initiating chemical carcinogens, tumor promoters and adenovirus in cell transformation. Teratogenesis Carcinogenesis Mutagenesis 1:245.

Fisher PB, Lee LS, Weinstein IB (1980b). Changes in epidermal growth factor receptors with adenovirus transformation, chemical carcinogen transformation and exposure to a phorbol ester tumor promoter. Biochem Biophys Res Commun 93:1160.

Fisher PB, Weinstein IB (1981a). In vitro screening tests for potential carcinogens. In Sontag JM (ed): "Carcinogens in Industry and the Environment," New York: Marcel Dekker Inc, Ch 6, p 113.

Fisher PB, Weinstein IB (1981b). Enhancement of cell proliferation in low calcium medium by tumor promoters. Carcinogenesis 2:89.

Fisher PB, Mufson RA, Weinstein IB, Little JB (1981a). Epidermal growth factor, like tumor promoters, enhances viral- and radiation-induced cell transformation. Carcinogenesis 2:183.

Fisher PB, Babiss LE, Weinstein IB, Ginsberg HS (1982a).

Analysis of type 5 adenovirus transformation with a cloned rat embryo cell line (CREF). Proc Natl Acad Sci USA 79:3527.

Fisher PB, Miranda AF, Mufson RA, Weinstein LS, Fujiki H, Sugimura T, Weinstein IB (1982b). Effects of teleocidin and the phorbol ester tumor promoters on cell transformation, differentiation and phospholipid metabolism. Cancer Res 42:2829.

Fisher PB, Weinstein IB, Goldstein NI, Young CSH, Carter TH (1982c). Modulation of adenovirus transformation and replication by chemical carcinogens and phorbol ester tumor promoters. In Rich MA, Furmanski P (ed), "Biological Carcinogenesis," New York: Marcel Dekker Inc, p 261.

Fisher PB (1983a). Chemical-viral interactions in cell transformation. Cancer Invest 1:495.

Fisher PB (1983b). Enhancement of viral transformation and expression of the transformed phenotype by tumor promoters. In Slaga TJ (ed), "Tumor Promotion and Cocarcinogenesis In Vitro, Mechanisms of Tumor Promotion," Fla: CRC Press Inc, p 57.

Fisher PB, Boersig MR, Graham GM, Weinstein IB (1983). Production of growth factors by type 5 adenovirus transformed rat embryo cells. J Cell Physiol 114:365.

Gallimore PH (1974). Interactions of adenovirus type 2 with rat embryo cells. Permissiveness, transformation and in vitro characteristics of adenovirus transformed rat embryo cells. J Gen Virol 25:263.

Ginsberg HS, Ensinger MJ, Kauffman RS, Mayer AJ, Lundholm U (1974). Cell transformation: a study of regulation with types 5 and 12 adenovirus temperature-sensitive mutants. Cold Spring Harbor Symp Quant Biol 39:419.

Goldstein NI, Fisher PB (1980). Surface properties of normal and adenovirus transformed rat embryo cells. J Cell Sci 45:87.

Graham FL, Abrahams PJ, Mulder C, Heijneker HL, Warnaar SO, DeVries FAJ, van der Eb AJ (1974). Studies on in vitro transformation by DNA and DNA fragments of human adenovirus and SV40. Cold Spring Harbor Symp Quant Biol 39:637.

Graham FL, Harrison T, Williams J (1978). Defective transforming capacity of adenovirus type 5 host-range mutants. Virol 86:10.

Hecker E (1975). Cocarcinogens and cocarcinogenesis. In Grundmann E (ed) "Handbuch der Allgemeinen Patholgie, vol IV/6, Gerswulste, Tumors II." Berlin,

Heidelberg: Springer Verlag, p 651.

Hiatt HH, Watson JD, Winsten JA (1977). Origins of Human Cancer. Cold Spring Harbor Conf on Cell Proliferation, vol 4, books A, B and C.

Houweling A, van der Elsen PJ, van der Eb AJ (1980). Partial transformation of primary rat cells by the leftmost 4.5% fragment of adenovirus 5 DNA. Virol 105:537.

Howard DK, Schlom J, Fisher PB (1983). Chemical carcinogen-mouse mammary tumor virus interactions in cell transformation. In Vitro 19:58.

Jones N, Shenk T (1979). Isolation of Ad5 host-range deletion mutants defective for transformation of rat embryo cells. Cell 15:205.

Kaplan PL, Topp WC, Ozanne B (1981). Simian virus 40 induces the production of a polypeptide transforming factor(s). Virol 108:484.

Kaplan PL, Ozanne B (1982). Polyoma virus-transformed cells produce transforming growth factor(s) and grow in serum-free medium. Virol 123:372.

Katze MG, Persson H, Philipson L (1981). Control of adenovirus gene expression: posttranscriptional control mediated by both viral and cellular gene products. Mol Cell Biol 1:807.

Katze MG, Persson H, Johansson BM, Philipson L (1983). Control of adenovirus gene expression: cellular gene products restrict expression of adenovirus host range mutants in nonpermissive cells. J Virol 46:50.

Mayer AJ, Ginsberg HS (1977). Persistence of type 5 adenovirus DNA in cells transformed by a temperature-sensitive mutant, H5ts125. Proc Natl Acad Sci USA 74:785.

Milo GE, Blakeslee JR, Hart R, Yohn DS (1978). Chemical carcinogen alteration of SV40 virus induced transformation of normal human cell populations in vitro. Chem Biol Interact 22:185.

Montell C, Courtois G, Eng C, Berk AJ (1984). Complete transformation by adenovirus 2 requires both E1a proteins. Cell 36:951.

Moses HL, Branum EL, Proper JA, Robinson RA (1981). Transforming growth factor production by chemically transformed cells. Cancer Res 41:2842.

Mufson RA, Fischer SM, Verma AK, Gleason GL, Slaga TJ, Boutwell RK (1979). Effects of 12-O-tetradecanoylphorbol-13-acetate and mezerein on epidermal ornithine decarboxylase activity, isoproterenol-stimulated levels of cyclic adenosine 3':5'-monophosphate, and induction of mouse skin tumors in vivo. Cancer Res 39:4791.

Nevins JR (1981). Mechanism of activation of early viral transcription by the adenovirus E1a gene product. Cell 26:213.

Ozanne B, Fulton RJ, Kaplan PL (1980). Kirsten murine sarcoma virus transformed cell lines and a spontaneously transformed rat cell line produce transforming factors. J Cell Physiol 105:163.

Price PJ, Freeman AE, Lane WT, Huebner RJ (1971). Morphological transformation of rat embryo cells by the combined action of 3-methylcholanthrene and Rauscher leukemia virus. Nature New Biol 230:144.

Rhim JS, Vass W, Cho HY, Huebner RJ (1971). Malignant transformation induced by 7, 12-dimethylbenz (a) anthracene in rat embryo cells infected with Rauscher leukemia virus. Intl J Cancer 7:65.

Slaga TJ, Sivak A, Boutwell RK (1978). Mechanisms of Tumor Promotion and Cocarcinogenesis. Carcinogenesis vol 2. New York: Raven Press.

Slaga TJ, Fischer SM, Nelson K, Gleason GL (1980). Studies on the mechanism of skin tumor promotion: evidence for several stages in promotion. Proc Natl Acad Sci USA 77:3659.

Solnick D, Anderson MA (1982). Transformation-deficient adenovirus mutant defective in expression of region 1A but not region 1B. J Virol 42:106.

Todaro GT, De Larco JE, Cohen S (1976). Transformation by murine and feline sarcoma viruses specifically blocks binding of epidermal growth factor to cells. Nature 264:26.

Twardzik DR, Todaro GJ, Marquardt H, Reynolds, FH Jr, Stephenson JR (1982). Transformation induced by Abelson murine leukemia virus involves production of a polypeptide growth factor. Science 216:894.

van der Eb AJ, Mulder C, Graham FL, Houweling A (1977). Transformation with specific fragments of adenovirus DNAs. I. Isolation of specific fragments with transforming activity of adenovirus 2 and 5 DNA. Gene 2:115.

Weinstein IB, Wigler M, Fisher PB, Sisskin E, Pietropaolo C (1978a). Cell culture studies on the biological effects of tumor promoters. In Slaga TJ, Sivak A, Boutwell RK (eds), "Mechanisms of Tumor Promotion and Cocarcinogenesis" vol 2, New York: Raven Press, p 313.

Weinstein IB, Wigler M, Yamasaki H, Lee LS, Fisher PB, Mufson A (1978b). Regulation of the expression of certain biologic markers of neoplasia. In Ruddon RW (ed), "Biological Markers of Neoplasia: Basic and Applied Aspects" New York: Elsevier North Holland Inc, p 451.

Weinstein IB, Yamasaki H, Wigler M, Lee LS, Fisher PB, Jeffrey A, Grunberger D (1979). Molecular and cellular events associated with the action of initiating carcinogens and tumor promoters. In Griffin AC, Shaw CR (eds), "Carcinogens: Identification and Mechanisms of Action", New York: Raven Press, p 399.

Molecular Basis of Cancer, Part A: Macromolecular
Structure, Carcinogens, and Oncogenes, pages 513–523
© 1985 Alan R. Liss, Inc.

TUMOR PROMOTERS — AN OVERVIEW OF MEMBRANE-ASSOCIATED ALTERATIONS AND INTRACELLULAR EVENTS

Charles E. Wenner, Ph.D., K. J. Leister, B.A.,
L. D. Tomei, Ph.D., Department of Experimental
Biology, Roswell Park Memorial Institute, Buffalo,
NY 14263 and Comprehensive Cancer Center, The
Ohio State University, Columbus, OH 43210

Pioneering studies of Berenblum helped establish our present concepts of initiation and promotion stages of carcinogenesis (for reviews see Berenblum, 1954, 1974). Tumor promoters lack carcinogenic activity by themselves but they can enhance the yield of tumors after administration of a low dose of an initiating carcinogen. It is reasonable to consider that initiating carcinogens damage DNA, which can lead to the subsequent emergence of an aberrant stem cell population. It is possible that the role of the tumor promoter is to inhibit normal death and promote proliferation of stem cells (Kanter et al, 1982; Kanter et al 1984) as well as to "turn on" their altered differentiation functions. Phorbol ester interaction with specific receptors that normally control the replication and differentiation of stem cells would then lead to a stable cell population which grows autonomously in the absence of tumor promoter.

Much of the available evidence to date indicates that tumor promoters act by epigenetic mechanisms, presumably by changes in events which are membrane associated. It is our view that the primary epigenetic mechanisms involve the following: 1) activation of cell cycle; 2) prevention of DNA breakdown.

It appears that tumor promoters are capable of altering the fundamental ability of cells to regulate their normal function. This subversion of the normal physiological pathways in many cell types involves activation of cell cycle but it is also evident that tumor promoters can influence differentiation. It can be inferred from such observations that the tumor promoter agent can subvert normal physiological regulatory pathways, perturb feedback regulatory systems, and under specific conditions associated with a primary carcinogenic insult, lead to the expression of neoplasia.

In the cells which we have studied most extensively, C3H 10T$\frac{1}{2}$ mouse fibroblasts, tumor promoting agents such as the phorbol esters and indole alkaloids, activate cell cycle. This is in accord with many studies which indicate, as a rule, tumor promoting agents are mitogenic (see Trewyn and Gatz, 1984). However, in other cell types such as human HL-60 cells, these same tumor promoting agents "push" cells into differentiation pathways, subverting G_1 regulatory systems. In either case, the epigenetic effects involve phenotypic changes.

In addition to effects on growth and differentiation, tumor promoting agents appear to be capable of blocking a cell suicide program referred to as apoptosis by Williams et al (1974). Apoptosis is the process by which cells initiate massive DNA fragmentation which preceeds cell death in response to diverse toxic stresses. These toxic stresses include beta-emission from incorporation of high specific activity tritiated thymidine into DNA, exposure to various toxic chemicals, and physiological stresses such as serum deprivation in vitro. Apoptosis is likely a result of specific gene expression since it is actinomycin- and cycloheximide-sensitive. We have observed that at least in one type of cell stress, tumor promoting agents can prevent this cell suicide program (Kanter et al, 1984). Therefore, we consider that two closely related epigenetic mechanisms may be involved in tumor promotion: 1) modification of phenotype and 2) retention into a viable compartment of a cell population otherwise destined for elimination following exposure to a cytotoxic insult. The consequence of these effects results in the emergence of a stable and transformed cell population.

The intent of this report is to briefly examine two aspects of tumor promoter-induced responses. 1) How tumor promoters bring about increase in DNA synthesis and cell divisions, and 2) how they exert protective effects in preventing cells from breaking down their DNA when cells are subject to stress conditions. Further, it focuses on the question Do these epigenetic processes occur at the cell membrane? Some of the earliest actions of tumor promoting agents involve membrane associated changes which entails binding of the promoter to membrane associated enzymes and changes in the regulation of specific ion movements.

We would like to initially discuss the basis for the study of tumor promoter stimulation of cell proliferation. First, several tumor promoting agents such as phorbolesters and indole alkaloids markedly amplify the proliferative effects of serum and other proliferative stimuli in vitro. Analogs which are inactive as tumor promoters are available which can serve as suitable controls to evaluate properties essential to tumor promotion. Second, tumor promoters activate protein kinase C whose activity is normally controlled by the products of phosphatidyl inositol metabolism associated with rapid cell proliferation (see Kikkawa, et al, 1983).

Recently protein kinase C has been found to be involved in signal transduction mediated by growth factors. Agonists interact at the cell membrane which initiates release of a new type of second messenger. This system is described in Fig. 1, and the possible bypass of the normal pathway by tumor promoters is outlined. Hydrolysis of phosphatidyl-inositols has been demonstrated to produce second messengers which act as modifiers of cell function (Downs and Michell, 1982). The effectors are namely diacylglycerol, and inositol 1,4,5-triphosphate which are associated with Ca^{2+} release. Oncogene products (such as those of the ros and src gene) have recently been demonstrated to enhance phosphorylation of phosphatidyl inositol which results in increased concentrations of these second messengers (Macara et al, 1984; Sugimito et al, 1984). Thus, oncogene products may have a regulatory role whereby pathways normally present in the cell are turned on. It is through these pathways that cell cycle is activated, and it is believed that by stimulating enzymes such as protein kinase C tumor promoters exert their pleiotropic effects.

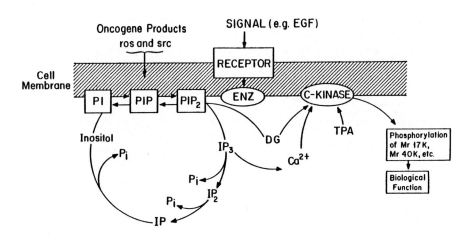

Figure 1

Do different classes of tumor promoters share similar structural moieties by which they interact with putative receptor sites?

The availability of a number of different types of tumor promoters has led to the question as to whether these agents share a common receptor. Phorbol esters are tetracyclic diterpene esters isolated from the Euphorbia plant species (Hecker, 1978), whereas teleocidins are indole alkaloids isolated from Streptomyces (Fujiki et al, 1981). Studies of structure-activity relationships by Weinstein and colleages have been based upon binding studies which involve displacement of or competition with ^{3}H-phorbol dibutyrate (^{3}H-PDBU). As pointed out by Horowitz et al (1983), the unsaturated keto group at C-3, a primary hydroxyl group at C-20, a hydroxyl group at C-4, and a lipophilic ester at C-12 are necessary for maximal activity. Similarly, carbonyl, amino, and hydroxyl groups in teleocidin, as well as the indole nitrogen may serve as analogous functional groups involved in the binding to its high affinity receptor (Fig. 2).

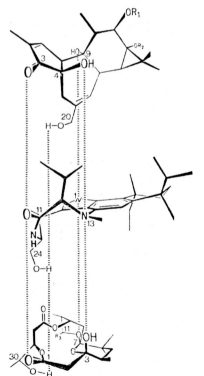

Figure 2. Perspective drawings of TPA (top), dihydrohydroteleocidin B (middle), and aplysiatoxin (bottom). The dotted lines connect heteroatoms whose spatial positions could correspond with one another (Weinstein et al, 1984). Permission of Dr. I.B. Weinstein and FASEB.

Despite substantial evidence that promoting agents such as phorbol esters, teleocidin, and aplysiatoxins bind to and act through a common set of receptors, there are some discrepancies. It appears that the polyacetate, debromoaplysiatoxin binds very weakly to the ^{3}H -PDBU receptor yet it is equipotent in stimulating release of ^{3}H - arachidonic acid from C3H 10T$\frac{1}{2}$ and ^{3}H -choline from CREF fibroblast (Horowitz et al, 1983). Further, debromoaplysiatoxin exerts biological effects at concentrations considerably less than that which it appears to bind to the above mentioned receptor. Therefore, it may be necessary to consider alternative explanations for the subtle difference between various classes of tumor promoting agents. One attractive view is that the effects of these agents are each dependent on perturbation of common membrane protein-lipid interactions, which are highly specific in view of the low concentrations required to exert biological effects.

It has been established that TPA interacts with phospholipid monolayers and bilayers (Jacobson et al, 1975; Wenner et al 1974). Dipalmityl phosphatidyl choline interacts with low mole fractions of TPA which results in a marked decrease in the heat of the minor phase transition as measured by differential scanning calorimetry (Jacobson et al, 1975). Dawson et al (1983) have also demonstrated recently that diacyl glycerol, an activator of protein kinase C when Ca^{2+} is present, facilitates hydrolysis by phospholipase A$_2$ (PLA$_2$) and phospholipase C of phospholipids such as phosphatidyl-choline (PC) or phosphatidyl-inositol, (PI). Presumably perturbation of the tightly packed bilayer structure by head group interaction makes the substrate accessible to the enzyme. Also, it could be demonstrated that 1,3 or 1,2 diolein reversed the inhibition of phospphatidylethanolamine hydrolysis by PLA$_2$ induced by PC to cause a hexagonal-to-bilayer conformation change in the structure of the hydrated substrate. As Dawson et al (1983) have proposed, it is possible that "insertion of the smaller hydrophilic head group of diacyl glycerol into the phospholipid bilayer allows better access of the active center of the enzyme to the susceptible bonds of the phospholipid." It is, therefore, feasible to propose that insertion of phorbol esters and related compounds behave in an analogous manner since "diacylglycerols" also induce inhibition of minor phase transitions. Thus, localized concentrations of TPA in a cell membrane or the presence of TPA at a specific membrane protein-lipid site may play a specific role in activating intracellular enzymes that are critical to proliferative and other biological events.

Correlation of tumor promoter–induced ouabain–sensitive ion movements with cell cycle activation

Studies in our laboratories have focused upon the role of ions in the proliferation of cells in vitro. It is not known whether promoter-induced ion movements are mediated by activation of protein kinase C. However, we have observed that tumor promoting agents induce striking changes in K^+ influx which we believe are essential to the expression of increased cell proliferation.

Interest in the regulation of cell proliferation has been renewed based upon results of studies which indicate that ion movements are intimately involved in G_1- S transitions. As described earlier, cell proliferation is normally controlled by the availability of endogenous growth factors and divalent cations have been implicated as a "second messenger" in this induced response (Boynton et al, 1982). These investigators demonstrate that the cell cycle state in which Ca^{2+} is involved is late G_1 just prior to S phase entry. The redistribution of Ca^{2+} plays an important role in the signal for DNA synthesis and tumor promoters apparently bypass or lessen the requirements for Ca^{2+}.

It was demonstrated by Quastel and Kaplan (1970) that ouabain could block S phase entry of lymphocytes stimulated by plant lectins implicating enhanced $(Na^+ - K^+)$-ATPase as a prerequisite for mitogenesis. Based on this, it was of interest to examine the role of Na^+/K^+ movements in tumor promoter-induced cell cycle activation. In our laboratory, we have found tumor promoters to be useful to follow advancement of cells through G_1 into the S phase. Cells staged in G_1 by serum deprivation or growth factor depletion can be demonstrated to move in synchrony in large number following cell cycle activation (Tomei et al, 1983). If tumor promoters were present during the staging, then re-activation of cell cycle revealed that a distinctly different state was associated with G_1 arrest compared with cells arrested by serum deprivation alone. It was then possible to compare the roles of $(Na^+ - K^+)$-ATPase in different G_1 states.

Earlier studies in both Swiss 3T3 and C3H-10T$\frac{1}{2}$ cells indicated that tumor promoters induced a rapid increase in $(Na^+ - K^+)$-ATPase activity (Wenner et al, 1981). Divergent responses have since been observed with tumor promoter-induced K^+ fluxes mediated by $(Na^+ - K^+)$-ATPase activity. However, we have found that the ability to consistently demonstrate direct stimulation of K^+ influx is quite dependent on maintenance of the following general conditions: a) Cells must be in the G_1 phase of the cell cycle since optimal $^{86}Rb^+$ uptake is observed immediately preceeding or at the point of S phase entry. b) Maximal responses are observed when cells are post-confluent quiescent (ie, G. phase arrest). An adequate basis for any proposal of a specific mechanism for the role of ion movements in mitogenesis requires study at intervals over an an extended time period. Single time point determinations without detailed knowledge of kinetics may be misleading.

After reaching a specific point in G_1 cells appear to be committed to DNA synthesis, and we have demonstrated that after cells progress to a certain stage in G_1, DNA synthesis becomes refractory to inhibition by ouabain (Leister et al, 1984). This state was found to be restricted to late G_1, two hours prior to S phase. Transition in ouabain-sensitivity has been observed using cultures which were initially low density, exponentially proliferating as well as high density, quiescent and by using two independent staging techniques. Therefore, the property of ouabain resistance is probably independent of growth state and density of the cell cultures.

It should be pointed out that this point in time for ouabain sensitivity transition is proximal to that of the "restriction point" described by Pardee (Pardee, 1974; Campisi et al, 1982). The control of growth in normal and neoplastic cells as proposed by Rossow et al (1979) is dependent on different rates of protein degradation. These authors have suggested that a regulatory protein with a half life of 2.5 h may be stabilized in transformed cells, and that a critical level of this protein is necessary for the commitment of cells to DNA synthesis.

The similarity between Pardee's "restriction point" with our "ouabain-sensitivity transition" leads to the question whether a critical factor for DNA synthesis may be dependent upon $(Na^+ = K^+)$-ATPase activity. With regard to the role of $(Na^+ - K^+)$-ATPase activity prior to this critical point in G_1, one may consider the following: 1) the ionic environment has a critical regulatory role in translational and/or transcriptional processes. 2) $(Na^+ - K^+)$-ATPase activity has been implicated in cell volume control; cells may need to reach a volume threshold level before S-phase entry can proceed. 3) $(Na^+ - K^+)$-ATPase activity has been shown to be tightly coupled to the bioenergetics of cells and in several cases, rapid growth has been associated with an increased rate of glycolysis.

The studies of Santalo and Wenner (1982) on the effects of variations of $(Na^+ - K^+)$-ATPase activity have indicated that the ionic environment has a critical regulatory role in translational and/or transcriptional processes. It has been shown that variations in the $(Na^+ - K^+)$-ATPase activity induced in human lymphocytes have a differential effect on protein and DNA synthesis. Concentrations of K^+ (0.1 - 0.3 mM) in the range of the apparent Km of $(Na^+ - K^+)$-ATPase induced incorporation of ^{3}H-uridine and ^{3}H-leucine but not ^{3}H-Thd into the acid-insoluble fraction. Only when the concentration of K^+ was increased to 0.7 mM was DNA synthesis observed. These findings suggested that the signal for DNA synthesis is different from that of RNA synthesis. Similar conclusions were later reached by Burns and Rozengurt (1984).

Further studies using various concentrations of ouabain led to considerable support for the role of K^+ movements in cell cycle regulation. Inhibition of DNA synthesis could be seen with 5×10^{-10}M ouabain (0.7 m M K^+), whereas, higher concentrations of 10^{-9}M or greater were required to inhibit protein and RNA synthesis. The same type of discrimination between synthesis of RNA and synthesis of DNA could be observed using cycloheximide. Cycloheximide (20 ng/ml) inhibited $(^3$H)-Thd incorporation but much greater concentrations (200-300 ng/ml) were required to decrease ^{3}H-uridine or ^{3}H-leucine incorporation. Similar responses were obtained with TPA or DHTB-induced activation of cell cycle in C3H 10T½ cells with the above-mentioned inhibitors used to vary $(Na^+ - K^+)$-ATPase (manuscript in preparation).

The similarity of results obtained with cycloheximide, low K^+ concentrations or low concentrations of ouabain supports a common inhibitory mechanism. This implies that a specific "initiator" protein (s) exists which is highly sensitive to a decreased activity of the cation pump or alternatively the requirement for its synthesis could be greater than that of other proteins. In either instance, the signal to enter the cell division cycle is dependent on the $(Na^+ - K^+)$-ATPase pump activity which can influence "initiator" protein synthesis.

**Relationship of tumor promotion to prevention of
  DNA fragmentation**

A number of cytotoxic effectors includng beta-irradiation, adriamycin, alkylating agents, and other chemical carcinogens lead to site specific DNA damage suggestive of an endonuclease I type activation (Kanter et al, 1982). The conclusion that endonuclease activities are involved is based on the non-random fragmentation pattern as indicated by the sharp peaks obtained in our gradient studies (Kanter et al, 1984) similar to those reported by Williams et al, 1974. Endonucleases can attack sites on nucleosomal linker regions but their regulation is not yet understood. It is relevant that tumor promoters in some cases can prevent genomic breakdown which is probably mediated by a DNAase I-type activity (Kanter et al, 1984). Apoptosis appears to be closely associated with regulation of DNAase I endonuclease and involves new protein synthesis. However, it is not clear whether tumor promoters affect a regulatory function of the endonuclease or alter the concentration and/or activity of the enzymes itself. There is the possibility that tumor promoters affect covalent modifications (phosphorylation) of the endonuclease target sites or perturb cytoskeletal entities (e.g. monomeric actin is an inhibitor of DNAase I) resulting in a direct modulation of endonuclease action. Each of these possibilities can arise from membrane-associated reactions. Non-repair associated DNA fragmentation may result in decreased cell survival and tumor promoters such as the phorbol esters and indole alkaloids may inbibit a generalized breakdown of the genome sufficiently to allow replication of even a small number of affected cells. Retention of cells which contain an inheritable transformed genome can lead to a stable, clonigenic population which has a transformed phenotype.

Berenblum, I (1954) A Speculatiave Review: The Probable Nature of Promoting Action and its Significance in the Understanding of the Mechanism of Carcinogenesis. Cancer Res 14:471

――― (1974) Carcinogenesis is a Biological Problem. Amsterdam: North Holland; New York: Elsevier.

Campisi J, Medrano, EE, Morreo G, Pardee AB (1982) Restriction Point Control of Cell Growth by a Labile Protein: Evidence for Increased Stability in Transformed Cells. Proc Natl Acad Sci 79:436

Dawson RMC, Hemington NL, Irvine RF (1983) Diacylglycerol Potentiates Phospholipase Attack Upon Phospholipid Bi-layers: Possible Connection with Cell Stimulation. Biochem Biophys Res Commun 117:196

Downes P, and Michell, RH (1982) Phosphatidylinositol 4-phosphate and Phosphatidylinositol 4,5-bis phosphate: Lipids in Search of a Function. Cell Calcium 3:467

Hecker, E (1978) Structure-activity Relationshlip in Diterpene Esters Irritant and Cocarcinogenic to Mouse Skin. In: Slaga TJ, Sivak A, and Boutwell lR (eds) Carcinogenesis: A Broad Critique Vol 2 p ll Raven Press

Horowitz AD, Fujiki H, Weinstein IB, Jeffrey A, Akin E, Moore, RE, Sugimura T (1983) Comparative Effects of Aplysiatoxin, Debromoaplysiatoxin, and Teleocidin on Receptor Binding and Phospholipid Metabolism. Cancer Res 43:1529

Jacobson K, Wenner CE, Kemp G, Papahadjopoulos, D (1975) Surface Properties of Phorbol Esters and their Interaction with Lipid Monolayers and Bilayers. Cancer Res 35:2991

Kanter PM, Tomei LD, Wenner CE (1982) TPA Suppression in Non-repair associated DNA Fragmentation in Murine and Human Cells. Proceedings 13th Int Cancer Congress Abstracts Sept 8-15, 1982, Seattle, WA p 542

Kanter PM, Leister KJ, Tomei LD, Wenner PA, and Wenner CE (1984) Epidermal Growth Factor and Tumor Promoters Prevent DNA Fragmentation by Different Mechanisms. Biochem Biophys Res Commun 118:392

Kikkawa V, Takai Y, Tanaka Y, Miyake R, and Nishizuka Y (1983) Protein Kinase C as a Possible Receptor Protein of Tumor-promoting Phorbol Esters. J Biol Chem 258:11442

Leister KJ, Tomei LD, and Wenner CE (1984) Correlation between Tumor Promoter-Induced Ion Movements and Cell Cycle Activation. Proc Am Assoc for Cancer Research 25:314

Macara IG, Marinetti GV, Balduzzi PC (1984) Transforming Protein of Avian Sarcoma Virus UR2 is Associated with Phosphatidylinositol Kinase Activity: Possible Role in Tumorigenesis. Proc Natl Acad Sci 81:2728

Pardee, AB (1974) A Restriction Point for Control of Normal Animal Cell Prolilferation. Proc Natl Acad Sci 71:1286

Quastel MR, and Kaplan JG (1970) Early Stimulation of Potassium Uptake in Lymphocytes Treated with PHA. Exptl Cell Res 63:230

Rossow PW, Riddle VGH, and Pardee AB (1979) Synthesis of Labile, Serum-dependent Protein in Early G1 Controls Animal Cell Growth. Proc Natl Acad Sci 76:4446

Burns CP and Rozengust E (1984) Extracellular Na$^+$ and initiation of DNA. Synthesis: Role of Intracellular pH and K$^+$. J Cell Biol 98:108

Santalo RC and Wenner CE (1982) Effects of low K$^+$ and Ouabain on Phytohemagglutinin-induced Macromolecular Synthesis in Human Lymphocytes. In International Workshop on Membranes in Tumor Growth. Instituto Italiano di Medicina Sociale - Rome p 209.

Sugimoto Y, Whitman M, Cantley LC, Erikson RL (1984) Evidence that the Rous Sarcoma Virus Transforming Gene Product Phosphorylates Phosphatidylinositol and Diacylglycerol. Proc Natl Acad Sci 81:2117

Tomei LD, Cheney JC, and Wenner CE (1981) The Effect of Phorbol Esters on the Proliferation of C3H 10T½ Mouse Fibroblasts: Consideration of both Stimulatory and Inhibitory Effects. J Cell Physiol 197:385

Trewyn, R and Gatz, HB (1984) Altered Growth Properties of Normal Human Cells Induced by Phorbol-12,13-Didecanoate. In Vitro 20:409.

Wenner CE, Cheney JC, Tomei LD (1981) Cell Cycle Activation and Ouabain-sensitive Ion Movements of 3T3 and C3H 10T½ Fibroblasts. J Supramol Struc and Cell Biochem 15:161

Weinstein IB, Gattoni-Celli S, Kirschmeier P, Hsiao W, Horowitz A, Jeffrey A (1984) Cellular Targets and Host Genes in Multistage Carcinogenesis. Fed Proc 43:2287.

Williams JR, Little JB, and Shipley WH (1976) Association of Mammalian Cell Death with a Specific Endonucleolytic Degradation of DNA. Nature 252:754

Molecular Basis of Cancer, Part A: Macromolecular
Structure, Carcinogens, and Oncogenes, pages 525–536
© 1985 Alan R. Liss, Inc.

SOME ELECTROSTATIC ASPECTS OF THE INTERACTION BETWEEN DNA OR
LIPIDS AND WR-2721 OR ITS METABOLITE WR-1065

Dan Vasilescu, Marie-Agnès Rix-Montel, Hubert Kranck,
Henri Broch and Eric Savant-Ros
Biophysics Laboratory, I.P.M., Nice University, Parc Valrose
06034 NICE CEDEX - France

INTRODUCTION

The phosphorylated aminothiol WR-2721 [S-2(3-aminopro-
pylamino) ethylphosphorothioic acid] is a multifunctional
drug. This molecule, derived from cysteamine, is known to be
the most effective radioprotector (Yuhas 1970) ; this drug
administrated to animals before irradiation with U.V., X or
γ rays is able to reduce the radiation injury. An other
aspect of WR-2721 is its intervention in cancer therapy
(Yuhas 1980). In vivo, this compound can protect normal and
malignant tissues in a differential manner (Yuhas, Storer
1969). It was shown that normal tissues absorb the drug readily while solid tumors do not (Yuhas and coll 1980 a).
Recently, phase I trials of WR-2721 were performed before
radiation therapy (Turrisi and coll 1983). On another hand
WR-2721 is able to increase the potentiality of chemotherapy
with cis-platin (Yuhas, Culo 1980 ; Yuhas and coll 1980 b).

In vitro studies have demonstrated that WR-1065 - the
free sulfhydryl part of WR-2721 - is the metabolic fraction
penetrating the cell membrane and able to interact with
nucleus (Harris, Phillips 1971 ; Purdie 1979). Consequently,
these drugs transport accross the cell membrane is also important (Purdie 1979, Ritter and coll 1982).

At the molecular level, it appears that DNA and lipids
are the most important targets for these molecules. In this
paper, we present some experimental and theoretical investigations related to the electrostatic properties of WR-2721
and WR-1065 themselves, and also, significant aspects of

these molecules interaction with DNA or with synthetic
lecithin.

ELECTROSTATIC PROPERTIES OF WR-2721 AND WR-1065

Dielectric Conductivity

When WR-2721 and WR-1065 (solid state forms are : WR-2721,
H_2O and WR-1065, 2HCl) are dissolved in water or neutral
salts such as NaCl, they take ionized forms. For WR-1065 we
obtain a bication :

$$NH_2-(CH_2)_3-NH-(CH_2)_2-SH, 2HCl \rightleftharpoons \overset{+}{N}H_3-(CH_2)_3-\overset{+}{N}H_2-(CH_2)_2-SH + 2Cl^-$$

and for WR-2721 the zwitterionic form :

$$NH_2-(CH_2)_3-NH-(CH_2)_2-S-PO_3H_2 \rightleftharpoons \overset{+}{N}H_3-(CH_2)_3-\overset{+}{N}H_2-(CH_2)_2-S-PO_3^{--}$$

The ionic conductivities of these drugs may be estimated by dielectric measurements in high frequency domain ; in
this case no electrode polarization occurs. The conductivity
of a liquid dielectric sample is expressed by :

$$\sigma = \sigma_i + \sigma_D$$

where σ_i is the ionic conductivity and σ_D the dielectric
relaxation contribution. At our frequency measurement (1MHz)
we are out of a relaxation zone and $\sigma_D \simeq 0$. Thus :

$$\sigma = \sigma_i = \varepsilon_0 K^{-1} R_p^{-1}$$

with : ε_0 = permittivity of free space ; K = cell measurement constant ; R_p = parallel resistance measured by impe-
dance bridge.

Thus the ionic conductivities of WR-1065 and WR-2721
are :

$$\sigma_{WR-1065, 2HCl} = \sigma_{WR-1065^{++}} + \sigma_{2Cl^-} = ne \left[(z\mu)_{WR-1065^{++}} + 2 \mu_{Cl^-} \right]$$

$$\sigma_{WR-2721} = ne (z\mu)_{WR-2721}$$

where : n = number of ions per cubic meter ; e = protonic
charge ; z = charge fraction ; μ = electrical mobility.

Figure 1 gives results obtained for the two compounds
dissolved in water. The observed linear behaviour of conductivity σ versus the drug concentration is in agreement with
the above equations. From these measurements we can deduce
the $(z\mu)$ values :

$$(z\mu)_{WR-2721} \simeq 2 \times 10^{-8} \, m^2 \, sec^{-1} \, volt^{-1} \quad and$$

$$(z\mu)_{WR-1065^{++}} \simeq 14 \times 10^{-8} \, m^2 \, sec^{-1} \, volt^{-1}$$

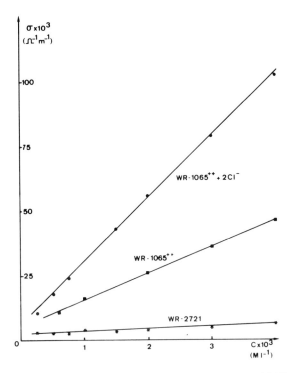

Fig. 1. Ionic conductivity of WR-2721 and WR-1065 in water versus drug concentration C at 1 MHz and 25°C.

We observe that a charge fraction $z \neq 0$ exists for the zwitterion WR-2721 ; this situation is probably correlated with the ionization state of the phosphate group. Concerning WR-1065[++], if we assume that $z \simeq 2$ for this bication, the resulting value of the electrical mobility $\mu \simeq 7 \times 10^{-8}$ m^2 sec^{-1} $volt^{-1}$ is similar to chloride anion one at the same temperature 25°C.

Quantum Mechanical Computations on WR-1065

Conformational energy computations and charge distribution have been conducted using PCILO and GAUSS-100 ab-initio methods. The nomenclature, geometries and angular definitions adopted for aminothiols are detailed in previous works (Broch

and coll. 1980 ; Broch and coll. 1982). We present here the
results concerning the Mulliken atomic net charge distribution (obtained by using minimal gaussian orbital bases con-
tracted into 5,2/3 for the first-row atoms and into 5,2,2/
3,2 for the sulfur atom) for the neutral and bicationic
forms of WR-1065 in their minimal energy conformations
(first determined by PCILO computations). From Mulliken atomic net charges, we can deduce the charges concentrated on
each chemical group like NH_2, CH_2, SH, etc ... We have also
calculated the electrostatic potential resulting from the
charge distribution on each molecule by using a program elaborated in our laboratory.

    The obtained results, for charge distribution in neutral
and bicationic forms of WR-1065, are represented in figure 2
which gives a perspective view of the molecules in their
minimal energy conformation.

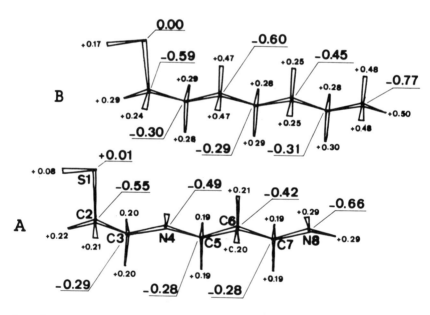

Fig. 2. Calculated ab-initio net charges (in proton unit)
for WR-1065. A : neutral form ; B : bicationic form.

We can observe the electrostatic transformation introduced
when charging positively the drug with a high concentration

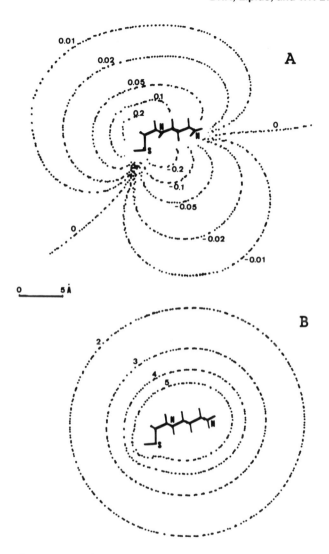

Fig. 3. Electrostatic potential due to charge distribution
for WR-1065. The isopotential lines are expressed in volts.
A : neutral form (plane parallel to S_1, C_2, C_3 plane ;
z = 2 Å). B : bicationic form (S_1, C_2, C_3 plane).

of cationic charge on NH_2 (+0.34)and NH_3 (+0.69) groups.
Three CH_2 groups located at C3, C5 and C7 are equally positively charged in the neutral molecule (+0.11 ; +0.10 ;+0.10)
and in the bicationic form (+0.27 ; +0.28 ; +0.27). The CH_2
group located at C6 position is zero charged in the two
cases. The sulfhydryl group SH which is slightly positive in
the neutral case (+0.09) begins more positive (+0.17) in the
bicationic form.

Figure 3 shows the electrostatic potential for the two
forms of the molecule. The isopotential lines of the neutral
form traduce the calculated dipole moment $|\vec{\mu}|$ = 1.45 debye.

INTERACTION OF WR-2721 OR WR-1065 WITH DNA OR WITH LECITHIN

Interaction of WR-2721 or WR-1065 with DNA

Previous studies dealing with DNA-cysteamine interac-
tion have shown a strong electrostatic interaction between
DNA phosphate sites and cysteamine NH_3^+ and SH groups. (Rix-
Montel and coll 1978 ; Broch and coll 1980).

A spectrophotometric study concerning interaction of DNA
with WR-2721 and WR-1065 has shown similar results (Vasilescu, Rix-Montel 1980). Figure 4 points out the variations of
the difference between the melting point (T_m) of the complex
DNA + WR-2721 or DNA + WR-1065 and DNA alone versus concentration of added drug. We can observe that the action of the
two molecules on DNA is identical : elevation of T_m corresponding to a strong stabilization of DNA structure. The phenomenon is cooperative and we obtain a plateau of saturation
when added WR-2721 or WR-1065 concentration is higher than
half DNA phosphate sites concentration. This cooperative
electrostatic effect is also well shown by plotting DNA +
drug melting point variation versus drug concentration logarithm. Figure 5 shows that we obtain a straight line represented by the equation : T_m = a log c + b. This behaviour
is similar to those observed for metallic counterions-DNA
phosphate sites interaction (Schildkraut, Lifson 1965).

It is to be pointed out that the electrostatic interaction between DNA phosphate groups and WR-2721 or WR-1065
is so strong that for a DNA phosphate sites concentration
$P \simeq 10^{-3}$ Ml^{-1}, we observe a precipitation as for DNA-polya-
mines interaction.

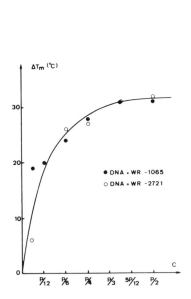

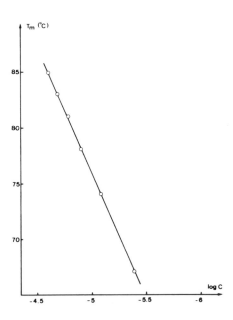

Fig. 4. Variation of the
melting point increment
($\Delta T_m = T_m$ (DNA + drug) −
T_m (DNA)) versus added
drug concentration C.
$P = 10^{-4}$ M.l^{-1} is the
DNA phosphate sites con-
centration.

Fig. 5. T_m variation of
DNA + WR −2721 or DNA +
WR − 1065 versus drug concen-
tration logarithm.

The interaction between anionic phosphate sites of DNA
and cationic groups of WR-2721 or WR-1065 is accompanied by
a counterion ejection out of phosphate sites. This phenomena
may be observed on figure 6 which shows the dielectric conductivity behaviour of a DNA solution versus the concentration of added WR-1065. The modellisation of the interaction
between DNA and WR-2721 or his metabolite may be introduced
as :
- interaction between cationic groups of the drug and adjacent phosphate sites situated on the same helical strand ;
- interaction by bridge-building between opposite phosphate
  groups on both sides of the minor groove region of DNA ;
  this second possibility resulting from the lengths ($\simeq$12-
  14 Å) and elongated conformations of these molecules
  (Broch and coll 1982).

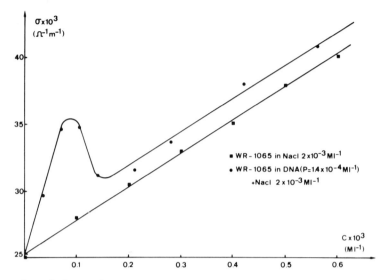

Fig. 6. Dielectric conductivity of WR-1065 and DNA+WR-1065 in NaCl 2 x 10^{-3} M 1^{-1}, versus WR-1065 concentration C at 1 MHz and 25°C.

Interaction of WR-2721 or WR-1065 with Synthetic Lecithin

We have studied - as model membranes - the interaction between dipalmitoylphosphatidylcholine (DPPC) and WR-2721 or WR-1065 (Rix-Montel and coll 1981). Smectic mesophases are a good model of liposomes in water ; these systems present two well defined thermal transconformations : a principal transition due to the melting of lipid aliphatic chains and a pretransition attributed to movements at the level of the polar head. By spectrophotometric measurements at the wavelength $\lambda = 450$ nm, we can observe change in lipid turbidity with temperature and then   determine the thermal transitions. Figure 7 shows results obtained for interaction of DPPC and WR-2721 or WR-1065. For the lipidic phase alone, the pretransition occurs at T ≃ 33°C and the principal transition at T ≃ 42°C. When WR-1065 interacts with lipid, the pretransition disappears and the principal transition is unchanged. For WR-2721, the pretransition exists but we observe a shift of 1-2°C to high temperatures ; the principal transition is not modified.

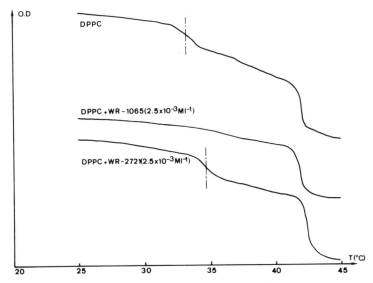

Fig. 7. Optical density of DPPC (8×10^{-4} M l^{-1}) alone or with added drug versus temperature at 450 nm. Vertical straight lines indicate the DPPC phase pretransition.

Dielectric conductivity measurements also reveal a difference between WR-2721 and his metabolite. Figure 8 indicates the obtained results. We observe an electrostatic interaction. In the case of WR-1065+lipid solution the conductivity σ increases until about DPPC concentration, then σ becomes a straight line parallel to the conductivity line of WR-1065 alone.

For WR-2721, the horizontal plateau indicates a strong electrostatic interaction (all the WR-2721 added is complexed to DPPC), then the conductivity line is parallel to the straight line corresponding to the free conductivity of WR-2721 itself. These conductivity measurements indicate that the addition of WR-2721 or WR-1065 to DPPC involves an interaction between ionized sites of the lipid polar head (phosphatidylcholine part) and ionized groups of the drugs.

In figure 9 we have made a modellisation of the situation for WR-2721. In the case of this molecule, three ionized groups NH_3^+, NH_2^+ and $PO3^{--}$, could interact respectively with the lone pairs of glycerol oxygens the phosphate and the trimethylammonium sites of the phosphatidylcholine.

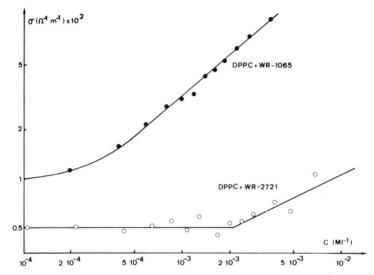

Fig. 8. Dielectric conductivity of DPPC (8×10^{-4} M l^{-1}) versus added drug concentration C at 1 MHz and 25°C.

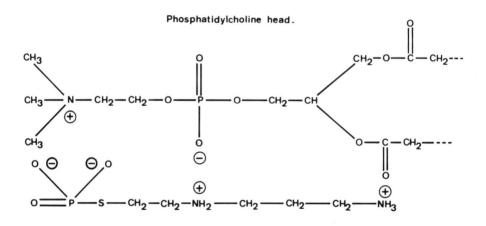

Fig. 9. Visualisation of electrostatic interaction between DPPC polar head and WR-2721.

AKNOWLEDGMENTS

The authors wish to thank Dr. D. Cabrol and Dr. H. Sentenac for stimulating discussions. This work was sponsored by grants n° 80/264 and n° 82/291 from DRET.

REFERENCES

Broch H, Cabrol D, Vasilescu D (1980). Quantum mechanical simulation of the interaction between radioprotector cysteamine and DNA. Int J Quantum Chem Quantum Biol Symp 7 : 283.

Broch H, Cabrol D, Vasilescu D (1982). Electrostatic properties of some sulfur-containing radioprotectors. Int J Quantum Chem Quantum Biol Symp 9:111.

Harris JW, Phillips TL (1971). Radiobiological and biochemical studies on thiophosphate compounds related to cysteamine. Radiat Res 46:362.

Purdie JW (1979). A comparative study of the radioprotective effects of cysteamine, WR-2721 and WR-1065 in cultured human cells. Radiation Res 77:303.

Ritter MA, Brown DQ, Glover DJ, Yuhas JM (1982). In vitro studies on the absorption of WR-2721 by tumors and normal tissues. J Radiation Oncology Biol Phys 8:523.

Rix-Montel MA, Kranck H, Vasilescu D (1981). Interaction between synthetic lecithin and various sulfur containing radioprotectors. Physiol Chem Phys 13:549.

Rix-Montel MA, Vasilescu D, Sentenac H (1978). Dielectric, potentiometric and spectrophotometric measurements of the interaction between DNA and cysteamine. Studia Biophys 69:209.

Schildkraut C, Lifson S (1965). Dependence of the melting temperature of DNA on salt concentration. Biopolymers 3:1965.

Turrisi AT, Kligerman MM, Glover DJ, Glick JH, Norfleet L, Gramkowski M (1983). Experience with phase I trials of WR-2721 preceding radiation therapy. In Nygaard OF, Simic MG (eds) : "Radioprotectors and Anticarcinogens", New York: Academic Press, p. 681.

Vasilescu D, Rix-Montel MA (1980). Interaction of sulfur-containing radioprotectors with DNA : a spectrophotometric study. Physiol Chem Phys 12:51.

Yuhas JM (1970). Biological factors affecting the radioprotective efficiency of S-2-3 (3-aminopropylamino) ethylphosphorothioic acid (WR-2721), LD 50(30) doses. Radiat Res 44:621.

Yuhas JM (1980). On the potential application of radiopro-
    tective drugs in solid tumor radiotherapy. In Sokol GH,
    Maickel RP (eds) : "Radiation-Drug Interactions in the
    Treatment of Cancer", New York : Wiley, p. 113.
Yuhas JM, Culo F (1980). Selective inhibition of the nephro-
    toxicity of cis-dichlorodiammineplatinium (II) by WR-2721
    without altering its antitumor properties. Cancer Treat
    Rep 64:57.
Yuhas JM, Storer JB (1969). Differential chemoprotection of
    normal and malignant tissues. J Natl Cancer Inst 42:331.
Yuhas JM, Spellman JM, Culo F (1980 a). The role of WR-2721
    in radiotherapy and/or chemotherapy. Cancer Clin Trials
    3:211.
Yuhas JM, Spellman JM, Jordan SW, Pardini MC, Afzal SMJ,
    Culo F (1980 b). Treatment of tumors with the combination
    of WR-2721 and cis-dichlorodiammineplatinium (II) or cy-
    clophosphamide. Br J Cancer 42:574.

Molecular Basis of Cancer, Part A: Macromolecular
Structure, Carcinogens, and Oncogenes, pages 537–547
© 1985 Alan R. Liss, Inc.

ADHESIVE PROPERTIES OF THE B16 MELANOMA

Paul Elvin, B.Tech., Ph.D. and Clive W. Evans,
B.Sc., Ph.D.
Department of Anatomy and Experimental Pathology
University of St. Andrews
St. Andrews KY16 9TS
Scotland.

The pioneering studies of Ludford (1932), Cowdry (1940)
and Coman (1944) were among the first to suggest that tumour
cells display decreased adhesive characteristics relative to
normal cells and thus that a relationship may exist between
decreased adhesiveness and the expression of tumorigenic or
metastatic potential. It is clear, however, that both
tumorigenesis and metastasis reflect complex cellular events
and that changes in cell adhesiveness may represent only one
aspect of these complex phenomena.

Analysis of the metastatic process suggests several
levels at which changes in cell adhesiveness may contribute
to metastasis. A decrease in mutual (homotypic) adhesiveness, for example, may facilitate the detachment of tumor
cells from the primary site. During both growth in the
primary and dissemination of tumor cells, decreased heterotypic adhesion might prove advantageous through the avoidance
of contact with host defense cells. Yet, during hemagenous
spread, if the tumor cell is to extravasate from the blood
vessels in which it is transported then it would seem that
some form of increased heterotypic adhesion would be
advantageous. This may not prove necessary, however, if
tumor cell lodgement could be established through fibrin or
platelet clotting (Gasic et al 1973) or through the formation
of homotypic emboli (Fidler 1973). If both increased
detachment from the primary and the formation of homotypic
emboli are to be involved in the promotion of metastasis,
then the adhesiveness of tumor cells must be envisaged to
change from low to high values at different stages of the
metastatic process (i.e. from detachment to lodgement). The

basis for such changes in adhesiveness may be related to cell
division, since it has been shown that cell adhesiveness
varies with different phases of the cell cycle. Substrate
adherent cells round up during M phase (Terasima, Tolmach
1963) presumably as a result of decreased interaction with
a substrate bridging moiety such as fibronectin, which is
found at lower levels on the cell surface during M phase
(Stenman, Wartiovaara, Vaheri 1977). The adhesiveness of
suspended cells does not necessarily correlate with that of
substrate adherent cells, however, since M phase cells are
actually significantly adherent when studied by aggregation
methods (Elvin, Evans 1983). Nevertheless, variations in
cell adhesiveness may provide the necessary mechanism by
which metastatic cells could detach from the primary tumor
and yet still be capable of adhesion at a remote site. The
possibility that changes in cell adhesiveness may influence
the organ localization of cells was shown in early studies
on lymphoid cell traffic (Evans, Davies 1977). It is
important to emphasize, however, that most techniques for
measuring adhesion provide information on average values
for a population of cells (Evans, Proctor 1978). Such
populations are unlikely to be homogenous as shown for
lymphoid cells (Evans, Davies 1977; Kellie, Evans 1981) and
in fact a wide variation in cell adhesiveness is likely to
exist. Thus at any one time a population of potentially
metastatic cells is almost certain to contain within it
cells which display the requisite adhesiveness hypothesised
for successful metastatic spread, although whether the
appropriate adhesive changes are found at the appropriate
time in cells which are capable of metastasizing remains to
be shown.

     Using a rigorously defined adhesion assay based on
aggregation within a cone and plate viscometer (Elvin, Evans
1982) we have shown that the B16 malignant melanoma variants
differ markedly in their adhesiveness. Contrary to other
reports (Nicolson, Winkelhake 1973), we have found that the
B16F10 variant which has significant lung colonizing ability
is less adhesive than the B16F1 variant which has poor lung
colonizing ability (Elvin, Evans 1984). Clearly, these
results do not argue for a significant contribution of
homotypic adhesion in the metastatic process at the lodgement stage, although they may be used in support of a role
for increased detachment of metastatic cells from the
primary. Such interpretations, however, are almost certainly
too simplistic given the inherent variation likely within

each cell line.   One distinct possibility where adhesion
may play a significant role in metastasis is in selective
organ colonization which is seen in the organotropic behavior
of certain human and animal tumors.   Thus the lung colonizing
ability of B16F10 cells may reflect the selective trapping
of these cells in the lungs rather than in other organs.
We have tested for this possibility by analysis of aggregate
composition following mixed aggregation of B16 variants
with syngeneic lung or liver cells.   The B16F10 variant
was found to adhere more to lung cells than did the B16F1
variant.   This was not the case with adhesion to liver
cells, thus reflecting the pattern of metastatic distribution
(Elvin, Evans 1984).   A similar study with the mouse
lymphoma L5178Y cell line (using a rosette-forming assay
system) showed that those variants which metastasized to
the liver formed more rosettes with hepatocytes than did
low metastatic variants (Cheingsong-Popov et al 1983).
These results argue against a significant role for non-
specific trapping in certain instances of metastasis,
although they do not necessarily exclude it.

Cells	Aggregation Index[a] ±SEM	Lung Colonies[b] mean (range)
B16F1	0.14 ± 0.01	27 (3-41)
B16F10	0.48 ± 0.02	138 (15-221)
B16F10B5	0.57 ± 0.01	19 (5-57)
B16F10C11	0.13 ± 0.01	189 (36->250)

Table 1.   Adhesiveness and lung colonizing ability of B16
cells and clones.
a)   Cells aggregated at a shear rate of 90sec^{-1}.   Index
     represents ratio of particle number after 10 min to
     particle number at start.
b) 2×10^5 cells i.v. Colonies counted at 14 days. n = 6.

The relevance of homotypic adhesiveness in the metastatic process has now been questioned further following the isolation of a number of clones of the B16F1 and F10 variants. The adhesiveness of the clones as assessed by aggregation techniques was found to vary markedly and no correlation with metastatic ability was discernible (Fig. 1). When two B16F10 clones (F10B5 and F10C11) of varying adhesiveness (Table 1) were tested by analysis of aggregate composition for their relative ability to adhere to lung or liver cells (Fig. 2), the aggregate composition profile of the parent B16F10 variant (Elvin, Evans 1984) was found for both of them. Thus there was a tendency for both clones to form more mixed aggregates with lung cells but not with liver cells, particularly when two cell aggregates are considered. This suggests that both of the clones have retained the selectivity of organ interaction typical of the B16F10 parent, even though one of them (F10B5) has a lowered ability to colonize the lungs. Thus although a particular clone of cells may show a selective adhesive interaction with one particular organ, this is clearly not enough to guarantee growth within that organ. Nevertheless, if a clone of cells otherwise has the necessary attributes for invasion and growth within the lungs, then selective adhesiveness to the lung tissue may promote the colonization of that organ. These results confirm the complexity of the metastatic phenomenon and argue for the involvement of a number of discrete events in the process overall.

The molecular mechanisms underlying the adhesive inter-actions of B16 melanoma cells remain to be elucidated. Interactions via terminal sialic acid groups may be one mechanism by which adhesion could be effected. B16F10 cells have been shown to have marginally more cell surface sialic acid when compared to B16F1 cells (Yogeeswaran, Stein, Sebastian 1978) and treatment with neuraminidase decreases the aggregation ability of B16F10 cells (Raz et al 1980). Normal B16F10 cells in culture express a 66Kd sialylglyco-protein which is poorly expressed in B16F1 cells (Yogeeswaran, Stein, Sebastian 1978) but it is still unknown, however, as to whether there is any direct involvement of the sialic acid moiety in adhesion. In a study of the basic homotypic adhesive properties of B16 cells we have shown the process to be Ca^{++} and Mg^{++} sensitive, inhibited at $4°C$ or by glutaraldehyde fixation, and promoted by some component in serum (Table 2). Despite a considerable amount of effort the serum component is as yet unidentified,

Treatment[a]	Aggregation Index ± SEM	
	B16F1	B16F10
CMEM 37°C (control)[c]	0.15 ± 0.01	0.40 ± 0.02
4°C	1.07 ± 0.02	1.07 ± 0.04
0.1% trypsin[b]	0.52 ± 0 03	0 80 ± 0.03
3% glutaraldehyde[d]	0.98 ± 0.03	0.99 ± 0.03
EMEM (serum free)	0.25 ± 0.02	0.62 ± 0.02
PBS	0.59 ± 0.02	0.90 ± 0.01
CMF-PBS	0.97 ± 0.01	0.95 ± 0.01

Table 2. Effects of various treatments on the aggregation of B16 melanoma cells.
a) Cells harvested with 2 mM EDTA (1 min, room temp.), except b.
b) 2 mM EDTA, 0.1% trypsin, 5 min at 37°C. Aggregation conditions as in control.
c) Eagle's Minimum Essential Medium (EMEM) + 10% FCS.
d) 3% glutaraldehyde in HEPES-buffered PBS, pH 7.1; 60 min at 4°C.
Other details as in Fig 1 and text.

Treatment[a]	Cells	Aggregation[b]	Lung colonies[c]	
			5×10^4	2×10^5
Control	B16F1			1(0-9)
2mM cysteine		106		7(4-13)
1mM CPDS		117		9(0-21)
Control	B16F10		13(0-35)	159(13->250)
2mM cysteine		233		
1mM CPDS		300	47(1-155)	229(124->250)

Table 3. Effects of cysteine and CPDS on aggregation and lung colony formation by B16 melanoma cells.
a) 20 min at 37°C; 10^6 cells ml^{-1}.
b) percentage of control aggregation index.
c) mean (range) n = 6.
Other details as in Fig 1 and text.

although it clearly is not fibronectin which has no significant effects on B16 cell aggregation (unpublished results). Homotypic adhesion is also sensitive to proteolytic enzymes such as trypsin, which necessitates cell harvesting by cation chelation. The effects of trypsin suggest a role for a cell surface determinant(s), although whether trypsin acts directly on a molecule involved in cell adhesion or has more general effects (such as on cell surface charge) remains to be determined.

A number of monoclonal antibodies against B16F1 cells have been prepared, some of which depress cell-substrate adhesion (Vollmers, Birchmeier 1983a,b). Following intraperitoneal preinjection of the host, at least three of these antibodies depress lung colonisation by B16 melanoma cells. Two of these active antibodies react with antigens of molecular weights between 40-50Kd which are found on both murine and human tumor cells but not on normal adult cells. From these studies it appears that more than one determinant might be involved in cell adhesion, although the precise relationship between antibodies which depress adhesion to plastic in vitro and their effects on adhesion to lung components in vivo is yet to be established.

It has been suggested that cell adhesion may be mediated through sulfhydryl groups since blocking such groups with various agents (e.g. N-ethylmaleimide) may lead to inhibition of adhesion (Grinnell, Srere 1971; George, Rao 1975). Many such agents are likely to be toxic, however, especially when tested in colony growth assays rather than by dye exclusion techniques (unpublished observations). We have found that treatment of B16 melanoma cells (20min) with 1 mM 6, 6' - carboxypyridine disulfide (CPDS) is non-toxic and that such treatment promotes adhesion (Table 3). Pretreatment with CPDS also promotes lung colony formation following intra-venous injection of either B16F1 or B16F10 cells into C57BL6 recipients. The promotory effects of CPDS on cell adhesion are particularly marked when B16F10 cells are considered, since the aggregation of B16F1 cells is near maximal under control conditions. When intraperitoneal injections of CPDS (2mg per mouse) were given to Swiss mice at 4 hr intervals for 7 days following an intracerebral injection of 2×10^5 Ehrlich ascites tumor cells, a significant reduction in the number of lung metastases was reported (Grassetti 1970). Comparison of these two experiments is difficult, but in the earlier study (Grassetti 1970) it is likely that

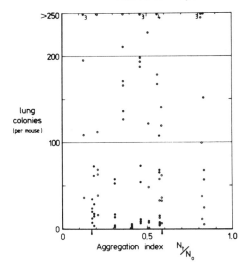

Fig. 1. Relationship between cell adhesion and lung colonization.

   ● B16F1 clones   o B16F10 clones
    Ⅰ adhesiveness of B16F1 parent   Å B16F10 parent
Details as in Table 1.

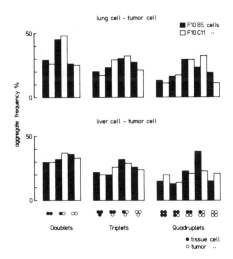

Fig. 2. Aggregate composition following heterotypic aggregation of two B16F10 clones with syngeneic lung or liver cells.
Conditions for aggregation and analysis as in Elvin,Evans (1984).

the CPDS reacted with more than the tumor cells, and indeed
there is no evidence to suggest that even this was the case
Thus simple blocking of sulfhydryl groups does not always
inhibit cell adhesion and may infact incur a protective
effect for tumor cells against host defense mechanisms.
We have found similar results to the stimulatory effects
seen with CPDS following pretreatment of B16 melanoma cells
with 2mM cysteine (Table 3).   Both CPDS and cysteine may
be expected to bind to sulfhydryl groups but their effects
on cell adhesion and metastasis could be generated through
the addition of an extra carboxyl group and not primarily
through their blocking activity.   Further studies are
required to discriminate between these two possibilities.

Recent studies with Rous sarcoma virus (RSV) have
shown that transformation is associated with the expression
of the 60Kd phosphoprotein pp60^{src}.   This src gene product
has been found localised within substratum adhesion plaques
and on the cytoplasmic side of cell-cell junctions of RSV
transformed NRK cells, where it may influence adhesiveness
and other cell behavioral properties through its effects on
cytoskeletal proteins such as vinculin (Shriver,
Rohrschneider 1981).   Despite its location in adhesive
sites the precise role of pp60^{src} in cell adhesion is
unknown, although it is unlikely to mediate adhesion
directly.   Infection of rat cerebellar cell lines with the
RSV mutant LA90, which is temperature sensitive for
transformation, leads to a failure in expression of the
neural cell adhesion molecule N-CAM at the permissive
temperature and a corresponding decrease in cell aggregation
(Greenberg, Brackenbury, Edelman 1984).   Since neuronal
tumours are not normally metastatic the role of such
adhesive changes in tumour spread cannot be evaluated fully.
It is clear from such studies, however, that adhesive
changes need not correlate with metastatic ability as argued
earlier.

The assumption is generally made that tumour cells are
less adhesive than normal cells.   Such a generalization has
major shortcomings, however, given the variability in
adhesion of a population of tumour cells as discussed above
and elsewhere (Elvin, Evans 1982).   Differences in technique
between different laboratories are also likely to contribute
to variations in adhesiveness, particularly when divergent
procedures are used for quantifying the adhesive process.
This is perhaps nowhere more marked than in studies of the

B16 melanoma itself where some groups have found the B16F10 variant to be more adhesive than the B16F1 (e.g. Nicolson, Winkelhake 1975) while others have found the opposite (Elvin, Evans 1984). Tao and Burger (1977) also found that non-metastasizing variants of the B16 cell line displayed greater homotypic adhesiveness and others have reported on this inverse correlation between homotypic adhesion and metastasis for different cell lines (Hausman 1983). These divergent results from different groups highlight the complexity of the adhesive process and suggest that any relationship between metastasis and homotypic adhesion in a single study may not have general applicability and could even be fortuitous. Studies aimed at clarifying the role of heterotypic adhesiveness in the organ selective distribution of certain tumours may ultimately prove to be more rewarding, although it should always be borne in mind that adhesiveness is but one event in the complex phenomenon of metastasis.

ACKNOWLEDGEMENTS

We are grateful to the National Foundation for Cancer Research (USA) for supporting our studies.

REFERENCES

Cheingsong-Popov R, Robinson P, Altevogt P, Schirrmacher V (1983). A mouse hepatocyte carbohydrate-specific receptor and its interaction with liver-metastasizing tumour cells. Int J Cancer 32:359.
Coman DR (1944). Decreased mutual adhesiveness, a property of cells from squamous cell carcinomas. Cancer Res 4:625.
Cowdry EV (1940). Properties of cancer cells. Arch Pathol 301:1245.
Elvin P, Evans CW (1982). The adhesiveness of normal and SV40 transformed Balb/c 3T3 cells: effects of culture density and shear rate. Eur J Cancer Clin Oncol 18:669.
Elvin P, Evans CW (1983). Cell adhesiveness and the cell cycle: correlation in synchronized Balb/c 3T3 cells. Biol Cell 48:1.
Elvin P, Evans CW (1984). Cell adhesion and experimental metastasis: a study using the B16 malignant melanoma model system. Euro J Cancer Clin Oncol 20:107.
Evans CW, Davies MJD (1977). The influence of cell adhesiveness on the migratory behaviour of murine

thymocytes. Cell Immunol 33:211.

Evans CW, Proctor J (1978). A collision analysis of lymphoid cell aggregation. J Cell Sci 33:17.

Fidler IJ (1973). The relationship of embolic homogeneity, number, size and viability to the incidence of experimental metastasis. Eur J Cancer 9:223.

Gasic GJ, Gasic TB, Galanti N, Johnson T, Murphy S (1973). Platelet-tumor cell interaction in mice. The role of platelets in the spread of malignant disease. Int J Cancer 11:704.

George JV, Rao KV (1975). The role of sulfhydryl groups in cellular adhesiveness. J. Cell Physiol 85:547.

Grassetti DR (1970). Effect of 6,6' -dithiodinicotinic acid on the dissemination of Ehrlich ascites tumor. Nature 228:282.

Greenberg ME, Brackenbury R, Edelman GM (1984). Alteration of neural cell adhesion molecule (N-CAM) expression after neuronal cell transformation by Rous sarcoma virus. Proc Natl Acad Sci 81:969.

Grinnell F, Srere PA (1971). Inhibition of cellular adhesiveness by sulfhydryl blocking agents. J Cell Physiol 78:153.

Hausman RE (1983). Increase in homotypic aggregation of metastatic Morris hepatoma cells after fusion with membranes from non-metastatic cells. Int J Cancer 32:603.

Kellie S, Evans CW (1981). Changes in lymphocyte adhesiveness during contact sensitization. Br J exp Path 62:158.

Ludford RJ (1932). Differences in the growth of transplantable tumors in plasma and serum culture media. Proc R Soc Lond 112:250.

Nicolson GL, Winkelhake JL (1975). Organ specificity of bloodborne metastasis determined by cell adhesion? Nature 255:230.

Raz A, Bucana C, McLellan W, Fidler IJ (1980). Distribution of membrane anionic sites on B16 melanoma variants with differing lung colonizing potential. Nature 284:363.

Shriver K, Rohrschneider L (1981). Organization of pp60[src] and selected cytoskeletal proteins within adhesion plaques and junctions of Rous sarcoma virus transformed rat cells. J Cell Biol 89:525.

Stenman S, Wartiovaara J, Vaheri A (1977). Changes in the distribution of a major fibroblast protein, fibronectin, during mitosis and interphase. J Cell Biol 74:453.

Tao T-W, Burger MM (1977). Non-metastasizing variants selected from metastasizing melanoma cells. Nature 270: 437.

Terasima T, Tolmach LJ (1963). Growth and nucleic acid synthesis in synchronously dividing populations of HeLa cells. Exp Cell Res 81:31.

Vollmers HP, Birchmeier W (1983a). Monoclonal antibodies inhibit the adhesion of mouse B16 melanoma cells in vitro and block lung metastases in vivo. Proc Natl Acad Sci 80:3729.

Vollmers HP, Birchmeier W (1983b). Monoclonal antibodies that prevent adhesion of B16 melanoma cells and reduce metastases in mice: crossreaction with human tumor cells. Proc Natl Acad Sci 80:6863.

Yogeeswaran G, Stein BS, Sebastian H (1978). Altered cell surface organization of gangliodsides and sialylglyco-proteins of mouse metastatic melanoma variant lines selected in vivo for enhanced lung implantation. Cancer Res 38:1336.

Molecular Basis of Cancer, Part A: Macromolecular
Structure, Carcinogens, and Oncogenes, pages 549–559
© 1985 Alan R. Liss, Inc.

THE COMPUTATION OF CONCENTRATION AND DIELECTRIC PROFILES IN
INTERFACIAL INHOMOGENEOUS REGIONS, AND THE RELATION BETWEEN
SURFACE CHARGE DENSITY AND SURFACE POTENTIALS

V. S. Vaidhyanathan, Ph.D.
Department of Biophysical Sciences
School of Medicine
State University of New York at Buffalo
Buffalo, New York 14214

1. INTRODUCTION

It may be reasonably stated that the surface properties
of malignant cells are in some respects different from the
surface properties of normal cells, which may account for
the difference in their growth rates. The interfacial
aqueous region near the cell surfaces play an important role
in the transport of nutrients into the cells. In this manner, one may justify the subject matter of this paper, which
is concerned with properties of interfacial regions, as being relevant to the subject matter of this conference, which
is the molecular basis of cancer.

One of the unsolved problems of interfacial region systems, consisting of a surface with charges and an electrolyte of known composition, is the lack of a reliable expression, existing between the electric potential at surface in
relation to the electric potential of the bulk solution,
(potential far from interface) and the surface charge density. For the case of a symmetrical ion systems, (1-1 electrolyte), an expression for this relation is presented by
Grahame (1947). This relation, known as the Gouy equation,
is

$$\sinh \{e\phi_0/2kT\} = A \ S/C^{1/2} \tag{1}$$

where ϕ_0 is the value of electric potential at the surface,
with reference to potential in bulk homogeneous solution, S
is the surface charge density. A is a constant, and C is
the concentration of 1-1 electrolyte, in aqueous solution.
e is the protonic charge, k is the Boltzmann constant and T

is the temperature in Kelvin scale. Equation (1) is derived
from Gauss equation and its validity is restricted to the
case of symmetrical 1-1 valence electrolyte and when the dielectric coefficient, ε, is not a function of position variable in interfacial regions. A general equation for unsym-
metrical many ion system, generally present in biological
systems, is not available. In this paper, an approximate
relation, which enables one to compute the surface charge
density, S, (charge per unit surface are) from knowledge of
composition of aqueous electrolyte and electric potential
difference, is presented. The method of computation of dielectric profile (which must exist in the inhomogeneous
region), is also included.

Our analysis of the inhomogeneous region near a biological cell membrane surface, is based on the assumed validity
of three basic postulates: these are, 1) the chemical potential of an ionic species, σ, in the inhomogeneous region is
described adequately by equation (5), where contributions to
chemical potential arising from the presence of different
nonelectrolyte molecules have been neglected, and contributions arising from ion-ion interactions energy terms are included. 2) The extent of the interfacial region is finite,
and its magnitude, d, is determined in a self-consistent
manner by the system itself. 3) Within the inhomogeneous region, which extends from x=0 to x=d, the electric potential,
$\emptyset(x)$, the dielectric coefficient $\varepsilon(x)$, the concentration of
different ionic species, $C_\sigma(x)$, are functions of position
variable x, and these become independent of x, for values of
x greater than d, where the system is homogeneous. The position variable x, is defined as normal to the yz plane of the
interfacial surface.

The original intent of our analysis was to introduce
the contributions from ion-ion interaction energy terms, as
correction to the classic limiting expression for the electrochemical potential of ions in solution, and to investigate the implications of the resultant. Such a modification
of the expression for chemical potential of an ion in inhomogeneous interfacial region, leads to certain (unexpected)
surprising results, which are at variance with the conclusions of classical equations. The two main conclusions
arising from our analysis are: 1) a dielectric profile must
exist in the inhomogeneous interfacial regions, which should
not be neglected; and 2) the electric potential profile and
concentration profiles of positively charged ions must have

schematically similar profiles in inhomogeneous regions at
equilibrium.

The dielectric coefficient, ε, is in general a function
of position variable, since it is dependent on field, concentration of ions and other properties of the system. In
order to overcome the lack of knowledge of dependence of the
dielectric coefficient on these variables, and to simplify
the mathematical aspects of the nonlinear problem, one assumes in general, that one may neglect the positional dependence of $\varepsilon(x)$. It can be shown exactly, that this assumption is quite untenable.

Once the basic set of nonlinear differential equations
were formulated (Vaidhyanathan, 1982, I), the solutions were
sought in Taylor series. This procedure is of utility, if
and only if, one could evaluate the various Taylor coefficients. The assumption of validity of a second order polynomial for dielectric profile (Vaidhyanathan, 1983,1984),
and the truncation of the Taylor series beyond the leading
seven terms, led to certain results, which are controversial,
including the existence of an extremum in charge density
profile.

In this paper, the results of an investigation, with a
very simple modest objective, namely, computation of charge
density profile $Y(x)$, on the assumption that the Taylor expansion of the electric potential profile, $\phi(x) = \sum_i \phi_i x^i$;
$(i!)\phi_i = (d^i\phi/dx^i)_{x=0}$, can be truncated with the leading six
terms, are presented. In addition to providing support for
many of our evidently controversial conclusions, the feasibility of calculation of the dielectric profile, including
its value at interface is presented.

2. THEORY

In general, the surface charge density, S, is related
to the value of the Gauss integral,

$$\int_o Y(x)\ dx = -\ \varepsilon(o)\ \phi'(o) = -\ S$$

$$Y(x) = (d/dx)\ \{\varepsilon(x)\phi'(x)\} = -\ 4\pi e \sum_\sigma Z_\sigma\ \sigma(x)$$

$$\phi'(x) = (d\phi(x)/dx), \tag{2}$$

The upper limit of integration in eq. (2) can be set as

either infinity, or d, where d is the extent of region in
which there exists lack of microscopic electroneutrality.
$\emptyset'(d) = 0$. $\emptyset(x)$ is the electric potential felt by a unit
charge at x. If the electric potential profile in inhomogeneous region is known, $\emptyset'(o)$ is known. If the charge density profile, $Y(x)$ is known or can be computed from the properties of the system, one can in principle perform the integration of   equation (2), thereby obtaining the values of
S and $\varepsilon(o)$, the value of dielectric coefficient at x = 0.

If the concentration of an ion of kind, σ, C_σ, with
valence charge number z_σ, at location x, in interfacial region is given by the expression,

$$C_\sigma(x) = C_\sigma(d) \exp\{z_\sigma \beta(x)\}; \quad \sum_\sigma C_\sigma(d) z_\sigma = 0$$

$$K(x) = \eta^2(x) \quad \varepsilon(x) = (4\pi e^2/kT) \sum_\sigma z_\sigma^2 C_\sigma(x) \tag{3}$$

where $\eta^2(x)$ is the local value of Debye-Huckel parameter,
and one imposes the condition that for values of x = d, ele-
ctroneutrality condition prevails, $\sum_\sigma z_\sigma C_\sigma(d) = 0$, $C_\sigma(d)$ being
the concentration of σ at x = d, and for values of x > d,
then one may verify that for any electrolyte system, of any
composition, K(x) is always greater than K(d) for most
values of β. For a 2-1 electrolyte system, the exception
to above statement occurs when β assumes values between 0
and -1. For three or more ion systems with a divalent cation, the exception to above statement occurs for smaller
range of values of β, when β is negative.

It should be recalled that the classic equation for the
electrochemical potential, μ_σ, of an ion of kind σ,

$$\mu_\sigma(x) = \mu_\sigma^*(T,P) + kT \ln C_\sigma(x) + z_\sigma e\emptyset(x)$$

$$= \text{a constant, independent of x at} \\ \text{equilibrium} \tag{4}$$

results from the relation for entropy of mixing of ideal
solutions, in which the mole fraction is replaced by concentrations of solute, when the solution is dilute, and where-
in the influence of an external field, is included in a
phenomenological manner by the addition of the last term of
eq. (4). At equilibrium, eq. (4) requires that as $C_\sigma(x)$ increases, for ions with positive charge, $\emptyset(x)$ must decrease.
Thus, one comes to the conclusion that if a surface is positively charged, then the potential at this surface is
negative (?).

When ion-ion interaction energy terms are included, one obtains the expression for electrochemical potential of charged species, σ, in inhomogeneous region as

$$\mu_\sigma(x) = \mu_\sigma^*(T,P) + kT \text{ in } C_\sigma(x) + Z_\sigma e \, F(x)$$

$$= \text{a constant, independent of } x, \text{ at equilibrium}$$

$$F(x) = \emptyset(x) - (H/4\pi) \, Y(x); \quad Y(x) = -(4\pi e) \sum_\sigma Z_\sigma C_\sigma(x) \qquad (5)$$

In equation (4) and (5), $\mu_\sigma^*(T,P)$ is the composition independent part of chemical potential. H denotes the ion-ion interaction energy term contribution to chemical potential of an ion of kind σ, which is absent in eq. (4). Since $Y(d)=O$, and microscopic electroneutrality is assumed to prevail in homogeneous electrolytes, $\sum_\sigma Z_\sigma C_\sigma = O$, the presence or absence of the last term $(H/4\pi)Y(x)$, in the expression for $F(x)$, did not create a controversy in analysis of aqueous electrochemical systems. As before the validity of equation (5) demands that as $C_\sigma(x)$ for positive ions increases, $F(x)$ must decrease. This requirement is satisfied when $\emptyset(x)$ and $C_\sigma(x)$, for Z_σ equals a positive integer, have similar schematic profiles, provided that the magnitude of $Y(x)/\{K(d)\}$ is greater than the magnitude of $\emptyset(x)$ for every value of x, in the inhomogeneous region, and that the value of $Y(x)$ has a sign opposite to the sign of $\emptyset(x)$. It is shown elsewhere that $-(4\pi/H) = K(d)$ for many ion system, provided that the electric potential satisfies the boundary conditions $\emptyset''(d)=\emptyset'''(d) = O$. In this paper, appropriate number of primes are utilized to indicate the differentials of appropriate order. Thus, $\emptyset'''(d) = (d^3\emptyset/dx^3)_{x=d}$.

From equation (5), it follows that the concentration of σ, at x, $C_\sigma(x)$ is related to the bulk average concentrations of ion σ, $C_\sigma(d)$, by the relation,

$$C_\sigma(x) = C_\sigma(d) \, \exp\{Z_\sigma \beta(x)\}$$

$$\beta(x) = (e/kT) \, \{F(d) - F(x)\}; \quad \beta(d) = O \qquad (6)$$

When $\beta(x) = (kT/e) \, mx$, one has the exponential concentration profiles for univalent ions and the potential is linear. Equation (6) reduces to the Nernst equilibrium expression when H terms of equation (5) are absent, or when $Y(x) = O$. Thus, validity of equation (5) leads to the stationary state Nernst-Planck analog equation (5), viz.,

$$C_\sigma'(x) + (Z_\sigma e/kT)C_\sigma(x)F'(x) = -(J_\sigma/D_\sigma) \text{ for steady state,}$$
$$= 0, \text{ for equilibrium} \qquad (7)$$

Equation (7) reduces to familiar Nernst-Planck equation when H terms are absent. In eq. (7), J_σ is the stationary state flux, and D_σ is the diffusion coefficient of ion of kind σ. One of the main conclusions to which the general Nernst-Planck analog equation, in which ion neutral molecule interactions are included, in which flux of uncharged species are zero, and concentration gradients of uncharged species are zero, is that $\emptyset'''(x)$ must be a constant, and thus $\emptyset(x)$ can at best be a fourth order polynomial in this case. This significant conclusion lends support and credance to the Taylor expansion approach. (Vaidhyanathan, 1979, eq. 55).

One obtains the following results which are exact, from equations (5) and (6).

$$K(x)\emptyset'(x) = Y'(x) \quad \{1 - (K(x)/K(d)\}$$

$$4\pi kT\, K(x)A'(x) = Y'(x)Y(x); \quad A(x) = \sum_\sigma C_\sigma(x)$$

$$Y'(x) = -\emptyset'(x)\{K(x)K(d)/(K(x) - K(d))\}$$

$$\beta(x) = (e/kT)\,\{\emptyset(d) - \emptyset(x) + (H/4\pi)Y(x)\}$$

$$= (e/kT)\,\Delta\emptyset(x) + \sum_\sigma C_\sigma(x)Z_\sigma/\sum_\sigma C_\sigma(d)Z_\sigma^2$$

$$= m(d-x) + (n/2)(d^2-x^2) + (p/3)(d^3-x^3) + \ldots \quad (8)$$

3.   COMPUTATION OF DIELECTRIC PROFILE

The basic postulates of this paper, if valid, require that the system parameters determine the dielectric profile. If one knows the electric potential profile, the value of distance parameter, d, and the values of ion concentrations $C_\sigma(d)$ and Z_σ one should be able to specify the Taylor expansion coefficients of dielectric profile, ε_0, ε_1, ε_2, etc. Such a calculation is presented in this section for a system, with aqueous electrolyte of three kinds of ions, one divalent ion of kind, δ, and two monovalent kinds of ions. The bulk homogeneous concentrations of the ions are specified as $C_\delta = 1$, $C_+ = 3$ and $C_- = 5$ ($\times 10^{-5}$ moles cm^{-3}). For electrolytes with concentrations of this order, it was shown elsewhere (Vaidhyanathan, 1983), that d equals about

21×10^{-8}cm. The cited calculation of d involved certain approximations, and for numerical illustrative example, we assume that $d = 25 \times 10^{-8}$cm. The value $\Delta\emptyset$ is assumed to equal $- 100$ mV $= -3.31373 \times 10^{-4}$esu/cm. For this system, from equation (8), the values of $\beta(x)$ are given by the solution of equation

$$12 \ \beta(x) - 3e^{\beta} - 2e^{2\beta} + 5e^{-\beta} = - 12 \ (e\emptyset(x)/kT) \qquad (9)$$

The values of $Y(x)$ are known from the relation,

$$Y(x) = - 4\pi e \ N \ \{3e^{\beta} + e^{2\beta} - 5e^{-\beta}\} \times 10^{-5} esu/cm^{3}$$

$$N = 6.02486 \times 10^{23}/mole. \qquad (10)$$

When one retains only the leading six terms of Taylor expansion of $\emptyset(x)$, one has, when $\emptyset(d) = 0$,

$$\emptyset_{o} = \emptyset_{4}d^{4}(1 + 4R); \ \emptyset_{1} = - \emptyset_{4}d^{3}(4 + 15R);$$

$$\emptyset_{2} = 2 \ \emptyset_{4}d^{2}(3 + 10R); \ \emptyset_{3} = - \emptyset_{4}d^{3}(4 + 10R)$$

$$R = (\emptyset_{5}d/\emptyset_{4}) \qquad (11)$$

For illustrative purposes, if one assumes $R = - 0.2$, the electric potential profile, i.e., value of $\emptyset(x)$ for any specified x, in the interfacial region is known. Eq. (9) enables one to compute $\beta(x)$ and eq. (10) enables one to compute $Y(x)$. One also can compute $C_{\sigma}(x)$, $K(x)$ and $\emptyset'(x)$. Thus, one knows $Y'(x)$ using eq. (8). Thus, the values of Y_{o} and Y_{1} are precisely known, once one specifies d and $\emptyset(x)$. The Taylor expansion of $Y(x)$ is given by

$$Y_{o} = 2\varepsilon_{o}\emptyset_{2} + \varepsilon_{1}\emptyset_{1}; \ Y_{1} = 6 \ \varepsilon_{o}\emptyset_{3} + 4 \ \varepsilon_{1}\emptyset_{2} + 2 \ \varepsilon_{2}\emptyset_{1}$$

$$Y_{2} = 12 \ \varepsilon_{o}\emptyset_{4} + 9 \ \varepsilon_{1}\emptyset_{3} + 6 \ \varepsilon_{2}\emptyset_{2} + 3 \ \varepsilon_{3}\emptyset_{1} \qquad (12)$$

Assuming the values, $T = 293.15^{O}$K, and $\varepsilon(d)$ equals 80.36. The computed values of $\emptyset(x)$, $K(x)$, $\beta(x)$, $Y(x)$ and $Y'(x)$ in the interfacial inhomogeneous region, is presented in Table 1, for the system specified in the foregoing. In Figure 1 are presented the resultant profiles of $\beta(x)$, $\emptyset'(x)$ and $Y'(x)$. One observes that the ratio of $(\emptyset'(x)/Y'(x))$ is negative definite for all values of x. For any many ion electrolyte system, one may verify that β must have a sign

Figure 1. Computed values of Ø(x), Ø'(x) Y(x), Y'(x) and
K(x) for the system. (Scales in y-axis vary: cf Tables 1
and 2).

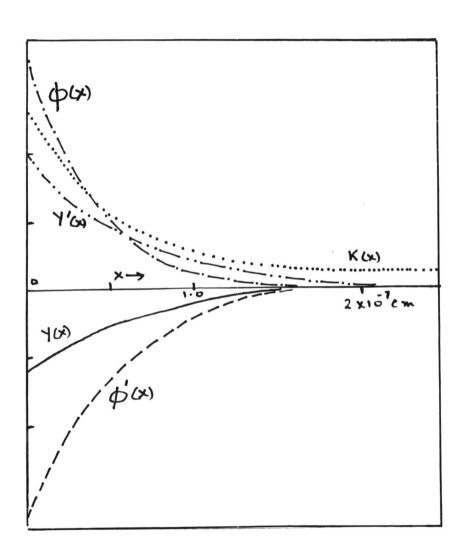

opposite to the sign of Y_o and that β should have a sign similar to the sign of $\emptyset(\mathring{o})$. These conclusions are in disagreement that one may obtain from the implications of equation (4).

For the system parameters specified, one obtains the Taylor expansion coefficients of $Y(x)$, which are presented in Table 2. Retention of leading seven terms of Taylor coefficients of $Y(x)$ and performing the integration yields the values of $\varepsilon_o \emptyset_1$. Since $\emptyset_1$ is known, one can evaluate ε_o the value of dielectric coefficient at interface. Since Y^o, ε_o, $\emptyset_1$ and $\emptyset_2$ are known, one may evaluate the second Taylor coefficient of $\varepsilon(x)$, viz., ε_1 from equation (12). Similarly, the expression for Y_1 will now yield ε_2, since $\emptyset_3$ is known. From the knowledge of ε_o, ε_1, ε_2 and the value of $\varepsilon(d)$, one can evaluate the contributions for $\varepsilon(d)$ from the rest of the Taylor coefficients. Imposition of the boundary condition that $\varepsilon'(d) = 0$, enables one to evaluate ε_4 and ε_5. The values obtained in this matter are also presented in Table 2.

Table 1. Computed values of various profiles, with assumed values of R, $\emptyset_o$, d and C_σ.

x	$\emptyset(x)$	$\beta(x)$	$Y(x)$	$K(x)$	$Y'(x)$
0.00	3.3137	1.6330	-242.877	522.893	380.976
0.25	1.9569	1.4125	-162.983	349.483	264.380
0.50	1.0858	1.1852	-107.960	233.702	180.619
0.75	0.5569	0.9556	- 70.546	158.689	122.340
1.00	0.2577	0.7302	- 45.210	111.636	82.981
1.25	0.1036	0.5177	- 25.953	83.203	56.823
1.50	0.0339	0.3287	- 16.101	66.835	39.036
1.75	0.0080	0.1741	- 8.009	57.996	25.987
2.50	0.0000	0.0000	0.000	51.791	0.000

Values of $\emptyset(x)$ are in 10^{-4} esu/cm, values of $Y(x)$ are in 10^{10} (esu/cm^3), values of $K(x)$ are in 10^{-14} cm^{-2} and $Y'(x)$ are in 10^{17} (esu/cm^4). The values of x are in 10^{-7} cm. 0.3313733×10^{-4} esu/cm equals 10 millivolts.

Table 2. Computed values of Taylor expansion coefficients of Charge Density Profiles and Dielectric Profile.

$$Y_o = -242.87689 \times 10^{10} \qquad \emptyset''(o) = 10.619 \times 10^{10} \, esu/cm^3$$
$$Y_1 = 380.97583 \, r \qquad \varepsilon(d) = 80.36$$
$$Y_2 = -265.53252 \, s \qquad \varepsilon(o) = 20.540348$$
$$Y_3 = 95.823458 \times 10^{31} \qquad \varepsilon_1 = 69.51159 \times 10^7$$
$$Y_4 = -13.600049 \, t \qquad \varepsilon_2 = 62.757635 \, w$$
$$\varepsilon_3 = -68.257837 \times 10^{21}$$
$$\varepsilon_4 = 14.344555 \times 10^{28}$$

$$r = 10^{17}; \ s = 10^{24}; \ t = 10^{38}; \ w = 10^{14}; \ y = 10^{28}$$

4. CONCLUSIONS

The results presented in this paper indicate the feasibility of computation of dielectric profile, from knowledge of electric potential profile. If the dielectric coefficient is not a function of x, then the Taylor coefficients of $Y(x)$, Y_o and Y_1 should equal, respectively, $2 \varepsilon_o \emptyset_2$ and $6 \varepsilon_o \emptyset_3$. Thus, the signs of Y_1, $\emptyset_3$ and $\emptyset_1$ should be the same. The ratio, $(\emptyset_1/Y_1)$ should be positive definite, when dielectric coefficient is a constant. When ion-ion interaction energy contributions are included, as in eq. (5), eq. (8) results, which is exact. Since $K(x)$ is always greater than $K(d)$, for most electrolyte systems, when ion-ion interaction terms, H, is included, it is necessary that the ratio of $\{\emptyset'(x)/Y'(x)\}$ is negative definite. This condition demands the existence of a dielectric profile.

For the system with three ions, whose concentrations are specified in the text, when $\emptyset_o$ assumes the values of 50, 100, 150, 200, 400 and 800 mV, the computed values of $\beta(o)$ are respectively, 1.346, 1.633, 1.812, 1.9433, 2.2703 and 2.60815. If $\emptyset_o$ assumes the values of - 100 and -59 mV, $\beta(o)$ can be computed to equal - 2.78224 and - 2.44136, respectively. Thus, one observes that concentrations of ions near surface does not increase in proportion to change in surface potentials. If the extent of inhomogeneous region, d, is dependent only on the bulk electrolyte concentrations, (d is a constant) and $\emptyset(x)$ can be expressed as a finite polynomial in x, the value of $\emptyset_1$ will double, if the value of $\emptyset_o$ is doubled. In order that the surface charge does not increase in proportion to change in $\emptyset_o$, it is imperative that the value of ε_o decrease with increase in $\emptyset_o$. This conclusion, which follows when ion-ion interaction energy terms are in-

cluded in eq. (5) is not evident from classical electrochemical expression (4). One may also verify that the
values of $\{Y(x)/K(d)\}$ is always greater than the magnitude
of values of $\emptyset(x)$.

5. REFERENCES

Grahame D. C., (1947) 'The Electrical Double Layer and the
Theory of Electrocapillarity'. Chem. Revs., 41, 441-501.
Vaidhyanathan V.S. (1982) 'Inhomogeneous Interfacial Regions
in Biological Systems, I. Basic Differential Equations'. J.
Biological Physics, 10, 153-165.
Vaidhyanathan V.S., (1982) ibid, II. Dielectric Profile and
Ion Distributions',p. 167-177.
Vaidhyanathan V.S., (1983) 'Ion Distributions in Inhomogen-
eous Regions', Colloids & Surfaces, 6, 291-306.
Vaidhyanathan V.S., (1979)'Nernst-Planck Analog Equations
and Stationary State Membrane Potentials'. Bull. Math.
Biology, 41, 365-385.
Vaidhyanathan V.S., (1984) 'Ado & Additional Comments on the
Interfacial Inhomogeneous Regions Near a Biological Mem-
brane'. Bioelectrochemistry & Bioenergetics, 00, 0000.

Index

PROGRESS IN CLINICAL AND BIOLOGICAL RESEARCH

Series Editors

Nathan Back
George J. Brewer
Vincent P. Eijsvoogel
Robert Grover

Kurt Hirschhorn
Seymour S. Kety
Sidney Udenfriend
Jonathan W. Uhr